T0291603

CAMBRIDGE PUBLIC HEALTH SERIES

UNDER THE EDITORSHIP OF

G. S. GRAHAM-SMITH, M.D., F.R.S., *University Lecturer in Hygiene and Secretary to the Sub-Syndicate for Tropical Medicine*

AND

J. E. PURVIS, M.A. *University Lecturer in Chemistry and Physics in their application to Hygiene and Preventive Medicine, and Secretary to the State Medicine Syndicate*

THE CHEMICAL EXAMINATION
OF WATER, SEWAGE, FOODS
AND OTHER SUBSTANCES

THE CHEMICAL EXAMINATION

OF

WATER, SEWAGE, FOODS

AND OTHER SUBSTANCES

BY

J. E. PURVIS, M.A.

University Lecturer in Chemistry and Physics as applied
to Hygiene and Public Health
St John's and Corpus Christi Colleges, Cambridge

AND

T. R. HODGSON, M.A.

Public Analyst for the County Boroughs of Blackpool and Wallasey
and the Municipal Boroughs of Bacup and Stalybridge
Formerly of Christ's College, Cambridge

SECOND & ENLARGED EDITION

CAMBRIDGE
AT THE UNIVERSITY PRESS
1922

CAMBRIDGE
UNIVERSITY PRESS

University Printing House, Cambridge CB2 8BS, United Kingdom

Cambridge University Press is part of the University of Cambridge.

It furthers the University's mission by disseminating knowledge in the pursuit of
education, learning and research at the highest international levels of excellence.

www.cambridge.org
Information on this title: www.cambridge.org/9781107494732

© Cambridge University Press 1922

First edition 1914
Second edition 1922
First published 1922
Re-issued 2015

A catalogue record for this publication is available from the British Library

ISBN 978-1-107-49473-2 Paperback

EDITORS' PREFACE

IN view of the increasing importance of the study of public hygiene and the recognition by doctors, teachers, administrators and members of Public Health and Hygiene Committees alike that the *salus populi* must rest, in part at least, upon a scientific basis, the Syndics of the Cambridge University Press have decided to publish a series of volumes dealing with the various subjects connected with Public Health.

The books included in the Series present in a useful and handy form the knowledge now available in many branches of the subject. They are written by experts, and the authors are occupied, or have been occupied, either in investigations connected with the various themes or in their application and administration. They include the latest scientific and practical information offered in a manner which is not too technical. The bibliographies contain references to the literature of each subject which will ensure their utility to the specialist.

It has been the desire of the editors to arrange that the books should appeal to various classes of readers: and it is hoped that they will be useful to the medical profession at home and abroad, to bacteriologists and laboratory students, to municipal engineers and architects, to medical officers of health and sanitary inspectors and to teachers and administrators.

Many of the volumes will contain material which will be suggestive and instructive to members of Public Health and Hygiene Committees; and it is intended that they shall seek to influence the large body of educated and intelligent public opinion interested in the problems of public health.

AUTHORS' PREFACE TO FIRST EDITION

THIS book is intended for the use of students who are attending courses of instruction for diplomas and degrees in Public Health, and for those who are studying the chemistry of water, sewage, sewage effluents, foods, disinfectants, etc. during their ordinary laboratory practice. It will probably be also useful to those who are engaged as public analysts or in public health matters generally.

It does not give an exhaustive account of all the available methods of examination, but it describes those which have been used and tested by the authors both in laboratory instruction and in the daily work of a public analyst. Full references are given in the text to the sources of the different methods, and, at the end, there is a short bibliography of some of the more important works which discuss the various subjects. No illustrations have been introduced, as the apparatus, as well as the appearance and characters of the substances which require the use of a microscope, can only be fully understood and appreciated in the actual practical work of the laboratory.

A considerable number of typical analyses have been introduced to illustrate the variations which may occur in the composition of the articles themselves. We desire to convey our grateful thanks to those who have allowed us to insert the results of their own work and which we have acknowledged by name in the appropriate places.

The methods employed in the bacteriological examination of water, sewage, foods, air, etc. is the subject of a separate volume in this series by Dr W. G. Savage.

J. E. P.
T. R. H.

CAMBRIDGE,
July, 1914.

PREFACE TO THE SECOND EDITION

THE success of the first edition has given an opportunity to the authors to make the book still more useful to students. They have included in this edition a considerable amount of fresh matter and newer methods of analysis. The chapters on water and milk have been expanded, and a more detailed account is described of the methods of analysis of foods and beverages. A chapter has been added containing an outline of elementary toxicological analysis.

The helpful criticisms by reviewers of the first edition have been carefully considered and their suggestions have usually been incorporated and developed in this enlarged edition.

J. E. P.
T. R. H.

CAMBRIDGE,
January, 1922.

CONTENTS

CHAP.   PAGE

I. WATER—SEWAGE—SEWAGE EFFLUENTS—RIVER-WATER AND SEWAGE—SEA-WATER AND SEWAGE—WORKS EFFLUENTS 1

II. MILK—CREAM—DRIED MILK—CONDENSED MILK . . 100

III. BUTTER—MARGARINE—LARD, DRIPPING, SUET—CHEESE, CREAM CHEESE—EDIBLE OILS 141

IV. TEA—COFFEE—CHICORY—COCOA 176

V. WHEAT FLOUR, SELF-RAISING FLOUR, BAKING POWDER —BREAD—RICE—PEARL BARLEY—STARCHES—INFANTS' FOODS 194

VI. PEPPER, CAYENNE, MUSTARD—NUTMEG, CINNAMON, GINGER 213

VII. CANE SUGAR—GOLDEN SYRUP AND TREACLE—HONEY—JAM 220

VIII. ALCOHOLIC BEVERAGES—WHISKEY, RUM, GIN, BRANDY—BEER—CIDER 228

IX. VINEGAR—LIME AND LEMON JUICE 238

X. MEAT AND MEAT PRODUCTS 245

XI. POISONOUS METALS IN FOODS 252

XII. PRESERVATIVES—DISINFECTANTS 260

XIII. AIR—COAL GAS—OTHER GASES 273

XIV. RAG FLOCK—URINE 291

XV. TOXICOLOGY 302

APPENDIX 314

BIBLIOGRAPHY 315

ADDENDA. TABLE OF ATOMIC WEIGHTS. ALCOHOL TABLE. VOLUMES OF OXYGEN AND NITROGEN ABSORBED FROM THE ATMOSPHERE BY DISTILLED WATER AND SEA-WATER. MILK TABLES. CONVERSION OF ALCOHOLIC STRENGTH. SPECIFIC GRAVITY OF ALCOHOL. FACTORS FOR USE IN VOLUMETRIC ANALYSIS. TABLE OF SOME USEFUL CONSTANTS 316–325

INDEX 327

CHAPTER I

WATER—SEWAGE—SEWAGE EFFLUENTS—RIVER-WATER AND SEWAGE—SEA-WATER AND SEWAGE —WORKS EFFLUENTS

WATER

CHEMICALLY pure water does not occur in nature. All water supplies are obtained ultimately from rain water, which contains various substances, both organic and inorganic, dissolved by the water during its passage through the air, soil, subsoil, etc.; and, it may be, by contamination with sewage material and trade wastes.

An analysis of water is undertaken with the object of estimating these impurities and of deciding whether the water is of sufficient purity to be used for domestic purposes. The value of this analysis depends on the accuracy of the results, and, in a large measure, on careful and proper sampling.

Method of sampling. The sample should be collected in a "Winchester Quart," having a ground glass stopper. Stone jars should not be used, and care should be taken to see that the bottle has not been previously used for storing ammonia and ammonium salts. Before collecting the sample, the bottle should be well rinsed at least three times with the water.

If the sample is to be taken from a stream, the bottle should be completely immersed in the stream, as near the centre as possible, and care should be taken not to disturb any mud.

If the sample is to be taken from a well, at least ten gallons should be allowed to run to waste before filling the bottle, and the water should then be allowed to flow directly into the bottle; in no case should a funnel be used.

When the sample is to be collected from a tap, at least ten gallons should be allowed to run to waste; and the sample should then be collected directly from the tap.

When a sample of water is submitted for analysis, the largest possible amount of information regarding it should be forwarded at the same time. In order to assist the analyst in arriving at his opinion, information on the following points is essential and should always be supplied: (*a*) risk of pollution; (*b*) nature of the surface and subsoil, *e.g.* clay, chalk, gravel, sand, etc.; (*c*) if the water comes from a well the approximate depth of the well.

Physical characters. A careful preliminary examination of a water is of great importance.

(*a*) Test the water with blue and red litmus papers, and notice if the reaction is acid or alkaline. Most drinking waters are slightly alkaline or neutral in reaction. Peaty waters and waters from upland surfaces are often acid, as well as waters from chemical works and breweries. Waters which are contaminated with sewage are usually alkaline. Waters which contain carbon dioxide give a slightly acid reaction.

(*b*) Warm a portion in a test-tube and notice if any smell is produced. Polluted water may give off sulphuretted hydrogen.

(*c*) Place a portion in a two-foot glass tube and examine it downwards in a good light. Notice if it is clear and bright or turbid. Pure water has a bluish tinge; polluted waters may be yellow or brown; peaty waters and upland surface waters are usually coloured yellow or brown.

(*d*) Allow a portion of the water to stand for an hour or two in a conical shaped tube, and collect the sediment. Mount a little of the sediment on a glass slide, and examine it carefully with a microscope to see if it is mineral matter, such as sand or chalk or oxide of iron; or vegetable matter, such as vegetable cells, starch granules, cotton or linen or silk fibre, yeasts, moulds, bacteria, diatoms and other water organisms; or animal refuse such as worms, insects, hairs, fish scales, animal fibre, etc.

(*e*) Also notice if it is well aerated, by shaking a portion of it in a glass bottle and noticing the liberation of gas bubbles.

Free and saline ammonia

Solutions required:
Nessler's solution. Weigh out

35 grams of potassium iodide,
13 grams of mercuric chloride,
120 grams of caustic potash,

dissolve each separately in water, and gradually add the potassium iodide solution to the solution of mercuric chloride, a precipitate of mercuric iodide appears at first which is afterwards redissolved in the excess of potassium iodide; the caustic potash solution is then added gradually; and, afterwards, a saturated solution of mercuric chloride drop by drop, until a very slight precipitate, which will not redissolve, is formed. The whole is then finally made up to 1000 c.c. and allowed to stand until the precipitate settles; the solution should always be kept in contact with the precipitate.

Ammonium chloride solution (strong): weigh out 3·147 grams of pure dry ammonium chloride, dissolve it in water and make up to 1000 c.c.

Ammonium chloride solution (dilute): measure out 10 c.c. of the strong ammonium chloride solution and add ammonia-free distilled water to 1000 c.c. 1 c.c. of this solution = 0·00001 gram of ammonia.

Estimation of free and saline ammonia. The most convenient apparatus for this determination is a 1500 c.c. round-bottomed distilling flask, with a ground glass stopper, having a fused-in delivery tube, bent at right angles, this delivery tube is fitted into a double surface condenser.

It is necessary first to free the apparatus from ammonia; and, in order to do this, 200 c.c. of distilled water and about one gram of solid sodium carbonate, which has been fused in a platinum dish to drive off any ammonium salts, are placed in the distilling flask and boiled; the distillate is collected in a Nessler cylinder, and the boiling continued until the distillate gives no colour with 2 c.c. of the Nessler solution. As soon as the apparatus has been freed from ammonia, 500 c.c. of the sample are added to the contents of the distilling flask and the boiling continued; the distillate being collected in Nessler cylinders, 50 c.c. at a time; to the contents of each cylinder, 2 c.c. of the Nessler solution are added and the colour obtained is compared with the standard colours.

Standard colours are obtained by placing known quantities of the dilute ammonium chloride solution (*e.g.* 0·5 c.c., 1·0 c.c., 1·5 c.c., etc.) in a Nessler cylinder, filling up to the mark with distilled water free from ammonia, and adding 2 c.c. of the

Nessler solution. In some cases it may be found that the colour obtained with the first glass of the distillate is too deep to be compared with a standard solution, the contents of the glass are therefore diluted to 250 c.c. and then compared with the standard; or an aliquot portion may be taken and diluted with ammonia-free water to 50 c.c. and then compared with the standard. The amount of ammonia obtained in the distillation is calculated from the known strength of the dilute ammonia solution.

In this process the sodium carbonate decomposes any ammonium salts in the water, and the ammonia so obtained, together with any free ammonia in the water, passes over and is collected in the distillate. Ammonia is one of the first products of the decomposition of animal matter and its presence in water in very large quantities must be looked upon with suspicion; but it must be remembered that ammonium salts are not in themselves harmful and their presence in water does not necessarily render the sample unfit for drinking purposes.

Albuminoid ammonia

Solution required:

Alkaline permanganate solution. Weigh out

8 grams of potassium permanganate,
200 grams of caustic potash,

dissolve these together in about 1200 c.c. of distilled water and evaporate the solution to about 900 c.c., add 200 c.c. of distilled water and again evaporate the solution to 1000 c.c.; the solution, which will be found to be free from ammonia, is kept in a glass stoppered bottle.

Estimation of albuminoid ammonia. To the remainder of the water in the distilling flask, after the estimation of free and saline ammonia, add 50 c.c. of the alkaline permanganate solution, which has been previously heated to boiling, and continue the boiling; the ammonia is estimated colorimetrically as before.

The nitrogen in organic combination (as urea, uric acid, indol, skatol, and other proteid substances) is oxidized by the action of the alkaline solution of permanganate to ammonia.

The amount of ammonia obtained is, therefore, a measure of the organically combined nitrogen present in the sample.

Estimation of total solid matter

Measure out 100 c.c. of the sample into a weighed platinum dish, and evaporate it to dryness on a water bath; then place the dish in a water oven at 100° C. for three hours; cool in a desiccator and weigh; the increase in weight represents the total solid matter in 100 c.c. of the water. Each mgm (= 0·001 of a gram) of solid matter represents one part per 100,000.

Chlorine as chlorides

Solutions required:

Silver nitrate solution. Weigh out 2·4 grams of pure dry silver nitrate, and dissolve it in distilled water and make up to 1000 c.c. 1 c.c. of this solution = 0·0005 gram of chlorine; or when working on 50 c.c. 1 c.c. = 1 part of chlorine per 100,000.

Potassium chromate solution. Weigh out 10 grams of potassium chromate, free from chloride, and dissolve it in 100 c.c. of distilled water.

Estimation of chlorine as chlorides. Place 50 c.c. of water in a porcelain dish; add three drops of the potassium chromate solution, and run in the silver nitrate solution from a burette, with constant stirring, until a slight but permanent red brown colour is obtained; then read off the number of c.c. of silver nitrate solution used. The silver nitrate precipitates the chlorine present in the water, as silver chloride; and, as soon as all the chloride is precipitated, a reddish insoluble compound of silver chromate is formed.

Oxygen absorbed from potassium permanganate solution

(1) *Solutions required:*

Potassium permanganate solution. Weigh out 0·395 gram of pure potassium permanganate; dissolve it in distilled water and make up to 1000 c.c. 1 c.c. of this solution = 0·0001 gram of available oxygen.

Oxalic acid solution. Weigh out 0·7875 gram of crystallized

oxalic acid; dissolve it in distilled water and make up to 1000
c.c. 1 c.c. of this solution = 1 c.c. of the permanganate solution.

Sulphuric acid solution. Measure out 33 c.c. of pure concentrated sulphuric acid, and add it gradually, with constant
stirring, to 66 c.c. of distilled water; allow it to cool; to the
cold solution add, drop by drop, potassium permanganate
solution until a faint pink colour remains after keeping the
solution at 80° F. for four hours.

Estimation of the oxygen absorbed. Into each of two conical
flasks, of about 800 c.c. capacity, pour a small quantity of
concentrated sulphuric acid and thoroughly rinse, taking care
that the sulphuric acid comes in contact with the whole of the
inside of the flask; wash out the flasks thoroughly first with
tap water and afterwards with distilled water.

Into one flask measure out 250 c.c. of the sample; into the
other flask 250 c.c. of distilled water; and to each add 10 c.c.
of the potassium permanganate solution from a pipette, and
10 c.c. of the sulphuric acid solution; raise the temperature to
80° F. and maintain it at this temperature for four hours; if,
at any time, the pink colour disappears a further quantity of
10 c.c. of the potassium permanganate solution must be added.
At the end of four hours titrate the solution in each flask with
the oxalic acid solution; the difference in the two titrations
multiplied by 0·0001 will give the amount of oxygen absorbed
by 250 c.c. of the sample.

(2) *Potassium iodide and sodium thiosulphate method.*

Solutions required:

Standard solution of potassium perman-⎫ prepared as
ganate.   ⎬ described
Dilute sulphuric acid solution.   ⎭ above.

Potassium iodide solution; 10 grams of KI are dissolved in
1000 c.c. of water.

Standard sodium thiosulphate solution; 1 gram of pure re-
crystallized sodium thiosulphate is dissolved in 1000 c.c. of water.

Starch solution; 1 gram of pure potato starch is mixed into
a smooth paste with a small quantity of water; and 200 c.c.
of boiling water are then carefully added with constant stirring
and the solution allowed to cool.

The process. The actual determination is carried out exactly
as described above, except that after standing for four hours
at 80° F. a few drops of the potassium iodide solution are
added to each flask, when a brown solution will be obtained
owing to the reaction of the potassium iodide with the excess
of potassium permanganate and the liberation of free iodine;
the standard solution of sodium thiosulphate is then run in
from a burette with constant shaking until a straw yellow
colour is obtained; a few drops of starch solution are then
added, producing a deep blue colour, and the titration with
the thiosulphate solution continued until the blue colour is
discharged.

Example. A blank experiment required 34 c.c. of the thiosulphate solution, and 250 c.c. of a water required 31·3 c.c.

$$400 \times 0{\cdot}001 \times \frac{34 - 31{\cdot}3}{34} = 0{\cdot}032 \text{ parts of oxygen absorbed per}$$

100,000 parts of water.

The purer natural waters, as a rule, contain only very small
quantities of oxidizable organic substances of vegetable origin;
this process, therefore, is a measure of the oxidizable organic
substances of animal origin in the water.

With a view of coming to a provisional conclusion more
rapidly than can possibly be done in all bacteriological tests,
and to a certain extent with chemical tests, Sir A. C. Houston,
in his 5th Report (1911) and 7th Report (1913) to the London
Metropolitan Water Board, made a considerable number of
detailed experiments to correlate the oxygen absorbed from
potassium permanganate in *five minutes*, as compared with
that absorbed in three hours, both at 80° F. He found that,
taking the arbitrary figure 0·1 per 100,000 as the basis for ob-
jecting to a water in a three hours' test, the comparable figure
for the five minutes' test was somewhat less than 0·038, the
ratios varying slightly with different waters. When a water is
appreciably worse than 0·1 in the three hours' test, the five
minutes' test will be usually above 0·038; and when a water is
appreciably better than 0·1 in the three hours' test, the five
minutes' test may be nearly always trusted not to exceed
0·038. Dr Houston states that since April, 1910, the figure
0·038 has been adopted for the five minutes' test, and if on

the examination of a sample of water, the results reach or exceed this amount, a telephone communication is sent at once to the district concerned. The five minutes' method is of little use when the waters are very good, but when they are unsatisfactory, the parallelism between the two sets of results is very striking, although, of course, the *actual* results differ in the two cases.

Nitrogen as Nitrates

Estimation of nitrogen as nitrates. Nitrogen occurring as nitrates is determined by one of several methods:

(*a*) Gasometric method.
(*b*) Colorimetric method.
(*c*) Ammonia method.
(*d*) Indigo method.
(*e*) Titanous Chloride method.

(*a*) *Gasometric method.* The residue from the determination of the total solid matter is dissolved in the smallest possible quantity of water, the sides of the dish being well scrubbed with a rubber-tipped glass rod; the solution is then poured into the cup of a Crum's nitrometer, filled with mercury and standing in a dish containing mercury, the tap is carefully opened and the solution allowed to run into the nitrometer; an equal volume of concentrated sulphuric acid is then poured into the cup and allowed to flow into the nitrometer in its turn, care being taken that no air is admitted; the bottom of the tube is closed with the thumb and the whole tube removed from the dish and well shaken, at an angle of 45° so that the mercury comes in contact with the mixture at the top of the tube; from time to time during the shaking the tube is replaced in the dish and the thumb removed to release the pressure; when the whole of the nitrate is decomposed the volume of gas obtained (nitric oxide) is noted, together with the temperature and pressure, and the volume is reduced to normal temperature and pressure. From the volume of the gas thus obtained the weight of nitrogen as nitrate in 100 c.c. of the water is calculated. The nitrogen present as nitrate is converted by the action of the sulphuric acid and mercury into nitric oxide (NO).

(b) *Colorimetric method.* *Solutions required:*

Phenol-sulphuric acid solution; weigh out 24 grams of pure phenol; dissolve it in 12 c.c. of distilled water and add 148 c.c. of pure concentrated sulphuric acid; heat the mixture on the water bath in a round bottomed flask for six hours; allow it to cool and preserve it in a tightly stoppered bottle.

Potassium nitrate solution; weigh out 0·722 gram of pure fused potassium nitrate; dissolve it in distilled water and make up to 1000 c.c. 1 c.c. of this solution = 0·0001 gram of nitrogen.

Place 25 c.c. of the water in a glass or porcelain dish and evaporate it to dryness on the water bath. 5 c.c. of the standard potassium nitrate solution are evaporated in another similar dish.

To each dish, when dry, 2 c.c. of phenol-sulphuric acid are added, and the contents of each dish thoroughly mixed with a glass rod while standing on the water bath; the contents are then washed with dilute ammonia solution into Nessler cylinders; excess of ammonia is added to each solution to the 50 c.c. mark. A deep yellow colour will appear in the standard solution and also in the water if nitrates are present; these colours are compared and the volume of the darker coloured solution equal in tint to 50 c.c. of the paler solution is noted. From this the amount of nitrate in 25 c.c. of the water is calculated, as 5 c.c. of the standard potassium nitrate solution, containing 0·0001 gram of nitrogen, were taken. When phenol-sulphuric acid acts upon a nitrate, picric acid is formed, and this with ammonia forms ammonium picrate, which has a deep yellow colour, clearly visible in even very dilute solutions.

The estimation of nitrates by this method shows a serious error in the presence of chlorine as chlorides, even when the chlorides are present in small quantities; and in order to overcome this error, Frederick (*Analyst*, 1919, XLIV, 281) proposes the following method, which is not affected by the presence of chlorides.

Solutions required:

Potassium nitrate solution containing 1·4434 grams of potassium nitrate in 1000 c.c.; 25 c.c. of this solution will contain 0·005 gram of nitrogen as nitrates; 10 c.c. of this solution are diluted to 100 c.c., and the resulting solution will contain 0·001 gram of nitrogen as nitrate in 25 c.c.

Phenol-sulphonic-sulphuric acid mixture. 4 grams of phenol are mixed with 4 c.c. of ammonia-free distilled water, 100 c.c. of pure sulphuric acid are then added and the mixture is heated for 6 hours at 80° to 85° C., cooled and made up to 500 c.c.; 300 c.c. of pure sulphuric acid are then mixed with 200 c.c. of ammonia-free water and added to the phenol-sulphonic acid solution, giving 1000 c.c. of the reagent.

The method. 25 c.c. of the sample are placed in a round-bottomed porcelain basin and 25 c.c. of the standard potassium nitrate solution are placed in a similar basin, 2 c.c. of the phenol-sulphonic-sulphuric acid mixture are added to each and thoroughly stirred with a glass rod. The basins are placed on a water bath and the contents are evaporated until no more water is expelled; during the evaporation, the liquid is occasionally stirred with a glass rod; the sides of the basin are washed with a very small quantity of water and the contents of the basin are again evaporated on the water bath, the residue is taken up with water and again evaporated; the final residue is taken up with water and washed into measuring glasses, the volume being brought up to about 95 c.c., 3 c.c. of ammonia (specific gravity 0·880) are then added and the volume is brought up to 100 c.c. with water. The colour in each glass is proportionate to the quantity of nitrate present. It is claimed that by this method the nitrogen as nitrates is accurately estimated, even in the presence of 100 parts of chlorine per 100,000, and further that the purity of the colours obtained is such that the matching with the standard solution is considerably simplified.

(c) *Ammonia method. Preparation of copper-zinc couple.* A small piece of zinc foil is immersed in a solution of copper sulphate containing 3 per cent. of the dissolved crystallized salt; a deposit of copper is left upon the zinc; the deposition of the copper should not be allowed to proceed too far, otherwise it will not adhere firmly to the zinc; the couple is well washed with distilled water.

250 c.c. of the sample are made acid with 0·5 gram of crystallized oxalic acid; the wet couple is added; the whole

placed in a water bath of cold water and the temperature
gradually raised to and maintained at 60° C. for one hour; the
ammonia formed is then distilled off in the ammonia distilling
apparatus and estimated colorimetrically with Nessler solution in the usual way.

The copper-zinc couple decomposes the water with the
formation of hydrogen, which reacts on the nitrate to form
nitrite; and this, in its turn, is further reduced by the hydrogen, forming ammonia.

Although this method is described it should be stated that
it has been proved by Purvis and Courtauld[1] that the method
is only reliable provided the waters contain merely inorganic
substances in solution, and little or no substances of an organic
nature. When sewages, or sewage effluents, or waters polluted
by animal or vegetable refuse were examined for nitrates by
the copper-zinc couple method, it was proved by them that
the effect of the couple was to produce ammonia by the reduction of the dissolved organic substances. The oxygen
liberated by the couple, as well as the hydrogen, influenced
the decomposition and the degradation of the dissolved organic
compounds, and produced ammonia as one of the final products, in addition to a reduction of the nitrates, whereby a
higher value is given to the nitric nitrogen present in any
solution. The method must, therefore, be rejected, for the ammonia thus produced comes from the dissolved nitrogenous
compounds as well as from the nitrates and nitrites.

(d) *Indigo method* (*Maix-Trommsdorf method*).

Solutions required:

Dilute indigo solution; 1 gram of pure powdered indigo is
mixed with 5 to 10 c.c. of fuming sulphuric acid in a small
mortar and allowed to stand for two hours; the mixture is
then diluted with 300 c.c. of water and filtered. 10 c.c. of this
solution are diluted to 100 c.c. for use. This solution must be
kept in the dark.

Concentrated sulphuric acid free from nitrates.

Potassium nitrate solution. 0·0749 gram of potassium
nitrate is dissolved in 1000 c.c. of water; 25 c.c. of this solution contain 0·001 gram of N_2O_5.

---

[1] *Proc. Camb. Phil. Soc.* (1908), vol. XIV, p. 441.

To determine the strength of the indigo solution, 25 c.c. of the potassium nitrate solution are placed in a small flask together with 25 c.c. of the concentrated sulphuric acid, and the indigo solution is run in from a burette, with constant shaking, until a permanent green colour is obtained; a second experiment is then made with a further 25 c.c. of the potassium nitrate solution, but in this case the whole of the indigo solution required in the first experiment is run in at once and the mixture well shaken. Should the green colour not be permanent, further quantities of the indigo solution are added drop by drop until the permanent colour is obtained. From the second experiment the number of c.c. of indigo solution corresponding to 0·001 gram of N_2O_5 is obtained; this should be from 7 to 9 c.c.

The process for the sample of water is carried out exactly as described above, 25 c.c. of water being used instead of the potassium nitrate solution. The method is very rapid, but the results obtained are not absolutely accurate as they are affected by the presence of easily oxidizable organic matter, and also by the rapidity with which the determination is carried out.

When animal organic matter containing nitrogen is oxidized, nitrates are ultimately formed; the presence, therefore, of large quantities of nitrogen in the form of nitrates in a water indicates past pollution, unless it can be shown that such nitrates are obtained from the rocks in the well. For example, waters from the chalk contain as much as 0·7 part per 100,000 of nitric nitrogen.

(e) *Titanous chloride method*, Knecht (*Ber.* 1903, XXXVI, 166).

100 c.c. of the sample of water are treated in a copper flask with excess of sodium hydroxide solution, followed by 20 c.c. of commercial titanous chloride solution; the mixture is then immediately distilled and the ammonia is estimated colorimetrically with Nessler solution in the usual way. The order of addition of the reagents must be strictly adhered to, otherwise some of the nitrogen will be lost; it is also essential that the reagents should be free from ammonia and a blank experiment with the reagents should always be first carried out. The saving of time in the use of this method is considerable as the reduction of the nitrate to ammonia is instantaneous.

Nitrogen as Nitrites

(a) *Solutions required:*

Metaphenylene-diamine solution. Weigh out 2 grams of metaphenylene-diamine hydrochloride; dissolve it in distilled water and make up to 100 c.c.

Standard potassium nitrite solution. Weigh out 0·406 gram of pure silver nitrite; dissolve it in boiling distilled water, and add excess of pure potassium chloride; cool and make up to 1000 c.c.; allow the precipitate of silver chloride to settle, and take 100 c.c. of the clear solution and dilute to 1000 c.c.; one c.c. of this solution = 0·00001 gram of N_2O_3. This solution will not keep long and has to be renewed constantly.

Place 100 c.c. of the water in a Nessler cylinder; add to it 2 c.c. of the metaphenylene-diamine solution, and 2 c.c. of 25 per cent. sulphuric acid; allow it to stand for at least thirty minutes; if a colour is produced, compare it with the colour obtained by treating known volumes of the standard nitrite solution in a similar manner.

Metaphenylene-diamine reacts with nitrous acid to form aminoazo-benzene or Bismarck-brown, which is the cause of the colour obtained.

The colour in this method is only progressively developed; and, in consequence, an attempt should not be made to compare the colours unless they have been standing for about thirty minutes.

(b) *Ilosvay's method of estimating nitrites.*

Solutions required: Weigh 0·1 gram of α-naphthylamine; dissolve in 200 c.c. of dilute acetic acid (sp. gr. 1·04).

Dissolve 0·5 gram of sulphanilic acid in 200 c.c. of dilute acetic acid.

100 c.c. of the sample of water are placed in a Nessler glass; and in another glass are placed 99 c.c. of distilled water and 1 c.c. of standard nitrite of potassium, as made in the last method. To each of these solutions add 2 c.c. of the sulphanilic acid solution and 2 c.c. of the naphthylamine solution. Allow to stand about five minutes and then compare the pink tints. If the tints are not equal then abstract a definite amount of the darker solution with a pipette, and make up to the original

volume with distilled water. Suppose, for example, that the
sample was darker, and that 40 c.c. were removed, and the
bulk made up to the original volume of 100 c.c., when the tints
were exactly the same; then 60 c.c. of the original 100 c.c.
were equal to 1 c.c. of the standard nitrite solution. Suppose
1 c.c. of this solution = 0·00001 gram N_2O_3, the 60 c.c. of the
sample are equivalent to 0·00001 gram N_2O_3, and therefore
the amount of N_2O_3 in parts per 100,000 will be equal to

$$\frac{0·00001 \times 100,000}{60} = 0·0167 \text{ gram } N_2O_3$$

$$= 0·0097 \text{ gram of nitrous nitrogen.}$$

It should be mentioned that a slight pink colour is acquired
by the blank solution if it stands too long.

Nitrites should never be present in potable waters as they
usually indicate insufficient oxidation of the organic matter,
and indeed the actual presence of sewage; the presence of
nitrites must, therefore, always be looked upon with the
gravest suspicion. At the same time, it must not be forgotten
that nitrites are often found in the waters from the Lower
Greensand, the purity of which is unquestionable.

Hardness

Solutions required:

Clark's soap solution. Weigh out
150 grams of lead plaster,
40 grams of dry potassium carbonate;

thoroughly mix in a mortar, add a little methylated spirit and
continue the mixing until a uniform mass is obtained; add a
little more methylated spirit and allow it to stand for some
hours; decant off the clear liquid and dilute with a mixture
of methylated spirit and distilled water (1 vol. of water to
2 vols. of methylated spirit) until exactly 14·25 c.c. of the
solution are required to form a permanent lather with the
standard calcium chloride solution.

Clark's soap solution may also be prepared by scraping 10
grams of shavings from a new cake of Castile soap, which are
dissolved in 1000 c.c. of 35 per cent. alcohol, care being taken
to dissolve all the soap; the solution is then filtered and kept
tightly stoppered.

Standard calcium chloride solution. Weigh out 0·2 gram of pure Iceland Spar; dissolve it in dilute hydrochloric acid in a dish provided with a glass cover to prevent loss by spurting; evaporate the solution to dryness on the water bath; redissolve the residue in distilled water and evaporate three times to remove all the hydrochloric acid; and finally dissolve in water and make up to 1000 c.c.

Hardness is of two kinds, "Temporary Hardness," which is due to the solution in the water of the carbonates of calcium and magnesium, and which can be removed by boiling; and "Permanent Hardness," which is primarily due to the presence of calcium and magnesium sulphates and which cannot be removed by boiling.

Estimation of total hardness. Measure out 50 c.c. of the water into a stoppered bottle of about 200 c.c. capacity, and run the soap solution from a burette into the water in the bottle, at first 0·5 c.c. at a time and finally 0·1 c.c. at a time, until, on shaking the bottle vigorously, a lather is formed which remains unbroken on the surface for three minutes; the volume of the soap solution used is then read off on the burette. If more than 16 c.c. of the soap solution are used, 25 c.c. of the water

Table of hardness.

c.c. of soap solution used	$CaCO_3$ per 100,000	c.c. of soap solution used	$CaCO_3$ per 100,000	c.c. of soap solution used	$CaCO_3$ per 100,000
1·00	0·48	6·25	7·78	11·50	15·63
1·25	0·88	6·50	8·14	11·75	16·03
1·50	1·27	6·75	8·50	12·00	16·43
1·75	1·63	7·00	8·86	12·25	16·82
2·00	1·95	7·25	9·21	12·50	17·22
2·25	2·40	7·50	9·57	12·75	17·62
2·50	2·60	7·75	9·93	13·00	18·02
2·75	2·92	8·00	10·30	13·25	18·41
3·00	3·25	8·25	10·67	13·50	18·81
3·25	3·58	8·50	11·05	13·75	19·21
3·50	3·90	8·75	11·42	14·00	19·60
3·75	2·96	9·00	11·80	14·25	20·00
4·00	4·57	9·25	12·18	14·50	20·40
4·25	4·93	9·50	12·56	14·75	20·79
4·50	5·29	9·75	12·93	15·00	21·19
4·75	5·64	10·00	13·31	15·25	21·60
5·00	6·00	10·25	13·68	15·50	22·02
5·25	6·36	10·50	14·06	15·75	22·43
5·50	6·71	10·75	14·44	16·00	22·86
5·75	7·07	11·00	14·84		
6·00	7·43	11·25	15·22		

should be diluted with distilled water, freed from carbon dioxide by boiling, and this diluted solution titrated as before. The degree of hardness is found by reference to the table on p. 15.

Estimation of permanent hardness. Place 100 c.c. of the water in a beaker and boil to about one-third of its volume; wash out the contents of the beaker into a 100 c.c. graduated flask; cool and make up to the 100 c.c. mark with distilled water, freed from carbon dioxide by boiling; the salts which produce temporary hardness are precipitated by the boiling and filtered off: titrate 50 c.c. of the filtered solution with the soap solution as before. The permanent hardness thus obtained is subtracted from the total hardness, the result being the temporary hardness.

Water Softening

Occasionally, in very small areas, it is found that the only available water supply for public purposes consists of water which is exceedingly hard; and, as it is always inadvisable to use a very hard water for domestic purposes, it becomes necessary to add to it various chemicals, which have the effect of removing the hardness, at least partially. The chemicals most commonly used are lime and sodium carbonate; and the amount required can be calculated from the results of analysis. It is necessary for this purpose to know the amount of acidity (calculated as CO_2), calcium carbonate, magnesium carbonate, calcium sulphate, and magnesia (calculated as MgO) existing as sulphate, nitrate or chloride. The reactions taking place on the additions of the chemicals are represented by the following equations:

1. $CO_2 + CaO = CaCO_3$.
2. $Ca(HCO_3)_2 + CaO = 2CaCO_3 + H_2O$.
3. $Mg(HCO_3)_2 + 2CaO = 2CaCO_3 + MgO + H_2O$.
4. $CaSO_4 + Na_2CO_3 = CaCO_3 + Na_2SO_4$.
5. $MgSO_4 + Na_2CO_3 + CaO = MgO + Na_2SO_4 + CaCO_3$.

From these equations the amount of softening materials to be added can be calculated. The amount of lime to be added, in parts per 100,000, is obtained by adding together:

the parts per 100,000 of acidity (calculated as CO_2) × 1·273,
the parts per 100,000 of calcium carbonate × 0·56,
and the parts per 100,000 of magnesium carbonate × 1·33.

The amount of sodium carbonate to be added, in parts per 100,000, is obtained by adding together:
the parts per 100,000 of calcium sulphate × 0·779,
and the parts per 100,000 of magnesia (as sulphate, etc.) × 2·65.

These calculations will give the amounts of pure lime and pure sodium carbonate required to soften the water; but it must always be remembered that the lime and sodium carbonate of commerce are not pure, and, therefore, the amount of each required will vary with the degree of purity. Lime is usually added in the form of lime water; each gallon of lime water contains approximately 70 grains of lime.

A rough calculation of the amounts of lime and sodium carbonate required may also be made from the temporary and permanent hardness:

The number of degrees of temporary hardness multiplied by 0·08 will give the amount of lime to be added in pounds per 1000 gallons of water.

The number of degrees of permanent hardness multiplied by 0·112 will give the amount of sodium carbonate to be added in pounds per 1000 gallons of water.

Detection of hypochlorite in waters. Ling (*Analyst*, 1918, XLIII, 347). Waters containing organic matter are frequently treated with hypochlorite for the purpose of removing the organic matter; this treatment converts the ammonia compounds into chloramine- and chloramino-derivatives; and, in consequence, the amount of ammonia and albuminoid ammonia is not reduced. The following method has been devised for the purpose of detecting the treatment with hypochlorite: place 50 c.c. of the sample and 50 c.c. of distilled water in two Nessler cylinders; add to each 1 c.c. of N/1 sulphuric acid and 0·1 gram of potassium iodide (free from iodate); a hypochlorite-treated water rapidly turns brown, but the distilled water remains colourless.

Estimation of dissolved oxygen in waters

For the methods employed in this determination see p. 61.

Poisonous metals

The two poisonous metals of most importance are usually copper and lead; iron, zinc, tin, and arsenic come next in importance. To test for these metals qualitatively, the sample of water should be concentrated if necessary. Then place 50 c.c. of each in test glasses, add one drop of dilute hydrochloric acid, and then one drop of ammonium sulphide from the end of a glass rod; a brown colour will be produced from either lead, copper or iron; a white precipitate with zinc.

(1) When the colour is brown, divide the solution into two portions; to one portion add excess of hydrochloric acid; the colour will disappear if it is iron. Confirm the iron by taking a fresh portion of the concentrated solution, add a drop of nitric acid, and then a few drops of potassium ferrocyanide, when a blue colour will be produced.

(2) If it is not iron, take the other portion, add a few drops of potassium cyanide; if the colour is destroyed, it is copper. Confirm the copper by taking two fresh portions of the concentrated solution; to one portion add potassium ferrocyanide, when a bronze colour or precipitate is produced if it is copper; and to the other portion add ammonia, when a blue colour results which confirms copper.

(3) If the precipitate does not dissolve when potassium cyanide is added, it is very probably lead. To confirm lead, take two fresh portions of the concentrated solution; to one add a drop or two of clear potassium iodide solution, when a yellow precipitate or opalescence of lead iodide will appear; and to the other portion add potassium chromate solution which produces a yellow precipitate of lead chromate: thus confirming lead.

(4) If the precipitate is white, it may be caused by zinc. This may be confirmed by adding potassium ferrocyanide to a portion of the concentrated solution, when a white gelatinous precipitate is produced.

(5) When arsenic is in solution the colour of the sample of water becomes yellow on the addition of one drop of ammonium sulphide; a yellow precipitate may be produced if the arsenic is in sufficient quantity. It may be confirmed by

placing some zinc foil in a large test-tube, and boiling it with
sodium hydroxide; a few drops of the concentrated water containing the dissolved arsenic compound are added and boiled
again; at the same time, hold a piece of filter paper over the
mouth of the test-tube, on which there is a spot of silver
nitrate, and the latter becomes black or brown if arsenic is
present. A blank experiment should be done with the reagents
themselves, because the zinc may contain arsenic.

(6) If it is thought that tin is present in the water, the concentrated sample is reduced from the stannic to the stannous
condition, by adding some metallic copper and a little hydrochloric acid, and boiled well; then a few drops of mercuric
chloride are added, when a silky precipitate of mercurous
chloride is produced, which may be further reduced to dark
grey mercury, if tin is dissolved in the water.

Estimation of poisonous metals

Lead.

Standard lead solution. Weigh out 0·183 gram of pure lead
acetate; dissolve in distilled water and make up to 1000 c.c.
1 c.c. of this solution = 0·0001 gram of lead.

Saturated sulphuretted hydrogen solution. This solution is
obtained by passing hydrogen sulphide gas, from a Kipp's
apparatus, into distilled water to saturation.

For the estimation, place 50 or 100 c.c. of the water in a
Nessler cylinder and add to it six drops of acetic acid and then
two drops of the saturated sulphuretted hydrogen solution;
in the presence of lead a brown or black colour will be produced; or one drop of ammonium sulphide may be used instead.
If the colour is obtained, place in another cylinder a measured
quantity of the standard lead solution (0·5, 1·0, 1·5 c.c., etc.);
fill the cylinder with distilled water to the 50 or 100 c.c. mark;
add acetic acid and sulphuretted hydrogen solution, or ammonium sulphide, as before, and match the colours in the two
cylinders.

Copper.

Standard copper solution. Weigh out 0·393 gram of pure
crystallized copper sulphate; dissolve in distilled water and

make up to 1000 c.c. 1 c.c. of this solution = 0·0001 gram of copper.

A very dilute solution of potassium ferrocyanide.

Concentrate 1000 c.c. of the water, if necessary, by evaporation on the water bath to 100 c.c. and place it in a Nessler cylinder; and to the water add six drops of acetic acid and three drops of the potassium ferrocyanide solution; in the presence of copper a brown colour is obtained. It may happen that the colour will be produced in the water without any concentration: in which case, time will be saved. The brown colour is matched by treating measured volumes of the standard copper solution in another cylinder in a similar manner; and from the number of c.c. of the standard copper solution required, the amount of copper present in the sample is calculated.

Iron.

Standard iron solution. Weigh out 0·497 gram of pure crystallized ferrous sulphate; dissolve in distilled water and make up to 1000 c.c. 1 c.c. of this solution = 0·0001 gram of iron.

Evaporate 1 litre of the sample of water, if necessary, to 100 c.c.; place in a Nessler glass: add two or three drops of acetic acid, and then a drop of saturated sulphuretted hydrogen, a dark colour will be produced of ferrous sulphide. Place in another Nessler glass a measured quantity of the standard iron solution and repeat the process in the same way, and match the colours as before. The amount of iron can then be calculated.

Mineral analysis

Determination of alkalinity. Measure out 500 c.c. of the water into a large flask; add a few drops of methyl orange as an indicator; and run in from a burette N/100 hydrochloric acid until the yellow colour of the methyl orange just turns to pink; the number of c.c. of N/100 acid used multiplied by 0·0005 gives the alkalinity in terms of calcium carbonate.

Estimation of silica. One litre of the water is placed in a large porcelain dish with about 5 c.c. of concentrated hydrochloric acid; the whole is evaporated to small bulk on a water bath; the contents of the dish are then washed out into a platinum dish and evaporated to dryness; the residue is dried in the air oven. The dry residue is moistened with a few drops of concentrated hydrochloric acid; the acid is then evaporated on the water bath and the residue placed in an air oven at 150° C. for 30 minutes. After being in the air oven for 30 minutes, the residue is treated with water, filtered, and the filter well washed with hot water and dried in a water oven. The dried filter paper and residue are placed in a platinum dish and ignited over a Bunsen flame; as soon as a white or nearly white ash is obtained, the dish is placed in a desiccator, allowed to cool and weighed; the increase in weight of the dish, less the weight of the filter paper ash, represents silica.

Estimation of iron. To the filtrate from the silica determination, add a few drops of bromine and a small quantity of solid ammonium chloride, make alkaline with ammonia, boil and filter, well wash the filter with hot water, dry the filter paper with the iron oxide precipitate in the water oven, and, when dry, ignite it in a platinum dish and weigh the residue. The weight of the residue, less the weight of the filter paper ash, represents iron as Fe_2O_3.

Estimation of lime. If the filtrate from the iron determination is large, it must first be concentrated to about 250 c.c.; after this concentration, the solution is made alkaline with ammonia, and about 0·5 gram of solid ammonium oxalate is added, the whole is heated to boiling and then allowed to stand till cool. As soon as the solution is cool, it is filtered and the precipitate is well washed with hot water and dried in a water oven; when dry, the filter paper and precipitate are placed in a platinum dish and ignited over a blowpipe till the weight is constant; the increase in weight, less the weight of the filter paper ash, is calculated as CaO.

Estimation of magnesia. The filtrate from the lime determination is evaporated to small bulk and made strongly alkaline with ammonia, and 0·5 gram of solid ammonium phosphate added, and the solution stirred with a glass rod until a precipitate begins to appear; as soon as a precipitate begins to appear, the beaker is covered with a clock glass, set aside and allowed to stand overnight. On the following morning, the precipitate is filtered off, well washed with water containing ammonia, and dried in a water oven; when dry, the precipitate and filter paper are placed in a platinum dish and ignited first over a Bunsen flame and finally over a blowpipe till constant in weight. From the increase in weight of the platinum dish, the weight of the ash of the filter paper is subtracted, the remainder is magnesium pyrophosphate ($Mg_2P_2O_7$). The weight of magnesium pyrophosphate obtained multiplied by 0·3604 gives the weight of magnesia.

Estimation of alkalies. Measure out 500 c.c. of the water into a porcelain dish and evaporate it to dryness on a water bath; dissolve the residue in a small quantity of distilled water and filter; the filtrate is placed in a glass dish, three drops of dilute sulphuric acid are added and the whole is evaporated to dryness; the residue is dissolved in a small quantity of distilled water, two drops of barium chloride solution are added, followed by excess of baryta water, the whole is evaporated to dryness and allowed to stand for 30 minutes. After standing, the residue is dissolved in 50 c.c. of distilled water and filtered; the excess of barium salt in the filtrate is then precipitated with excess of ammonium carbonate; the precipitate is filtered off and the filtrate is evaporated to dryness and heated to 150° C. to remove the ammonium salts. When the ammonium salts have been removed, the residue is dissolved in distilled water and filtered; the filtrate is placed in a weighed platinum dish, a few drops of hydrochloric acid added, and evaporated to dryness, dried in the water oven and weighed; the residue consists of potassium and sodium chlorides. The weighed residue of the mixed chlorides is dissolved in water, a few drops of hydrochloric acid are added and an excess of a solution of platinum chloride; the solution is then evaporated to a syrupy consistency on a water bath in a porcelain basin; the contents of the basin are allowed to cool and are then treated with alcohol (specific gravity, 0·864), washed by decantation and the washings passed through a dried and weighed filter paper; the washing is continued until the alcohol is colourless; the precipitate is finally collected on the filter paper, washed with alcohol, dried in the water oven and weighed. The weight of potassium platino-chloride obtained multiplied by 0·3094

gives the weight of potassium chloride; the weight of sodium
chloride being obtained by subtracting this from the weight
of the mixed chlorides.

Estimation of sulphates. Measure out 500 c.c. of the water
into a beaker of about 800 c.c. capacity; place the beaker on a
sand bath and evaporate the water to about 150 c.c.; and to
the water while still hot, add 10 c.c. of concentrated hydrochloric acid and 25 c.c. of a boiling solution of barium chloride;
continue the boiling for a short time, and allow the precipitate
to settle in the beaker. As soon as the precipitate has settled,
collect it on a filter paper, specially prepared to retain barium
sulphate; wash with hot water until the washings give no
reaction for chlorides, and dry in a water oven; when the precipitate is dry, carefully transfer it from the filter paper to a
piece of glazed paper and cover it with a watch glass; fold up
the filter paper and incinerate it in a platinum dish over a
Bunsen flame; after the incineration of the paper, carefully
brush the precipitate into the dish and again ignite over the
Bunsen flame; allow the dish to cool in a desiccator, and weigh;
from this weight subtract the weight of the filter paper ash.
The weight of barium sulphate obtained multiplied by 0·34293
gives the weight of sulphate (as SO_3).

Notes on Water Purification

As many public water supplies undergo purification, before
being supplied to the general public, the following analyses of
the water supply of the County Borough of Stockport are of
interest. They represent weekly analyses of both the filtered
and unfiltered water over a period of twelve months and have
been kindly supplied by Messrs Bell Bros., of Manchester.
They also show the variation in the composition of the water
and the degree of purification after passing through the filters.
The average purification for the twelve months was: albuminoid ammonia, 89 per cent.; oxygen absorbed in 4 hours at
80° F., 85·3 per cent.; plumbo-solvency in a ½ in. × 3 ft. tube,
76·3 per cent.; the plumbo-solvency represents dissolved lead
after a second 24 hours' contact; U. is the unfiltered water and
F. is the filtered water.

	1		2		3	
	U.	F.	U.	F.	U.	F.
Free ammonia	0·006	0·006	0·006	0·005	0·0054	0·0054
Albuminoid ammonia ..	0·008	Trace	0·008	Trace	0·0064	Trace
Oxygen absorbed in 4 hours at 80° F.	0·358	0·033	0·337	0·031	0·281	0·035
Alkalinity	0·10°	0·0	0·10°	0·40°	0·20°	0·05°
Plumbo-solvency at 24 hours in ½ in. × 3 ft. tube ..	0·70	0·08	0·28	0·09	0·24	0·08

	4		5		6	
	U.	F.	U.	F.	U.	F.
Free ammonia	0·005	0·004	0·004	0·004	0·0036	0·0026
Albuminoid ammonia ..	0·0066	0·0016	0·006	0·0014	0·0064	0·001
Oxygen absorbed in 4 hours at 80° F.	0·285	0·055	0·277	0·084	0·248	0·061
Alkalinity	0·25°	0·45°	0·30°	0·05°	0·35°	0·10°
Plumbo-solvency at 24 hours in ½ in. × 3 ft. tube ..	0·20	0·06	0·24	0·04	0·18	0·06

	7		8		9	
	U.	F.	U.	F.	U.	F.
Free ammonia	0·002	0·002	0·003	0·002	0·0026	0·0036
Albuminoid ammonia ..	0·005	0·003	0·005	Trace	0·0054	0·001
Oxygen absorbed in 4 hours at 80° F.	0·242	0·056	0·253	0·028	0·262	0·030
Alkalinity	0·40°	0·40°	0·40°	0·40°	0·35°	0·10°
Plumbo-solvency at 24 hours in ½ in. × 3 ft. tube ..	0·20	0·10	0·40	0·06	0·20	0·06

	10		11		12	
	U.	F.	U.	F.	U.	F.
Free ammonia	0·002	0·0024	0·002	0·0026	0·001	0·0014
Albuminoid ammonia ..	0·005	0·001	0·005	0·001	0·0044	0·001
Oxygen absorbed in 4 hours at 80° F.	0·256	0·019	0·240	0·025	0·232	0·030
Alkalinity	0·35°	0·05°	0·30°	0·25°	0·45°	0·45°
Plumbo-solvency at 24 hours in ½ in. × 3 ft. tube ..	0·24	0·06	0·30	0·12	0·25	0·06

	13		14		15	
	U.	F.	U.	F.	U.	F.
Free ammonia	0·001	0·001	0·001	0·0016	Trace	0·001
Albuminoid ammonia ..	0·0048	0·001	0·005	0·001	0·008	0·001
Oxygen absorbed in 4 hours at 80° F.	0·214	0·034	0·222	0·022	0·238	0·019
Alkalinity	0·40°	0·15°	0·35°	0·30°	0·25°	0·50°
Plumbo-solvency at 24 hours in ½ in. × 3 ft. tube ..	0·28	0·04	0·28	0·12	0·16	0·04

	16		17		18	
	U.	F.	U.	F.	U.	F.
Free ammonia	Trace	Trace	Trace	Trace	Trace	Trace
Albuminoid ammonia	0·007	0·0014	0·0066	0·0014	0·0044	Trace
Oxygen absorbed in 4 hours at 80° F.	0·246	0·024	0·207	0·020	0·188	0·014
Alkalinity	0·25°	0·30°	0·20°	0·45°	0·25°	0·0
Plumbo-solvency at 24 hours in ½ in. × 3 ft. tube	0·22	0·07	0·14	0·04	0·20	0·08

	19		20		21	
	U.	F.	U.	F.	U.	F.
Free ammonia	Trace	Trace	Trace	Trace	Trace	0·002
Albuminoid ammonia	0·0048	Trace	0·0038	Trace	0·0046	0·001
Oxygen absorbed in 4 hours at 80° F.	0·182	0·021	0·176	0·021	0·249	0·024
Alkalinity	0·30°	1·00°	0·40°	0·8°	0·25°	0·45°
Plumbo-solvency at 24 hours in ½ in. × 3 ft. tube	0·18	0·04	0·12	0·04	0·30	0·04

	22		23		24	
	U.	F.	U.	F.	U.	F.
Free ammonia	0·002	0·002	0·002	0·002	0·0014	0·0014
Albuminoid ammonia	0·0034	0·001	0·0048	0·001	0·0036	Trace
Oxygen absorbed in 4 hours at 80° F.	0·201	0·020	0·174	0·022	0·155	0·019
Alkalinity	0·25°	0·35°	0·25°	0·75°	0·20°	0·75°
Plumbo-solvency at 24 hours in ½ in. × 3 ft. tube	0·32	0·04	0·20	0·05	0·36	0·04

	25		26		27	
	U.	F.	U.	F.	U.	F.
Free ammonia	0·0016	0·0014	0·001	0·0014	0·001	0·0014
Albuminoid ammonia	0·0034	Trace	0·0036	Trace	0·004	Trace
Oxygen absorbed in 4 hours at 80° F.	0·145	0·020	0·143	0·015	0·170	0·023
Alkalinity	0·30°	0·75°	0·45°	1·3°	0·45°	0·75°
Plumbo-solvency at 24 hours in ½ in. × 3 ft. tube	0·20	0·06	0·30	0·03	0·28	0·09

	28		29		30	
	U.	F.	U.	F.	U.	F.
Free ammonia	0·0014	0·0014	0·002	0·001	0·002	0·002
Albuminoid ammonia	0·004	0·001	0·0036	Trace	0·0046	Trace
Oxygen absorbed in 4 hours at 80° F.	0·154	0·026	0·145	0·023	0·160	0·027
Alkalinity	0·50°	0·75°	0·50°	0·60°	0·45°	0·85°
Plumbo-solvency at 24 hours in ½ in. × 3 ft. tube	0·26	0·06	0·16	0·05	0·20	0·06

	31 U.	31 F.	32 U.	32 F.	33 U.	33 F.
Free ammonia	0·0024	0·0028	0·0014	0·002	0·002	0·002
Albuminoid ammonia	0·004	Trace	0·004	Trace	0·0034	Trace
Oxygen absorbed in 4 hours at 80° F.	0·171	0·024	0·149	0·027	0·145	0·032
Alkalinity	0·35°	0·85°	0·55°	1·00°	0·50°	0·90°
Plumbo-solvency at 24 hours in ¼ in. × 3 ft. tube	0·26	0·06	0·20	0·04	0·18	0·04

	34 U.	34 F.	35 U.	35 F.	36 U.	36 F.
Free ammonia	0·001	0·0014	Trace	Trace	0·0014	0·0014
Albuminoid ammonia	0·004	Trace	0·0044	Trace	0·0038	Trace
Oxygen absorbed in 4 hours at 80° F.	0·157	0·025	0·151	0·012	0·170	0·024
Alkalinity	0·50°	1·20°	0·55°	1·15°	0·50°	1·15°
Plumbo-solvency at 24 hours in ¼ in. × 3 ft. tube	0·20	0·00	0·15	0·03	0·22	0·06

	37 U.	37 F.	38 U.	38 F.	39 U.	39 F.
Free ammonia	Trace	0·001	0·001	0·001	Trace	Trace
Albuminoid ammonia	0·0038	Trace	0·004	Trace	0·0038	Trace
Oxygen absorbed in 4 hours at 80° F.	0·154	0·020	0·150	0·027	0·147	0·024
Alkalinity	0·45°	1·20°	0·55°	1·05°	0·55°	1·40°
Plumbo-solvency at 24 hours in ¼ in. × 3 ft. tube	0·24	0·04	0·16	0·06	0·14	0·03

	40 U.	40 F.	41 U.	41 F.	42 U.	42 F.
Free ammonia	Trace	Trace	Trace	Trace	Trace	Trace
Albuminoid ammonia	0·0044	Trace	0·005	Trace	0·005	Trace
Oxygen absorbed in 4 hours at 80° F.	0·143	0·023	0·140	0·020	0·133	0·025
Alkalinity	0·75°	1·20°	0·65°	1·40°	0·70°	1·15°
Plumbo-solvency at 24 hours in ¼ in. × 3 ft. tube	0·22	0·04	0·14	0·03	0·15	0·04

	43 U.	43 F.	44 U.	44 F.	45 U.	45 F.
Free ammonia	Trace	0·001	Trace	0·0014	Trace	0·001
Albuminoid ammonia	0·0054	0·001	0·004	Trace	0·005	0·0014
Oxygen absorbed in 4 hours at 80° F.	0·116	0·026	0·116	0·029	0·117	0·018
Alkalinity	0·85°	0·60°	0·85°	1·15°	0·90°	1·45°
Plumbo-solvency at 24 hours in ¼ in. × 3 ft. tube	0·14	0·08	0·24	0·03	0·18	0·04

	46		47		48	
	U.	F.	U.	F.	U.	F.
Free ammonia	Trace	Trace	Trace	Trace	Trace	Trace
Albuminoid ammonia ..	0·0044	0·001	0·0034	Trace	0·004	Trace
Oxygen absorbed in 4 hours at 80° F.	0·114	0·016	0·122	0·029	0·127	0·029
Alkalinity	1·00°	1·30°	1·05°	1·75°	1·20°	1·85°
Plumbo-solvency at 24 hours in ¼ in. × 3 ft. tube ..	0·16	0·04	0·12	0·02	0·16	0·00

	49		50		51	
	U.	F.	U.	F.	U.	F.
Free ammonia	Trace	Trace	Trace	0·001	0·001	0·001
Albuminoid ammonia ..	0·003	0·001	0·003	Trace	0·004	0·001
Oxygen absorbed in 4 hours at 80° F.	0·132	0·032	0·139	0·030	0·142	0·032
Alkalinity	1·25°	1·85°	1·20°	1·75°	1·20°	2·20°
Plumbo-solvency at 24 hours in ¼ in. × 3 ft. tube ..	0·14	0·04	0·14	0·06	0·16	0·04

The purification of a water supply should always be considered from the standpoint of the impurity which has to be removed, e.g. suspended solids, solids (both mineral and organic) in solution, etc. A surface water is very liable to be turbid from the presence of suspended matter; and this, in periods of rain or flood, is generally very excessive. A surface water is also liable to contain acid dissolved out of the peaty matter over which it passes. Such waters are disastrous, when unpurified, owing to their solvent action on the lead pipes. Water from deep wells may possibly contain objectionable mineral matter in solution, such as salts of iron, lime and magnesia; and, although these in themselves may not be deleterious, their removal is necessary if the water is to be used for domestic purposes.

It is essential that a general public water supply should be free from suspended matter; it should be clear, bright, and odourless; it should be free from mineral matter detrimental to health, or which would render the water unfit for use in household utensils or boilers. Many public authorities still make use of the method of filtration by gravity over a large area of prepared filter beds. The incompleteness of this method in a number of areas is demonstrated by the large number of household filters found in such areas; these are usually of the old animal charcoal type and remove the suspended matter, some of the dissolved organic matter and also some of the hardness. But they are themselves liable to become contaminated by vegetable growths; with the result that, eventually, the filtered water is far more impure than the unfiltered supply. If efficient purification of the original supply were effected before the water was discharged into the service pipes, the use of the household filter would be superfluous. Many public authorities, also, who obtain their water from a supposed uncontaminated source, do not consider it necessary to purify the water at all and admit the water direct to the service pipe; such a practice cannot always be recommended.

In many cases the water is so hard that it necessitates the addition of chemicals for the purpose of removing the lime and other salts. The usual chemicals used are lime water or sodium hydroxide solution and sodium carbonate; these effect the removal of both the temporary and the permanent hardness, and also neutralize the peaty acids, thus removing the plumbo-solvency. In many cases also a small quantity of aluminium sulphate is added; this produces a gelatinous insoluble precipitate of aluminium hydroxide, which is deposited on the filtering media, causing the removal of the objectionable colour and also of suspended matter and materially assisting the removal of bacteria and micro-organisms.

Interpretation of results

The correct interpretation of the results of an analysis of a sample of water is exceedingly difficult. It is not possible to obtain an infallible knowledge of the subject from text-books; it requires a long and varied experience of actual samples. A few suggestions may, however, be made to give a general idea of the methods, by which a correct interpretation is obtained.

The interpretation of analyses is illustrated later by some typical examples.

Deep well water. A deep well water containing over 0·006 parts of albuminoid ammonia per 100,000 is suspicious, as this amount would indicate surface pollution. The nitrates in a deep well water may be disregarded unless they are present in excessive quantities with a low albuminoid ammonia. The oxygen absorbed should be low. The chlorine should be low unless the well is near a coal seam, or near to the sea or a brackish estuary. Nitrites may be produced by reduction of nitrate, as in the water from the Lower Greensand rocks, but they must be looked upon with suspicion. The amount of free ammonia in a water from the Lower Greensand is often very high.

Shallow well water. If the amounts of albuminoid ammonia and oxygen absorbed in a shallow well water are high, and there is no other indication of pollution, the organic matter present may be of vegetable origin. High nitrate and chlorine, whether or not accompanied by high free and albuminoid ammonias, undoubtedly point to past pollution with animal organic matter.

Moorland waters. Moorland waters are often yellowish brown in colour. Albuminoid ammonia and oxygen absorbed are usually high with a low nitrate, pointing to organic matter of vegetable origin. The reaction of these waters is of very great importance, as, if they are even slightly acid, they will probably have a plumbo-solvent action.

The proportion of total solids in a water is not of very great importance from a Public Health point of view; as it depends on the geological nature of the strata through which the water has passed.

Examples:

Free and saline ammonia. 500 c.c. of the sample were taken for the estimation, the first distillate was matched with 0·8 c.c. of the standard dilute ammonia solution, the second distillate with 0·2 c.c., the third distillate was free from ammonia.

0·8 + 0·2 = 1·0 c.c. of the standard dilute ammonia solution used. Therefore the free ammonia in the sample

$$= 1\cdot0 \times 2 \times 100 \times 0\cdot00001 = 0\cdot002 \text{ part per 100,000.}$$

Albuminoid ammonia. The first distillate gave a colour equal to 0·5 c.c. of the standard dilute ammonia solution, the second to 0·2 c.c., the third distillate was free from ammonia.

0·5 + 0·2 = 0·7 c.c. of the standard dilute ammonium chloride solution used.

$0 \cdot 7 \times 2 \times 100 \times 0 \cdot 00001 = 0 \cdot 0014$ part per 100,000 of albuminoid ammonia.

Total solid matter. 100 c.c. of the water were taken for the estimation.

The weight of the dish and solid matter was 34·444 grams.
The weight of the dish was.. .. .. 34·431 grams.
∴ The weight of the solid matter was.. .. ·013 gram.

$0 \cdot 013 \times 1000 = 13 \cdot 0$ parts per 100,000 of total solid matter.

Chlorides. 50 c.c. of a sample were titrated with the standard silver nitrate solution, and required 4·5 c.c. to produce a slight permanent red colour, using the potassium chromate solution as an indicator.

The amount of chlorine as chlorides in the sample therefore was 4·5 parts per 100,000.

Oxygen absorbed from potassium permanganate solution. 250 c.c. of a sample were used for an estimation, 10 c.c. of the standard potassium permanganate solution were added and at the end of four hours 8·7 c.c. of the standard oxalic acid solution were required to decolorize the solution.

The amount of potassium permanganate solution used by the sample was $10 \cdot 0 - 8 \cdot 7 = 1 \cdot 3$ c.c.

$1 \cdot 3 \times 0 \cdot 0001 \times 4 \times 100 = 0 \cdot 052$ part per 100,000 of oxygen absorbed.

Nitrates. (a) *Gasometric.* 100 c.c. of a sample were used for the estimation and the volume of gas obtained was 0·7 c.c. The temperature was 16° C. and the pressure 770 mm.

The volume of gas reduced to normal temperature and pressure

$$= \frac{0 \cdot 7 \times 273 \times 770}{289 \times 760} = 0 \cdot 67 \text{ c.c.}$$

1 c.c. of NO weighs 0·00134 gram.

Therefore $0 \cdot 67 \times 0 \cdot 00134 \times 1000 = 0 \cdot 898$ part per 100,000 of nitrogen as nitrate.

(b) *Colorimetric.* In a colorimetric determination it was found that the standard potassium nitrate solution gave a very much deeper colour than the water, and that 10 c.c. of the standard solution was equal in tint to the 100 c.c. of the water.

Therefore the nitrogen as nitrate in the 25 c.c. of water taken

$$= \frac{5 \times 10}{100} \times 0.0001 \times 4000 = 0.2 \text{ part per } 100,000.$$

(c) *Ammonia method.* The first distillate was matched by 4·7 c.c. of the standard solution, the second distillate by 0·5, the third by 0·1 c.c., the fourth distillate contained no ammonia.

4·7 + 0·5 + 0·1 = 5·3 c.c. of the standard solution used.

Now 17 grams of ammonia contain 14 grams of nitrogen, therefore the nitrogen as nitrate in the sample was:

$$\frac{5.3 \times 14}{17} \times 0.0001 \times 4 \times 100 = 0.174 \text{ part per } 100,000.$$

Nitrites. In an estimation of nitrites, 100 c.c. of the water gave a colour which was exactly matched with 0·5 c.c. of the standard nitrite solution.

The amount of nitrite as N_2O_3 therefore was

0·5 × 0·00001 × 1000 = 0·005 part per 100,000.

Lead. The colour obtained with 100 c.c. of the water was exactly matched with 15 c.c. of the standard lead solution.

The amount of lead in the water was

1·5 × 0·0001 × 1000 = 0·15 part per 100,000.

Copper. 1000 c.c. of water after concentration to 100 c.c. gave a colour which was matched with 0·7 c.c. of the standard copper solution.

The amount of copper in the water was

0·7 × 0·0001 × 100 = 0·007 part per 100,000.

Typical analyses

The following typical analyses are introduced to show the wide differences to be met with both in the inorganic and organic constituents of waters. The numbers are in parts per 100,000 except where specially mentioned. It should also be remembered that an analysis of the organic constituents need not be the final judgment of a water. It is necessary that the chemist should know some of the conditions to aid him in a sound judgment of the results of his analysis[1]. For this purpose (1) he should be acquainted with the geological nature of the district from which the water is obtained; and the general saline constituents of the geological strata, for an analysis may show high chlorides which have been dissolved from the rocks. This is particularly the case with wells near the sea coast and from the Lower Greensand rocks; (2) he should be acquainted with the gathering ground, the methods of storage and distribution of the water; (3) if the water is obtained from wells, he should visit the place himself to note any faults in the outlet, the surface drainage and in the covers of the wells; (4) he should know the amount of the rainfall before and after the analysis was made, for after a heavy rainfall the analysis often gives results which differ very considerably from one before the rainfall; and (5) in case of any doubt a bacterial analysis should be undertaken. A water may be chemically pure and still contain the germs of disease; and, on the other hand, a water may be bacterially pure, whereas chemically the constituents might indicate contamination.

Physical characters	(1) Well aerated, no smell or sediment, reaction slightly alkaline	(2) Slightly opalescent, but there was no smell
Free and saline ammonia ..	0·001	0·0860
Albuminoid ammonia	0·002	0·0055
Oxygen absorbed from potassium permanganate in four hours at 80° F.	0·007	0·0060
Chlorine	2·500	9·8000
Nitric nitrogen	0·600	nil
Nitrous nitrogen	nil	0·0050
Total solids	44	81
(a) Volatile solids	22	15
(b) Non-volatile solids (faint charring on incineration)	22	66 (faint charring on heating)
Total hardness (per 100 c.c.) ..	17°	11°
(a) Permanent hardness ..	5°	10·5°
(b) Temporary hardness ..	12°	0·5° (9 parts of iron per 100,000 were found)

Number (1) is a water obtained from a deep well in the Upper Chalk. Organically it is very pure; the only fault is

[1] See Purvis, *Journ. Roy. Sany. Inst.* (1905), vol. xxvi, p. 429.

the high degree of hardness, which could easily be remedied, as it is chiefly caused by the acid carbonate of calcium and in a less degree of the salt of magnesium. Number (2) is a water from the Lower Greensand. The high free ammonia and chlorine are noticeable: high figures are always obtained from such waters; but the albuminoid ammonia is comparatively low, and the figure for oxygen absorbed is also low: the absence of nitric nitrogen should be noticed, and the presence of nitrous nitrogen. The latter must not condemn the water. It has not been produced by bacteria, but by the reduction of the nitrates as a consequence of the iron salt, to which the colour of the Lower Greensand owes its origin, being partly oxidized to the ferric condition.

Physical characters	(3) Clear, no smell, no sediment, neutral reaction	(4) Slightly opalescent, no smell, light yellow brown colour
Free and saline ammonia ..	0·0010	0·0720
Albuminoid ammonia	0·0024	0·0240
Oxygen absorbed from potassium permanganate in three hours at 80° F.	0·0040	0·0170
Chlorine	4·0000	18·8000
Nitric nitrogen	0·7500	2·000
Nitrous nitrogen	nil	0·004
Total solids	46	128
(a) Volatile solids	10	45
(b) Non-volatile solids ..	36 (no charring on heating)	83 (blackened on heating)
Total hardness (per 100 c.c.) ..	22°	18°
(a) Permanent hardness ..	10°	12°
(b) Temporary hardness ..	12°	6°
	No poisonous metals	No poisonous metals

Number (3) is a water from a shallow well in the Magnesian Limestone. The outstanding figures are those for the chlorine and nitric nitrogen. The two ammonias and the oxygen absorbed figures are low. The water shows, therefore, signs of past contamination, and the potential danger is obvious. Such a well would have to be carefully watched, and should be bacterially analysed. Care should be taken to protect the water from any possible contamination.

Number (4) is a water from a shallow well. All the numbers are very high; and it must be condemned as quite unfit for drinking purposes. It shows unmistakeable signs of a high degree of pollution.

Physical characters	(5) Brown colour, sediment, slightly acid reaction, no smell	(6) Good
Free and saline ammonia ..	0·0960	trace
Albuminoid ammonia	0·0470	0·0574
Oxygen absorbed from potassium permanganate in three hours at 80° F.	0·3950	0·0050
Chlorine	3·2000	1·2000
Nitric nitrogen	trace	0·5000
Nitrous nitrogen	nil	nil
Total solids	22	31
(a) Volatile solids	14	12
(b) Non-volatile solids ..	8 (blackened on heating)	19 (very slight charring on heating)
Total hardness (per 100 c.c.) ..	6·5°	16°
(a) Permanent hardness ..	3·5°	4·5°
(b) Temporary hardness ..	3·0°	11·5°
	No poisonous metals	No poisonous metals

Number (5) is a water from a village pond and has been used for drinking purposes. The pollution was partly caused by vegetable growths; but a microscopic examination of the sediment showed the bodies and wings of various insects as well as vegetable cells and debris. The water must be wholly condemned for drinking purposes. The softness of the water is noticeable.

Number (6) is a water from a well in the Upper Chalk about 37 feet deep. The two outstanding figures are those for the albuminoid ammonia and the nitric nitrogen. The former is a little disconcerting; but the low chlorine and oxygen absorbed figures are in its favour. On the whole, the water must be watched carefully, and a bacterial analysis should be made. Care should also be taken that the mouth of the well is protected.

Physical characters	(7) Neutral reaction, clear, no sediment	(8) Neutral reaction, no smell, no sediment, clear
Free and saline ammonia ..	0·0420	0·0020
Albuminoid ammonia	0·2940	0·0100
Oxygen absorbed from potassium permanganate in three hours at 80° F.	0·1880	0·3000
Chlorine	32·0000	6·000
Nitric nitrogen	3·0000	7·000
Nitrous nitrogen	0·0090	nil
Total solids	255	—
(a) Volatile solids	50	—
(b) Non-volatile solids ..	205 (blackened on heating	—
Total hardness (per 100 c.c.) ..	34°	33°
(a) Permanent hardness ..	31°	—
(b) Temporary hardness ..	3°	—
	No poisonous metals	No poisonous metals

Number (7) is water from a shallow well. It is highly polluted with organic matter. Every item is high and the presence of nitrous nitrogen shows that bacterial action is going on. It must be condemned as a dangerous water: the high degree of hardness is also unfavourable to its use for other purposes.

Number (8) is also from a shallow well. All the figures are high except the free ammonia. The high nitrate and chlorine figures show considerable past pollution: and the high figures for the albuminoid ammonia and the oxygen absorbed show that the pollution is going on. It must be condemned for drinking purposes.

Physical characters	(9) Not very clear, poorly ærated, neutral reaction	(10) Slightly turbid, pale yellow colour (grains per gallon)
Free and saline ammonia ..	0·0060	none
Albuminoid ammonia	0·0056	·0217
Oxygen absorbed from potassium permanganate in four hours at 80° F.	0·0080	·1092
Chlorine	3·1000	9·200
Nitric nitrogen	3·5000	1·600
Nitrous nitrogen	nil	nil
Total solids	60	127
(a) Volatile solids	14	—
(b) Non-volatile solids ..	46 (slight charring on heating)	—
Total hardness (per 100 c.c.) ..	20°	—
(a) Permanent hardness ..	7°	—
(b) Temporary hardness ..	13°	—
	No poisonous metals	A microscopic examination of the slight deposit showed that it was organic matter

Number (9) is from a shallow well (20 feet deep) in the Chalk formation: it shows definite signs of past contamination, as indicated by the high nitric nitrogen and the comparatively high chlorine figure; the two ammonias and the oxygen absorbed figures are also higher than is usually found in deep wells from the Chalk; and for these reasons also it must be condemned.

Number (10) is from a well in the gravel above the Chalk. The numbers in No. 10 are in grains per gallon. With the exception of the free ammonia, all the constituents are high; and both the smell on heating and the microscopic examination of the sediment showed that the water was polluted with sewage, and was unfit for drinking purposes. We are indebted to Mr J. West Knights for this analysis.

	(11)	(12)	(13)	(14)	(15)
Free and saline ammonia ..	0·000	0·557	0·006	0·003	0·024
Albuminoid ammonia ..	0·004	0·550	0·008	0·004	0·004
Oxygen absorbed from potassium permanganate in four hours at 80° F. ..	0·170	0·871	—	—	—
Chlorine	0·800	3·570	8·700	6·800	22·95
Nitric nitrogen	nil	nil	6·350	3·800	0·220
Nitrous nitrogen	nil	nil	—	—	—
Total solids	6·000	42·5	112·5	220·2	194·0

Number (11) is an analysis of the Birmingham City Water Supply by Mr J. F. Liverseege, F.I.C., City Analyst. The gathering ground is near Rhayader in Wales; the geological formation is Silurian and consists of shales and flagstones, with some massive layers of conglomerate. None of the land is cultivated; the whole is occupied as rough hill pasture restricted to sheep farming; the water shows a complete absence of free and saline ammonia, low chlorine, and total solids and medium oxygen absorbed. (For the mineral analysis of Number (11) see p. 46.)

Number (12) is an analysis of a water from a shallow well with a cesspool at a short distance from it; the free and saline and albuminoid ammonias and the oxygen absorbed are exceedingly high; the water is grossly contaminated with fresh animal organic matter and must be condemned.

Numbers (13), (14) and (15) are analyses of Burton-on-Trent waters by Messrs F. E. Lott and C. G. Matthews (*Jour. Soc. Chem. Ind.* 1911, vol. xxx, p. 69). No. (13) consists partly of rain water in the Trent valley and partly of water from springs in the Marl bed underlying the gravel and shows a high nitrate, total solids and chlorine. No. (14) is from a bore hole in the Marl bed and No. (15) is from a bore hole in the Lower Keuper Sandstone and shows high chlorine, total solids, and free and saline ammonia, with a low nitrate. For the mineral analyses of numbers (13), (14) and (15) see p. 47.

	(16)	(17)	(18)
Free and saline ammonia	0·001	0·000	0·003
Albuminoid ammonia	0·001	0·005	0·002
Oxygen absorbed from potassium permanganate in four hours at 80° F.	—	0·107	0·002
Chlorine	1·800	1·420	2·230
Nitric nitrogen	0·250	0·110	0·300
Nitrous nitrogen	—	—	—
Total solids	30·000	28·250	16·200
Mineral solid matter	—	20·750	—
Organic solid matter	—	7·500	—

Number (16) is an analysis by Mr C. L. L. Claremont, B.Sc.,
F.I.C., of the Portsmouth Public Water Supply; it is taken
from a deep chalk spring in the western end of the South
Downs; every item is low and the water is satisfactory. For
the mineral analysis of number (16) see p. 48.

Number (17) is an analysis by Mr E. Russell, B.Sc., F.I.C.,
City Analyst, of the Bristol City Water Supply showing a
medium oxygen absorbed and a moderately high organic solid
matter.

Number (18) is an analysis by the late Professor J. Campbell
Brown of a water from a deep bore hole in the Keuper Sandstone in south-west Lancashire; every item is low and the
water is satisfactory.

	(19)	(20)	(21)	(22)
Free and saline ammonia	0·003	0·006	0·0006	traces
Albuminoid ammonia	0·009	0·017	0·0052	0·0034
Oxygen absorbed from potassium permanganate in four hours at 80° F.	0·840	0·296	0·1294	0·1150
Chlorine	1·500	0·600	0·9000	1·3000
Nitric nitrogen	trace	0·109	0·0066	0·0500
Nitrous nitrogen	—	—	—	—
Total solids	10·160	3·980	3·800	7·000
Mineral solids	—	—	3·080	4·600
Organic and volatile solids	—	—	·720	2·400
Total hardness	—	—	·630	3·000

Numbers (19) and (20) are analyses of the Liverpool City
Water Supply by the late Professor J. Campbell Brown
(*Engineering*, 1903, LXXVI, 472), Number (19) is from the Rivingstone Supply in the Millstone Grit formation and number (20)
from the Vyrnwy Supply. Both waters are quite satisfactory.

Number (21) is an analysis of the Glasgow Water Supply
from Loch Katrine by Mr F. W. Harris, F.I.C., City Analyst.
All the items are extremely low. The total solids and the hardness are low. The obvious drawback to the water is its great
softness. (See p. 49 for the mineral analysis.)

Number (22) is an analysis of the water supply of the County
Borough of Blackpool which C. Arthur, Esq., secretary to the
Fylde Water Board, has kindly placed at our disposal. The
water is an upland surface water, the gathering ground of
which is the Lancashire and Yorkshire Moors. The surface is
soft and peaty and is thoroughly safeguarded from all risks of
animal pollution. The water is exceedingly soft; there is no

temporary hardness; and the hardness, wholly "permanent,"
is only 3°; the water is so soft that it has an erosive action on
lead pipes; it is slightly brown and turbid (see p. 52 for mineral
analysis).

	(23)	(24)	(25)
Free and saline ammonia	0·004	0·005	0·002
Albuminoid ammonia	0·005	0·005	0·002
Oxygen absorbed from potassium permanganate in four hours at 80° F.	0·006	—	0·004
Chlorine	2·000	1·800	4·250
Nitric nitrogen	0·371	0·350	0·173
Nitrous nitrogen	—	—	—
Total solids	18·600	17·200	27·600

Numbers (23), (24) and (25) are analyses by the late Professor J. Campbell Brown (*Engineering*, 1903, LXXVI, 472) of
waters from the same bore hole at Newton in south-west Lancashire at different depths, number (23) at 60 ft., number (24)
at 130 ft., number (25) at 500 ft. The particular items to be
noticed are the decrease in the free and saline and albuminoid
ammonias and the nitrate, and the increase in the total solids
and chlorine, as the depth increases.

	(26)	(27)	(28)	(29)	(30)
Free and saline ammonia ..	0·060	0·875	0·120	0·100	0·080
Albuminoid ammonia ..	0·002	0·004	0·006	0·008	0·004
Oxygen absorbed from potassium permanganate in four hours at 80° F. ..	0·036	0·680	—	0·124	0·035
Chlorine	17·1	1491·0	142·0	10·7	4·8
Nitric nitrogen	0·0	0·0	0·0	0·055	0·055
Nitrous nitrogen	—	—	—	—	—
Total solids	59·5	2628·0	282·0	62·5	51·0

Numbers (26), (27), (28), (29) and (30) are analyses by Mr
J. White, F.I.C., County Analyst of Derbyshire, of samples of
water taken from a bore hole at Ilkeston in Derbyshire.

Number (26) is the water originally yielded by the bore hole.
Number (27) is an abnormal water which gained access to the
bore hole by the splitting of the steel lining tubes. Number (28)
is a sample collected from the pumping shaft after the abnormal water had appeared. Numbers (29) and (30) are from
the pumping shaft about 80 ft. below the surface before the
water was found.

The particular items to note are the enormous chlorine, total
solids and free and saline ammonia in the abnormal water.
The mineral analysis of this water should be noted (p. 48).

Physical characters	(31) Yellow, turbid, no smell	(32) Deep yellow, slightly turbid, no smell	(33) Deep yellow, turbid, no smell	(34) Slightly turbid, no smell
Free and saline ammonia	none	·0007	0·0028	trace
Albuminoid ammonia ..	·0112	·0371	·0119	·0035
Oxgyen absorbed from potassium permangan- ate in 15 *minutes* at 140° F.	·0616	·1680	·1624	·0252
Chlorine	3·400	11·400	7·700	1·800
Nitric nitrogen	1·100	4·000	1·500	·500
Total solids	44·00	96·00	87·00	30·00
	The sediment showed earthy matter on a micro- scopic examination	There was a deposit of or- ganic matter	There was a deposit of or- ganic matter	A slight de- posit of oxide of iron

The above analyses are kindly supplied by Mr J. West Knights, Public Analyst for Cambridge, and the numbers represent grains per gallon.

Number (31) is from a shallow well and shows that the albuminoid ammonia and oxygen absorbed figures are high; the total solids and chlorides are not very low; the nitrates are high and unsatisfactory; the microscopic examination was bad. The water was considered to be polluted with sewage, and unfit for drinking purposes.

Number (32) is also from a well and shows that the total solids, chlorides and nitrates are all very high; the high nitrate figure must be specially noticed: the albuminoid ammonia and the oxygen absorbed figures are also very high. The water was condemned as highly polluted with sewage and quite unfit for drinking purposes.

Number (33) is also from a shallow well. The total solids, chlorides and nitrates are very high and unsatisfactory; the albuminoid ammonia and the oxygen absorbed are both very high, and show the presence of much organic matter; the appearance and the microscopic examination were also bad. The water was considered to be polluted and unfit for drinking purposes.

Number (34) is from a well in the Chalk. The solids, chlorides and nitrates are fairly low and quite satisfactory; the two ammonias and the oxygen absorbed are all low and show the absence of organic matter. The water is unpolluted and fit for drinking purposes.

	(35)	(36)	(37)	(38)
Physical characters	Slightly turbid, no smell	Clear, no smell, no deposit	Very turbid, no smell	Clear, no smell
Free and saline ammonia	0·0007	0·0005	·0357	0·0238
Albuminoid ammonia ..	·0021	0·0005	·0014	·0007
Oxygen absorbed from potassium permanganate in 15 *minutes* at 140° F.	·0168	0·0084	·0140	·0112
Chlorine	2·000	1·500	5·800	1·600
Nitric nitrogen	·100	none	none	none
Total solids	28·00	24·00	65·00	18·00
		The slight turbidity was from a slight deposit of chalk		The turbidity was caused by a deposit of hydrated oxide of iron	

The above analyses have also been supplied by Mr J. West Knights. They show the differences between the water of the Chalk and the Lower Greensand as well as variations in the water from different parts of the Greensand. The numbers represent grains per gallon.

Number (35) is from a deep well in the Chalk, and shows that the solids, chlorides and nitrates are low and quite satisfactory; the two ammonias and the oxygen absorbed figures are all low, and show the absence of organic matter. The water was unpolluted and fit for drinking purposes.

Number (36) is from the Lower Greensand. The solids, chlorides, nitrates, the two ammonias and the oxygen absorbed are all very low. The water was unpolluted and quite fit for drinking purposes.

Number (37) is also from the Greensand. All the items are low: and the water is quite unpolluted. The deposit of the oxide of iron could be cleared by subsidence or filtration.

Number (38) is also from the Greensand. All the items are low, and the water is quite fit for drinking purposes.

	(39)	(40)	(41)
Free and saline ammonia.. ..	Nil	Nil	Nil
Albuminoid ammonia	0·00005	0·008	0·009
Total solid matter..	44·0	46·0	30·0
Organic matter	12·0	18·0	12·0
Mineral matter	32·0	28·0	18·0
Oxygen absorbed from potassium permanganate in four hours at 80° F.	0·03	0·033	0·084
Chlorine	9·6	8·3	5·0
Nitrogen as nitrate	0·26	0·46	0·26
Total hardness	16·0°	16·5°	9·3°
(a) Temporary	6·5°	7·5°	2·8°
(b) Permanent	9·5°	9·0°	6·5°

Numbers (39) and (40) are taken from two bore holes at
Liscard in the Wirral peninsula, the bore holes are 800 feet
deep in the Red Sandstone; number (41) shows the water as
supplied to the public in the County Borough of Wallasey and
consists of the water from the bore holes mixed with the
Liverpool public supply (Numbers (19) and (20)).

	(42)
Free and saline ammonia..	0·500
Albuminoid ammonia	Nil
Oxygen absorbed from potassium permanganate	
in four hours at 80° F...	0·304
Chlorine	680·0
Nitric nitrogen	Nil
Nitrous nitrogen	Nil
Total solids	1185·4
Total hardness	101·5°
(a) Temporary	25·2°
(b) Permanent	76·3°

This water (Number (42)), the analysis of which was kindly
supplied by Messrs Bell Bros., of Manchester, was taken from a
colliery in South Staffordshire. On exposure to air it rapidly
became turbid and rusty; note the excessive chlorine, total
solids and hardness; the water is quite unfit for domestic use.

	(43)
Free and saline ammonia..	0·004
Albuminoid ammonia	0·023
Oxygen absorbed from potassium permanganate	
in four hours at 80° F...	0·255
Chlorine	4·7
Nitric nitrogen	0·125
Total solids..	43·0
Organic matter	7·0
Mineral matter	36·0
Total hardness	14°
(a) Temporary	1°
(b) Permanent	13°

Number (43) is the water from a shallow well in the Salford
district; the albuminoid ammonia and the oxygen absorbed
are both very high; the total solids are high; the chlorine is
high but the nitric nitrogen is satisfactory; the pollution may
be due to organic matter of vegetable origin, which could be
removed by efficient filtration. But as it stands the water
must be condemned.

	(43 a)
Free and saline ammonia..	0·0193
Albuminoid ammonia	0·021
Oxygen absorbed from potassium permanganate in four hours at 80° F...	0·0383
Chlorine	0·9
Nitrogen as nitrates	Nil
Nitrogen as nitrites	Nil
Total solids	5·6
Organic matter	1·54
Mineral matter	4·06
Total hardness	3°
(a) Temporary	Nil
(b) Permanent	3°

Number (43 a) is the water supply of the County Borough of
Huddersfield; the ammonia figures and oxygen absorbed are
slightly high; the water is an upland surface water and has
practically no hardness.

	(44)	(45)	(46)	(47)
Free ammonia	0·0076	0·0119	0·0074	0·0103
Albuminoid ammonia	0·0018	0·0018	0·0012	0·0016
Total solid matter..	9·92	9·17	11·24	6·12
Organic matter	3·27	2·90	4·04	3·12
Mineral matter	6·42	6·07	7·08	6·12
Suspended matter..	0·23	0·20	0·12	0·08
Oxygen absorbed from potassium permanganate in four hours at 27° C.	0·008	0·008	0·011	0·010
Chlorine	1·4	1·4	1·4	1·4
Nitrogen as nitrate	0·078	0·075	0·083	0·089
Total hardness	3·67°	4·67°	5·6°	4·3°
(a) Temporary	0·17°	1·5°	2·5°	0·6°
(b) Permanent	3·5°	3·17°	3·1°	3·7°

Numbers (44), (45), (46) and (47) are analyses of the water
supplied by the Ashton-under-Lyne, Stalybridge and Dukinfield Waterworks Committee, kindly supplied by Messrs J.
Rowbottom, Borough Surveyor, and G. H. Raddin, B.Eng.,
Water Engineer. The water is collected partly in the Greenfield Valley in Saddleworth and partly in the Swineshaw
Valley, near Stalybridge; the total solid matter and hardness
are very low and there is occasionally a slight plumbo-solvent
action.

	(48)
Free and saline ammonia..	0·008
Albuminoid ammonia	0·014
Oxygen absorbed from potassium permanganate in four hours at 80° F...	0·036
Chlorine	1·1
Nitric nitrogen	Nil
Nitrous nitrogen	Nil
Total solids..	6·2
Total hardness	3°

Number (48) is an analysis of the Derwent Valley water at
Langley Mill; the albuminoid ammonia and oxygen absorbed
figures are very high; the hardness is very low (see p. 52 for
mineral analysis).

	(49)
Free and saline ammonia..	0·0006
Albuminoid ammonia	0·0026
Oxygen absorbed from potassium permanganate in four hours at 80° F.	0·024
Chlorine	1·40
Nitric nitrogen	0·02
Nitrous nitrogen	Nil
Total hardness	4·5°
(a) Temporary	0·5°
(b) Permanent	4·0°

Number (49) is the water supplied by a joint water board to
the County Borough of Bury, kindly supplied by Mr J. Woodhead Smith, A.M.I.C.E., the Water Engineer; all the numbers
are very low and the water is well suited for domestic purposes.

	(50)	(51)
Free and saline ammonia..	0·004	0·001
Albuminoid ammonia	0·013	0·010
Oxygen absorbed from potassium permanganate in four hours at 80° F.	0·018	0·018
Chlorine	1·9	2·1
Nitric nitrogen	Nil	Nil
Nitrous nitrogen	Nil	Nil
Total solid matter..	25·0	26·0
Organic and volatile matter	3·0	8·0
Mineral matter	22·0	18·0
Total hardness	11°	10°
(a) Temporary	5°	5°
(b) Permanent	6°	5°

Number (50) is from a shallow well in the Edmonton district,
and Number (51) is a surface water from the same district;
both are very much alike in character and would appear to be
the same water; all the figures are low except the albuminoid
ammonia and this is very probably due to vegetable matter
and would be removed by efficient filtration.

	(52)	(53)	(54)	(55)	(56)	(57)	(58)
Free and saline ammonia	0·004	0·002	0·004	0·002	0·004	0·004	0·002
Albuminoid ammonia ..	0·024	0·018	0·012	0·022	0·020	0·008	0·009
Oxygen absorbed from potassium permanganate in four hours at 80° F.	0·13	0·15	0·12	0·12	0·09	0·06	0·06
Chlorine	1·3	1·1	1·3	1·6	1·2	1·2	1·1
Nitric nitrogen	Nil	Nil	Nil	Nil	0·02	0·015	0·017
Nitrous nitrogen ..	Nil	Nil	Nil	Nil	Nil	Nil	Nil
Total solid matter ..	14·0	14·0	12·0	12·0	12·0	10·0	10·0
Organic and volatile matter..	4·0	4·0	2·0	2·0	1·0	2·0	2·0
Mineral matter	10·0	10·0	10·0	10·0	11·0	8·0	8·0
Total hardness ..	4°	4°	4°	4°	3°	3°	3°
(a) Temporary ..	Nil	Nil	Nil	Nil	Nil	Nil	Nil
(b) Permanent ..	4°	4°	4°	4°	3°	3°	3°

Numbers (52), (53), (54), (55), (56), (57) and (58) are taken from the different reservoirs of the Fylde Water Board; number (52) from the surface at the south end of the Gryzedale Lea reservoir; number (53) at a depth of two feet at the same place; number (54) from the surface at the outlet of the same reservoir; number (55) from the surface at the north end of the Gryzedale reservoir; number (56) from the surface at the intake of the North Barnacre reservoir; number (57) from the surface at the inlet culvert of the South Barnacre reservoir, and number (58) from the surface of the same reservoir. The water is an upland surface water and all the numbers are exceedingly low; there is no temporary hardness and in consequence the water is of great value for boilers and for domestic purposes.

	(59)	(60)
Free and saline ammonia..	0·03	0·02
Albuminoid ammonia	0·016	0·018
Oxygen absorbed from potassium permanganate in four hours at 80° F. ..	0·16	0·19
Chlorine	1·6	1·6
Nitric nitrogen	0·1	0·1
Nitrous nitrogen	Nil	Nil
Total solid matter	13·0	14·0
Organic and volatile matter	3·0	4·0
Mineral matter	10·0	10·0
Total hardness	4°	3·5°
(a) Temporary	Nil	Nil
(b) Permanent	4°	3·5°

Numbers (59) and (60) are from the River Etherow at Hollingworth, and show a slight difference in the two samples; both the ammonia figures and the figure for oxygen absorbed are high, these were due to the presence of vegetable organic matter, which could be removed by filtration; the hardness is extremely low, temporary hardness being completely absent (see p. 53 for mineral analysis).

	(61)
Free and saline ammonia..	0·019
Albuminoid ammonia	0·04
Oxygen absorbed from potassium permanganate in four hours at 80° F...	0·3
Nitric nitrogen	1·0
Nitrous nitrogen	Nil
Total solid matter..	46·0
Organic and volatile matter	12·0
Mineral matter	34·0
Total hardness	22°
(a) Temporary..	12°
(b) Permanent..	10°

Number (61) is the water from the River Ancholme, near Lincoln; all the figures are high and the water is very hard; it is contaminated with a considerable quantity of organic matter, probably of animal origin, and is quite unfit for use for domestic purposes.

	(62)
Free and saline ammonia..	0·0016
Albuminoid ammonia	0·025
Oxygen absorbed from potassium permanganate in four hours at 80° F...	0·33
Nitric nitrogen	0·06
Nitrous nitrogen	Nil
Total solid matter..	49·0
Organic and volatile matter	12·0
Mineral matter	37·0
Total hardness	15°
(a) Temporary..	3°
(b) Permanent..	12°

Number (62) is a shallow well water from Sale; the well was situated in a bend of the River Mersey at about 50 yards from the river; it is polluted with a considerable quantity of organic matter, probably from the river; the albuminoid ammonia and oxygen absorbed are high and the water is quite unfit for use for domestic purposes.

	(63)	(64)
Free and saline ammonia..	Nil	0·001
Albuminoid ammonia	0·004	0·005
Oxygen absorbed from potassium permanganate in four hours at 80° F.	0·032	0·15
Chlorine	12·3	5·2
Nitric nitrogen	0·01	0·006
Nitrous nitrogen	Nil	Nil
Total solid matter..	60·0	28·0
Organic and volatile matter	20·0	12·0
Mineral matter	40·0	16·0
Total hardness	15°	8°
(a) Temporary..	4°	2°
(b) Permanent..	11°	6°

Number (63) was taken from the same bore hole at Liscard as number (40), *after an interval of seven years*; there has been an increase in the total solid matter, organic and volatile matter, mineral matter and chlorine, and a decrease in the albuminoid ammonia, nitrogen as nitrate and hardness.

Number (64) consists of the same water mixed with the Liverpool Supply and is the same as number (41), except that the amount of the Liverpool Supply has been increased.

Mineral analyses

The following are a series of analyses of the mineral constituents of various waters. They show the great differences there are in waters from various localities. The numbers represent parts per 100,000.

	(1)
Carbonates (as CO_3)	1·44
Sulphates (as SO_4)	0·10
Chlorides (as Cl)	0·95
Silicates (as SiO_4)	0·43
Calcium (as Ca)	1·03
Magnesium (as Mg)	0·18
Iron (as Fe)	0·08
Potassium (as K)	0·14
Sodium (as Na)	0·53

The above, No. (1), supplied by Mr J. F. Liverseege, F.I.C., City Analyst, Birmingham, is a mineral analysis of number (11) (see the organic analysis, p. 36) and is an upland surface water from the Silurian formation. Every item is low.

	(2)
Calcium carbonate	25·00
Magnesium carbonate	9·80
Sodium sulphate	4·27
Sodium chloride	4·33

The water, No. (2), of which the above is the analysis of the dissolved salts, was taken from the Red Sandstone of Manchester. It is particularly interesting owing to the complete absence of calcium and magnesium sulphates. The sample also contained a very large amount of free carbon dioxide; and, unless the containing bottles had been immediately corked, a considerable proportion of it would have escaped.

The above analysis is published by permission of T. R. Wollaston, Esq.

(3)

Sulphates (as SO_3) ..	..	..	..	19·71
Chlorine (as Cl) ..	..	..	..	9·57
Nitrogen (as nitrate)	..	..	..	0·20
Lime (as $CaCO_3$) ..	..	..	..	24·62
Magnesium (as MgO)	..	..	..	0·38
Potassium (as K_2O)	..	..	..	0·54
Sodium (as Na_2O)	..	..	..	25·50
Silica (as SiO_2) ..	..	..	..	0·14
Alkalinity (as Na_2CO_3)	..	..	..	15·10

The above, No. (3), is an analysis of an alkaline water. The interesting points in this water are its high alkalinity, the small quantity of magnesium salts, and the appearance of the lime as carbonate with the consequent absence of permanent hardness.

			(4)	(5)	(6)
Magnesium carbonate	..	..	4·9	3·1	3·6
Magnesium sulphate	..	..	17·74	32·0	19·5
Magnesium nitrate ..	..	..	8·7	5·2	0·3
Magnesium chloride..	..	..	1·9	nil	nil
Calcium carbonate ..	..	..	20·2	20·0	17·8
Calcium sulphate	..	..	46·1	147·0	89·5
Sodium sulphate	..	..	nil	1·0	23·5
Potassium and sodium chlorides	..	12·0	11·2	37·8
Iron, silica and alumina	..	..	1·3	0·7	2·0

The above are the analyses of numbers (13), (14) and (15) (see the organic analyses, p. 36). They are due to Messrs Lott and Matthews. Number (4) is partly rain water from the Trent Valley and partly water from springs in the Marl bed underlying the gravel. Number (5) is from a bore hole in the Marl bed and number (6) from a bore hole in the Lower Keuper Sandstone. The proportion of calcium sulphate is high, especially in numbers (5) and (6). Number (6) shows the presence of sodium sulphate in moderately large quantity.

(7)

Magnesium carbonate	..	..	..	56·7
Magnesium sulphate	..	..	..	1·1
Magnesium chloride	..	..	..	24·0
Calcium carbonate ..	..	..	..	203·4
Potassium sulphate	..	..	..	4·3
Sodium chloride ..	..	..	..	34·3
Ferrous carbonate ..	..	..	..	1·5
Silica ..	..	..	..	14·5

Number (7) is an analysis by Muspratt of the water from the St Ann's well at Buxton and shows very high calcium carbonate, magnesium carbonate, sodium chloride and magnesium chloride. Note also the presence of ferrous carbonate. On being exposed to the air this water deposits hydrated ferric oxide, and it can be used as a natural purifying agent for the treatment of the Buxton sewage.

					(8)
Nitrogen as nitrates	..	..	..	..	0·25
Carbonates (as CO₂)	..	..	..	..	9·94
Sulphates (as SO₃)	..	..	..	..	0·48
Silica (as SiO₂)	..	..	..	..	0·60
Iron and alumina ..	..	..	..	..	0·30
Lime (as CaO)	..	..	..	..	12·80
Magnesia (as MgO)	..	..	..	..	0·50
Sodium (as Na)	..	..	..	..	0·31
Potassium (as K) ..	..	..	..	..	1·04

Number (8) is the analysis of the water number (16) (see organic analysis, p. 36) of the Portsmouth Public Water Supply from a deep chalk spring in the western end of the South Downs. The analysis is by Mr C. L. L. Claremont, B.Sc., F.I.C.

	(9)	(10)
Nitrogen as nitrate ..	trace	0·109
Alkalis	1·06	0·518
Magnesia	0·461	0·127
Lime..	1·735	0·706
Iron	0·016	0·99
Oxide of manganese	0·017	0·059
Sulphates (as SO₃) ..	2·144	0·600
Silica	0·463	0·214

Numbers (9) and (10) are the analyses by the late Professor Campbell Brown of the Liverpool City Supply (see organic analyses, numbers (19) and (20), p. 37). Number (9) is from the Rivingstone Supply in the Millstone Grit and number (10) from the Vyrnwy Supply. The item of exceptional interest is the presence of the oxide of manganese.

	(11)	(12)	(13)
Silica (as SiO₂)	0·0	0·0	1·0
Iron (as Fe₂O₃)	trace	4·5	1·2
Baryta (as BaO)	1·38	28·36	2·23
Lime (as CaO)	2·60	141·64	15·54
Magnesia (as MgO)	trace	42·16	4·32
Soda (as Na₂O)	0·0	1080·76	114·02

Numbers (11), (12) and (13) are the analyses of numbers (26), (27) and (28) (see organic analyses, p. 38) from a bore hole at Ilkeston. Number (11) is the original water, number (12)

the abnormal water, number (13) from the pumping shaft. All
these show the presence of soluble barium salts, a rare occur-
rence in a natural water in this country. A particular item to
note is the extraordinary amount of soda which accounts for
the very high chlorine in the organic analyses. The analyses
were made by Mr J. White, F.I.C. (*Analyst*, 1899, vol. XXIV,
p. 67).

The following, No. (14), is the analysis of the Ilkley Spa
water. (Analysis made by Mr B. A. Burrell, *Chem. News*, 1913,
p. 295.)

	(14)
Ferric oxide (Fe$_2$O$_3$)	0·023
Calcium carbonate (CaCO$_3$)	1·157
Calcium nitrate (Ca(NO$_3$)$_2$)	0·020
Calcium silicate (CaSiO$_3$)	2·936
Calcium sulphate (CaSO$_4$)	0·742
Magnesium carbonate (MgCO$_3$)	2·033
Magnesium sulphate (MgSO$_4$)	1·557
Potassium carbonate (K$_2$CO$_3$)	0·221
Sodium carbonate (Na$_2$CO$_3$)	1·246
Sodium chloride (NaCl)	1·650
Lithium chloride (LiCl)	0·118

The height of the well from which this water is drawn is
660 ft. above sea-level; the water issues from the middle or
third grits of the Millstone Grit series and is clear and free
from sediment.

	(15)
Lime	0·51
Magnesia	trace
Oxides of iron and alumina	0·34
Sulphates (as SO$_3$)	0·91
Sodium chloride	1·32

Number (15) is the analysis of the Glasgow City Water
Supply (see organic analysis, number (21), p. 37) by F. W.
Harris, Esq., City Analyst. As might be expected from the
low total solid matter, nearly half of the mineral matter is
sodium chloride. Note the complete absence of carbonates,
which explains the absence of temporary hardness.

	(16)
Calcium sulphate (CaSO$_4$)	2·47
Magnesium sulphate (MgSO$_4$)	0·84
Magnesium chloride (MgCl$_2$)	0·73
Sodium chloride (NaCl)	0·70
Iron, Alumina and Silica	0·36

Number (16) is an analysis of the Manchester tap water derived from Lake Thirlmere. The total hardness is 2°. Note the absence of carbonate with the consequent absence of temporary hardness. The water is a pure, very soft siliceous water well suited for domestic and industrial uses.

	(17)
Calcium sulphate ($CaSO_4$)	32·18
Calcium carbonate ($CaCO_3$)	15·80
Magnesium sulphate ($MgSO_4$)	12·70
Magnesium carbonate ($MgCO_3$)	3·94
Potassium sulphate (K_2SO_4)	9·53
Potassium chloride (KCl)	2·68
Sodium chloride ($NaCl$)	12·99
Iron carbonate ($FeCO_3$)	0·82
Silica (SiO_2)	0·99

Number (17) is a typical hard water from the Keuper Marl at Burton containing a large temporary and permanent hardness. It is not suitable for domestic purposes, but is well suited for brewing Burton pale ales and also for malting purposes.

	(18)
Calcium carbonate ($CaCO_3$)	26·97
Magnesium carbonate ($MgCO_3$)	0·40
Sodium chloride ($NaCl$)	2·77
Sodium sulphate (Na_2SO_4)	1·06
Potassium silicate (K_2SiO_3)	0·92
Potassium sulphate (K_2SO_4)	0·54
Potassium carbonate (K_2CO_3)	0·37
Silica (SiO_2)	0·08

Number (18) is an analysis of a water from a London Chalk well. In this case all the hardness is temporary and there is no permanent. The water would require careful softening before being used for domestic or industrial purposes.

	(19)
Calcium sulphate ($CaSO_4$)	16·70
Calcium carbonate ($CaCO_3$)	28·37
Magnesium sulphate ($MgSO_4$)	15·57
Magnesium carbonate ($MgCO_3$)	7·82
Sodium sulphate (Na_2SO_4)	6·37
Sodium chloride ($NaCl$)	16·73
Potassium chloride (KCl)	4·08
Silica (SiO_2)	0·68

Number (19) is an analysis of a well water from the Edinburgh district. It is excessively hard (both temporary and permanent) and is not suitable for domestic and industrial purposes unless it is carefully softened.

The following analyses were kindly supplied by Mr J. West Knights. The numbers represent grains per gallon. Number (20) is the analysis of the mineral constituents of a well in the Lower Greensand.

	(20)	(21)	(22)	(23)	(24)
Calcium carbonate	14·20	5·71	23·00	15·26	18·00
Magnesium carbonate	nil	2·56	—	—	—
Magnesium sulphate	9·00	nil	3·24	0·75	0·75
Sodium chloride	8·89	4·94	17·31	2·30	6·59
Sodium sulphate	19·91	8·34	—	0·40	—
Sodium carbonate	nil	3·45	—	—	—
Sodium nitrate	nil	nil	6·07	—	—
Calcium nitrate	—	—	—	—	5·85
Calcium sulphate	—	—	—	—	3·01
Not determined	—	—	4·38	0·29	—
Total solids	52·00	25·00	54·00	19·00	34·2

Number (21) is also from another well in the Lower Greensand.

Number (22) is from a shallow well in the Chalk.

Number (23) is from a deep well in the Chalk.

Number (24) is from a deep well near Newmarket.

	(25)
Calcium sulphate ($CaSO_4 2H_2O$)	11·954
Calcium carbonate ($CaCO_3$)	65·000
Calcium chloride ($CaCl_2$)	86·639
Magnesium chloride ($MgCl_2$)	44·760
Sulphate of iron ($FeSO_4$)	1·900
Silica (SiO_2)	1·000
Sodium chloride ($NaCl$)	974·133

Number (25) is the mineral analysis of number (42) p. 41, the presence of the extraordinary amount of sodium chloride accounts for the very high chlorine content and also for the very high total solid matter.

	(25)	(26)	(27)	(28)	(29)
Silica (as SiO_2)	3·2	9·8	0·3	1·2	4·0
Iron (as Fe_2O_3)	0·04	0·72	0·02	0·02	0·05
Alumina (as Al_2O_3)	0·16	0·28	0·28	1·18	1·95
Lime (as CaO)	3·60	0·20	0·70	0·20	9·60
Magnesia (as MgO)	0·13	0·13	0·13	0·13	0·13
Sulphates (as SO_3)	3·78	1·37	1·52	1·72	6·52
Chlorine (as Cl)	0·80	1·00	1·00	1·00	1·30
Nitrogen as nitrates	Nil	Nil	Nil	Nil	Nil

Numbers (25), (26), (27), (28) and (29) are samples of the Huddersfield water supply from the reservoir and before filtration; they were taken at different times and from different portions of the reservoir and show the variations in the mineral composition of the water.

4—2

(30)

Silica (as SiO₂)	..	..	..	..	0·76
Iron (as Fe₂O₃)	..	..	..	..	0·086
Alumina (as Al₂O₃)		..	..	..	0·03
Lime (as CaO)	..	..	..	..	1·56
Magnesia (as MgO)		..	..	..	0·50
Sulphates (as SO₃)..		..	..	..	2·34
Chlorine (as Cl)	..	..	..	..	1·1

Number (30) is a mineral analysis of the Derwent Valley Water at Langley Mill; for the organic analysis see number (48), p. 42.

(31)

Silica (as SiO₂)	..	..	..	..	0·8
Iron (as Fe₂O₃)	..	..	..	..	10·4
Alumina (as Al₂O₃)		..	..	..	0·4
Lime (as CaO)	..	..	..	..	11·6
Magnesia (as MgO)		..	..	..	0·58
Sulphates (as SO₃)..		..	..	..	18·95
Chlorine (as Cl)	..	..	..	..	10·6

Number (31) is a water from a 6-foot bore hole in the New Red Sandstone in the Ormskirk district; the iron, lime, sulphates and chlorine are all very high; and, as might be expected, the permanent hardness is very high (17° Clark).

(32)

Silica (as SiO₂)	..	..	..	..	2·4
Iron (as Fe₂O₃)	..	..	..	..	1·2
Alumina (as Al₂O₃)		..	..	..	Nil
Lime (as CaO)	..	..	..	..	5·2
Magnesia (as MgO)		..	..	..	0·08
Sulphates (as SO₃)..		..	..	..	10·63
Chlorine (as Cl)	..	..	..	..	4·9

Number (32) is a water from a river in the Colne Valley district; the sulphates are rather high and the sample was coloured a deep blue from the effluent from a neighbouring chemical works; the sample was not intended to be used for domestic purposes, but as a boiler feed water, for which purpose it is well suited.

(33)

Silica (as SiO₂)	..	..	..	..	0·8
Iron (as Fe₂O₃)	..	..	..	..	0·32
Alumina (as Al₂O₃)		..	..	..	0·02
Lime (as CaO)	..	..	..	..	0·68
Magnesia (as MgO)		..	..	..	0·12
Sulphates (as SO₃)		..	..	..	0·71
Chlorine (as Cl)	..	..	..	..	1·3

Number (33) is the mineral analysis of number (22) (see organic analysis, p. 37); it is an upland surface water, supplied by the Fylde Water Board to the County Borough of Blackpool; every item is very low.

	(34)	(35)
Silica (as SiO_2)	1·2	2·8
Iron (as Fe_2O_3)	0·6	0·6
Alumina (as Al_2O_3)	Nil	Nil
Lime (as CaO)	3·0	2·2
Magnesia (as MgO)	0·4	0·4
Sulphates (as SO_3)	3·4	2·4
Chlorine (as Cl)	1·6	1·6

Numbers (34) and (35) are the mineral analyses of numbers
(59) and (60) (see organic analysis, p. 44); they are samples of
water from the River Etherow; all the items are very low.

	(36)	(37)	(38)
Silica (as SiO_2)	6·0	6·0	14·8
Iron (as Fe_2O_3)	3·6	4·9	1·3
Alumina (as Al_2O_3)	1·2	1·1	Nil
Lime (as CaO)	21·6	12·0	4·8
Magnesia (as MgO)	5·1	2·6	4·5
Sulphates (as SO_3)	222·5	166·2	195·1
Chlorine (as Cl)	245·0	142·0	175·0

Numbers (36), (37) and (38) are river waters from Muestra
in India; the hardness of each was 18°, 24° and 22° respectively; the total solid matter was for number (36), 894·0, number
(37), 588·0 and number (38), 708·0 parts per 100,000; the sulphates and chlorides are exceedingly high, due to the presence
of sodium sulphate and sodium chloride, and render the
samples quite unfit for use for either domestic or industrial
purposes.

	(39)	(40)
Silica (as SiO_2)	0·8	50·0
Iron (as Fe_2O_3)	1·0	54·0
Alumina (as Al_2O_3)	Nil	Nil
Lime (as CaO)	1·2	10·0
Magnesia (as MgO)	0·2	20·9
Sulphates (as SO_3)	3·1	37·1
Chlorine (as Cl)	1·6	44·2

Number (39) is a sample of water taken from the river at
Stalybridge; and number (40) is a sample of the same water
after it has been in a works boiler for some time; the solids in
the latter were mostly in the suspended state; it is interesting
to note the very large increase in all the figures in water from
the boiler.

By the courtesy of Sir A. C. Houston, the Director of Water
Examinations, London Metropolitan Water Board, we are permitted to quote (on p. 54) some of the results of the chemical

This table contains the average results of the chemical examination of the London water for the year 1911-12.

	Thames (raw water, 238 samples)	Lee (raw water, 238 samples)	New River (raw water, 338 samples)	New River (filtered water, 245 samples)	East London, Clapton (filtered water, 246 samples)	Chelsea (filtered water, 243 samples)
Ammoniacal nitrogen	0·0073	0·0106	0·0029	0·0017	0·0003	0·0002
Albuminoid nitrogen	0·0155	0·0156	0·0090	0·0033	0·0056	0·0059
Oxidised nitrogen	0·2600	0·3200	0·3100	0·2800	0·2400	0·2500
Chlorine	1·7600	2·1400	1·6200	1·7100	2·0800	1·7000
Oxygen absorbed from potassium permanganate in 3 hours at 80° F.	0·2062	0·2102	0·0920	0·0439	0·0719	0·0892
Total hardness	21·670	24·870	24·890	22·680	22·990	21·000
Permanent hardness	5·620	6·81	4·970	5·070	7·160	6·090

The table below contains the results of the mineral analyses of some of the London waters. The numbers are in parts per 100,000.

	Thames (raw water, Nov. 15/09)	Lambeth (filtered water, Nov. 15/09)	Kent wells		Lee Valley wells	
			(Deptford Garden well, Nov. 4/09)	(Darenth well, Jan. 11/10)	(Park well, Nov. 4/09)	(East Ham well, Jan. 14/10)
Calcium carbonate	23·00	21·64	24·20	23·23	17·57	8·66
Magnesium carbonate	nil	nil	nil	0·10	3·07	6·67
Sodium carbonate	nil	nil	nil	nil	nil	7·80
Calcium sulphate	3·28	3·47	9·20	nil	nil	nil
Magnesium sulphate	2·39	2·30	2·09	0·96	5·79	nil
Sodium sulphate	0·43	0·44	nil	0·67	3·90	11·06
Magnesium chloride	nil	nil	nil	nil	nil	nil
Chlorine as NaCl (+a little KCl)	2·82	2·93	3·43	2·24	3·28	12·10
Calcium nitrate	nil	nil	nil	nil	nil	nil
Magnesium nitrate	nil	nil	1·47	nil	nil	nil
Sodium nitrate	1·70	1·63	1·46	2·43	nil	nil
Sesquioxides of iron and alumina	0·06	0·01	0·12	nil	0·06	0·06
Silica	1·06	1·24	1·20	1·00	1·42	0·92
	34·74	33·66	43·17	30·63	35·09	47·27

examination of the London water. The numbers represent parts per 100,000; and give the averages for the year 1911-12 of a considerable number of analyses.

The series of County Memoirs issued by the Geological Survey dealing with the water supplies derived from underground sources are of great importance to public health authorities. They contain a large amount of information relative to the geological nature of water-bearing strata, together with a considerable number of detailed analyses of waters both of the organic and the mineral constituents obtained from such strata. Each memoir has also a complete bibliography.

SEWAGE

In sampling a crude sewage, care must be taken to obtain a representative sample and it must be proportional to the rate of flow.

The person taking the sample should be instructed to take a portion of the inflow every hour; the contents of the various Winchester quarts collected during 24 hours should be mixed and a representative sample taken from the mixed portions. In order that the sample may represent the true sewage a sample should be taken on each of ten consecutive days.

Free and albuminoid ammonia in sewage and sewage effluents are estimated in accordance with the directions for water analysis (pp. 2, 3, 4) except that for the determination 5 c.c. of the sample are mixed with 500 c.c. of ammonia-free distilled water.

Nitrogen as nitrates and nitrites, total solid matter and chlorine are also determined as directed under water analysis (pp. 5-14).

Oxygen absorbed test in four hours at 80° F. The methods described on pp. 5-7 may be used, but 10 or 20 c.c. of the sewage (or sewage effluent) are taken and diluted to 250 c.c. with ammonia-free water before placing it in the bottle.

Oxygen absorbed in three minutes at 80° F. *Solutions required:*

Strong potassium permanganate solution. Weigh out 3·95 grams of pure potassium permanganate; dissolve in distilled water and make up to 1000 c.c. 1 c.c. of this solution = 0·001 gram of available oxygen.

Sulphuric acid solution prepared as directed under water analysis (p. 6).

Oxalic acid solution. Weigh out 7·875 grams of crystallized oxalic acid; dissolve in distilled water and make up to 1000 c.c. 1 c.c. of this solution = 1 c.c. of the strong potassium permanganate solution.

For the estimation, measure out 10 c.c. of the well-shaken sample into a conical flask after rinsing with concentrated sulphuric acid; add 240 c.c. of distilled water and 10 c.c. of the sulphuric acid solution; raise the temperature on the water bath to 80° F., and add 10 c.c. of the strong potassium permanganate solution (at 80° F.) from a pipette and maintain the temperature at 80° F. for three minutes.

At the end of three minutes, titrate the solution with the oxalic acid solution until the pink colour just disappears; the difference between the number of c.c. of oxalic acid solution used in a blank experiment and in the sewage multiplied by 0·001 gives the amount of oxygen absorbed by 10 c.c. of the sewage in three minutes.

Example:

Sewage taken	10 c.c.
Strong potassium permanganate solution added	10 c.c.
Oxalic acid used for the blank	10·0 c.c.
Oxalic acid used for sewage	7·5 c.c.
	2·5 c.c.

2·5 × 0·001 = 0·0025 part of oxygen absorbed by 10 c.c. of sewage = 25·0 parts of oxygen absorbed per 100,000.

Estimation of suspended matter. 250 c.c. of the well-shaken sample are filtered through a dried and weighed filter paper, the suspended matter on the paper is washed with water, dried in the water oven, and weighed, the weight of the filter paper subtracted from the total weight gives the weight of suspended matter in 250 c.c. of the sample. The filter paper containing the suspended matter is then placed in a platinum dish and incinerated; from the weight of the ash is subtracted the weight of the filter paper ash, giving the weight of mineral matter in suspension.

Example:

Weight of filter paper, weighing bottle and
suspended matter   ..   ..   20·133
Weight of filter paper and weighing bottle ..   19·999
Weight of suspended matter   ..   ..   ..   ·134

0·134 × 4 × 100 = 53·6 parts of suspended matter per 100,000.

Weight of dish, mineral matter and filter paper
ash   ..   ..   48·4470
Weight of dish   ..   ..   48·4440
Weight of mineral matter and filter paper ash   ·0030
Weight of filter paper ash   ..   ..   ..   ·0005
Weight of mineral suspended matter   ..   ..   ·0025

0·0025 × 4 × 100 = 1·0 part of mineral suspended matter per 100,000.

Estimation of total organic nitrogen. *Solutions required:*
Phenol sulphuric acid solution.
Weigh out 200 grams of phosphoric anhydride.
          40 grams of phenol.
Measure out 1000 c.c. of concentrated sulphuric acid.
Dissolve the phosphoric anhydride in part of the sulphuric acid and the phenol in the remainder, cool the two solutions and mix them.

The process used for the estimation is the Kjeldahl-Jodlbaur method, in which 250–500 c.c. of the crude sewage are evaporated with 25 c.c. of the phenol-sulphuric acid in a 700 c.c. Kjeldahl flask; three grams of zinc dust and one gram of mercury are then added and the mixture allowed to stand for a short time, in order to allow the nitrates to be reduced. After the nitrates have been reduced, the flask is heated until the contents are colourless, the flame being allowed to play directly on the flask. When the contents of the flask are colourless, the flame is removed and the flask allowed to cool; when quite cold the contents are washed out into a 1000 c.c. boiling flask with distilled water and made alkaline with caustic soda solution; 20 c.c. of a 10 per cent. potassium sulphide solution are added, to precipitate the mercury; a few pieces of pipeclay are placed in the flask, which is then connected to a condenser and the ammonia distilled off and collected in an excess of a normal solution of sulphuric acid, placed in the receiver. As soon as all the ammonia has been distilled over, the excess of acid in the receiver is titrated with normal caustic soda solution; the number of c.c. of acid taken, less the number of c.c. of soda solution used, multiplied by 0·014 gives the total nitrogen in the volume of sewage taken.

A blank experiment should be performed with the materials used in order to determine the amount of nitrogen present in them, and the nitrogen so obtained should be subtracted from the total nitrogen.

Example:

500 c.c. of the sample taken for the estimation gave the following results:

Normal sulphuric acid placed in receiver ..	10·0 c.c.
Normal soda solution used to neutralize excess of acid	6·5 c.c.
	3·5 c.c.
Less acid used in the blank experiment	·3 c.c.
Acid neutralized by the ammonia from the sewage	3·2 c.c.

3·2 × 0·014 × 200 = 8·96 parts of total nitrogen per 100,000.

Strength of sewage. The strength of a sewage can be calculated with a fair degree of accuracy by McGowan's formula (*Royal Commission on Sewage Disposal, 5th Report,* p. 16, also appendix IV to this Report), which is:—the organic nitrogen plus the ammoniacal nitrogen multiplied by 4·5 plus the oxygen absorbed in four hours multiplied by 6·5 gives a figure upon which the strength is based (or Ammon. N. + Org. N.) × 4·5 + (oxygen absorbed in four hours × 6·5). For example a sewage may be graded as follows:

Weak is .. under 60
Medium is .. 50–100
Average is .. 100–175
Strong is .. above 175

A rough guide to the strength of a crude sewage may also be obtained from the figure for the oxygen absorbed test in four hours at 80° F.: for example:

Weak .. .. .. 7–8 parts per 100,000
Average .. .. .. 10–12 ,, ,,
Strong .. .. .. 17–25 ,, ,,

Typical Analyses of a crude sewage in parts per 100,000.

Free ammonia	7·31	4·43	5·0	10·61	16·58
Albuminoid ammonia ..	1·52	1·07	1·8	1·42	2·21
Oxygen absorbed in three minutes at 80° F... ..	—	3·51	12·8	5·30	9·50
Oxygen absorbed in four hours at 80° F.	17·81	13·99	24·0	19·81	21·19
Total solid matter	—	—	178·9	—	—
Chlorine	10·30	9·88	15·2	16·28	17·12
Nitrogen as nitrate	nil	nil	nil	nil	nil
Suspended matter	17·6	46·5	86·0	49·50	62·1

A typical Analysis of a crude sewage containing trade waste.

parts per 100,000

Free ammonia	2·3
Albuminoid ammonia	3·7
Oxygen absorbed in three minutes at 80° F.	50·7
Oxygen absorbed in four hours at 80° F. ..	69·2
Total solid matter	216·0
Chlorine	48·0
Nitrogen as nitrate	nil
Suspended matter	40·0

Analyses of crude sewage obtained from the same source on seven consecutive days showing variations in the composition.

Free ammonia	3·5	3·5	5·4	3·2	4·4	4·0	4·0
Albuminoid ammonia ..	1·4	1·8	1·3	1·8	2·4	1·9	1·6
Oxygen absorbed in three mins. at 80° F. ..	4·7	8·4	9·7	6·4	14·4	8·8	7·2
Oxygen absorbed in four hours at 80° F. ..	14·9	20·6	26·6	25·5	29·5	21·6	21·5
Total solid matter	120·0	144·0	184·0	140·0	172·0	136·0	110·0
Chlorine ..	10·0	14·4	16·8	12·7	18·8	13·2	12·4
Nitrogen as nitrate	nil	nil	nil	nil	nil	nil	nil
Suspended matter	40·0	52·0	90·0	48·0	52·0	36·0	80·0
Strength ..	average	average	strong	strong	strong	average	average

SEWAGE EFFLUENTS

It is important from a Public Health point of view that a stream should not be polluted with a sewage or sewage effluent, which might be harmful to the animal life contained therein, or which might produce a nuisance or cause disease to be carried to the towns and villages near which the stream passes on its way to the sea.

An enormous amount of work has been performed on sewages and their effluents by the officers of the Royal Commission on Sewage Disposal and the results of this work are published in the various reports of the Commission. A large number of analyses of all kinds of sewages and sewage effluents are contained in these reports.

In the *8th Report*, vol. I of the Commission, a standard is formulated, with which it is recommended that all effluents should comply before being poured into a stream. In the suggested standard a normal sewage effluent should not contain more than three grams per 100,000 of suspended matter and should not take up more than two grams of dissolved oxygen per 100,000 at 65° F. in five days: but the Report also discusses cases where, owing to the relatively small volume of the river, which is the receiver of sewage effluents, a more stringent standard is necessary: and, on the other hand, conditions of dilution which indicate that a relaxation of the normal standard may be allowed. Methods of determining the suspended matter and the dissolved oxygen absorbed are also given. (*8th Report*, vol. II, appendix.)

Determination of suspended matter

Preparation of the asbestos; a considerable quantity of asbestos floss is well washed with water, digested with hydrochloric acid, and, afterwards, thoroughly washed with water until all traces of hydrochloric acid are removed.

The process. Sufficient of the washed asbestos is placed in a Gooch crucible to form a layer 0·2 cm. deep; the crucible is fixed to a pressure filter flask and the pump turned on; the asbestos is spread evenly over the bottom of the crucible and well rammed down; a gentle stream of water is run through the crucible all the time. After the asbestos has been well packed in the crucible, 250 c.c. of tap water are run through, to remove all loose particles, and finally a few c.c. of distilled water; the crucible is then dried in the air oven at 105° C., ignited and weighed.

The amount of effluent taken for the determination of the suspended matter varies considerably, but the average is 200 c.c. A small quantity of this 200 c.c. is used to moisten the asbestos; the pump is then turned on very gently and as much as possible of the liquid is run through under this gentle pressure; the pressure is increased towards the end until the 200 c.c. have passed through the crucible; the contents of the crucible are now washed with distilled water; dried in the air oven at 105° C. and weighed regularly till the weight is constant; the increase in weight of the crucible represents the total suspended matter in 200 c.c. of the effluent.

The crucible is now ignited at a low red heat, allowed to cool and reweighed; the loss in weight is due to volatile matter, and this subtracted from the total gives the mineral matter. The determination should always be made in duplicate.

Example: 200 c.c. of a sewage effluent were taken for the estimation; the increase in weight of the crucible was 0·0812 gram. The total suspended matter therefore was

0·0812 × 500 = 40·6 parts per 100,000.

After ignition the crucible had lost in weight 0·052 gram, the volatile matter was 0·052 × 500 = 26·0 parts per 100,000, 40·6 − 26·0 = 14·6 parts per 100,000 of mineral matter.

Determination of the dissolved oxygen

Winkler's method (*Ber.* 1888, XXI, p. 2843) as modified by Rideal and Stewart (*Analyst*, 1901, XXVI, p. 141); see also *8th Report*, vol. II, Appendix of the Royal Commission on Sewage Disposal, p. 97. The principle on which it depends is the oxidation in an alkaline liquid of manganous oxide to a higher oxide of manganese, the subsequent liberation of iodine from potassium iodide by this in the acidified solution, and the titration of the liberated iodine by sodium thiosulphate.

Solutions required:

Concentrated sulphuric acid.

Concentrated hydrochloric acid (free from chlorine).

N/8 potassium permanganate solution (3·94 grams $KMnO_4$ per litre).

A 2 per cent. solution of potassium oxalate ($K_2C_2O_4 + H_2O$ —crystals).

A 33 per cent. solution of manganous chloride ($MnCl_2 + 4H_2O$—crystals).

A solution containing 70 grams of caustic potash and 10 grams of potassium iodide per 100 c.c.

A solution of N/20 sodium thiosulphate (12·4 grams per 1000 c.c.).

The estimation is made in bottles of 340 to 360 c.c. capacity, with well-fitting ground glass stoppers; in cold weather the bottles are warmed to 18° C. (65° F.).

Shake the bottle containing the effluent thoroughly well in order to bring the dissolved oxygen content to something near that of the diluting water; measure out into a flask of ample size one volume of the effluent and four volumes of tap water at 18° C.; mix these well and fill four of the bottles completely with the mixture; the bottles, which must be filled quietly and quickly, are then left unstoppered to remove any air bubbles; at the end of five minutes, the stoppers are replaced in the bottles and two of the bottles are placed in the incubator at 18° C. (65° F.) for five days, the other two being used for the determination at once.

To each bottle add 0·9 c.c. of the concentrated sulphuric acid; then sufficient of the potassium permanganate solution to leave a slight pink colour (1 to 2 c.c. is usually enough); mix the contents of the bottles and allow them to stand for 20 minutes with the stoppers in the bottles; this is to oxidize any nitrites to nitrates; at the end of 20 minutes, about 1 c.c. of the potassium oxalate solution is added to each bottle in order to destroy the excess of potassium permanganate, the bottles are at once restoppered and the contents well mixed.

As soon as the contents are colourless, the stoppers are removed and 1 c.c. of the manganous chloride solution is run into each bottle from a pipette, the tip of the pipette being at the bottom of the bottle; immediately afterwards 4 c.c. of the caustic potash-potassium iodide solution are added, again at the bottom of the bottle; the stoppers are inserted and the bottles turned over once or twice, and after a few minutes again turned over; the bottles are then allowed to stand for a few minutes to allow the hydroxides of manganese to settle. After standing, 5 c.c. of strong hydrochloric acid are run into each bottle from a pipette, again at the bottom; the bottles are restoppered and kept in a dark place for ten minutes, being rotated occasionally; after standing for ten minutes, 20 c.c. of the contents are pipetted out of each bottle and rejected; the remainder of the contents in the bottle is titrated with the sodium thiosulphate solution till colourless; using a clear starch solution as an indicator towards the end. The oxygen equivalent of the sodium thiosulphate being known, the amount of the dissolved oxygen is easily calculated. The mean of the two determinations is taken.

After five days' incubation, the oxygen remaining in solution in the other two bottles is determined in the same way; the difference between the two determinations represents the dissolved oxygen absorbed by the effluent in the interval.

The dissolved oxygen is calculated as follows:

N = the number of c.c. of the sodium thiosulphate solution used.

S = the strength of the sodium thiosulphate solution in grams of oxygen per c.c.

v = the volume of the bottle in c.c.

$$\therefore \text{the dissolved oxygen in parts per 100,000} = \frac{100,000 \times N \times S}{v}.$$

Winkler (*Zeit. Anal. Chem.* 1914, LIII, 665, and *Analyst*, 1915, XL, 299) modifies this method as follows: to the bottle containing the water, manganous chloride solution and potassium hydroxide solution are added in the usual way; a current of carbon dioxide is then passed in for about 10 minutes, thus converting the manganous hydroxide into manganous carbonate and manganous bicarbonate; the liquid is filtered and the precipitate is washed with a 2 per cent. solution of potassium carbonate, and then dissolved in hydrochloric acid, containing potassium iodide; the liberated iodine is then titrated with sodium thiosulphate solution.

Another method employed by the Royal Commission on Sewage Disposal (5th Report, appendix VI, pp. 221–226) for estimating the amount of oxygen dissolved in water gives excellent results. It is described by Letts and Blake (Proc. Roy. Dublin Soc. vol. IX (N.S.), pt. 4, No. 33) and has been used by the New York Metropolitan Sewage Commission (Report, 1912, p. 303).

Reagents required: standard ferrous sulphate is prepared by dissolving 144 grams of the pure crystallized salt in distilled water; add 15 c.c. of strong sulphuric acid: dilute the whole to three litres.

Standard sodium carbonate. Dissolve 100 grams of the crystals of pure sodium carbonate in one litre of water.

Standard sulphuric acid. Dissolve one part of concentrated sulphuric acid in an equal volume of distilled water.

Standard potassium permanganate. Dissolve 25·4 grams of pure potassium permanganate in distilled water and dilute to 4·5 litres with distilled water.

Method of testing. The volume of the separating flask is first measured by filling it with distilled water; replace the stopper and then run the water into a measuring cylinder. The flask is afterwards filled with the water to be analysed. Six c.c. of the standard ferrous sulphate solution and 4 c.c. of the sodium carbonate solution are added by means of a pipette and delivered near the bottom of the flask; replace the stopper and shake the contents. The dissolved oxygen in the presence of the sodium carbonate oxidizes a portion of the ferrous sulphate which is precipitated. Allow to stand five minutes: then invert the flask, and introduce 10 c.c. of the standard sulphuric acid through the small bulb of the flask, by means of the stopcock. The acid is allowed to mix thoroughly with the other contents of the flask, and it is allowed to stand until the mixture is almost colourless. The contents of the flask are then emptied into a dish and titrated in the usual way with the standard potassium permanganate solution. A blank sample is then analysed. In this case the flask is filled with the water as before; 10 c.c. of the standard sulphuric acid are added and the whole shaken well; add 6 c.c. of the standard ferrous sulphate and shake again; empty the flask into a dish and titrate with the standard potassium permanganate solution. The addition of the acid in this part of the experiment prevents the dissolved oxygen from acting upon the ferrous sulphate.

Subtract the result of the titration of the first sample from that of the second and the amount of the ferrous sulphate oxidized by the oxygen dissolved in the water is thus obtained. The results should be stated in terms of the number of c.c. of dissolved oxygen in one litre of water. Suppose for example 1 c.c. of the potassium permanganate solution is equal to 1·009 c.c. of oxygen at 0° C. and 760 mm. pressure, the amount of the difference between the two titrations is multiplied by 1·009 and by 1000 and divided by the volume content, in c.c.'s, of the analysing flask. If it is required to determine the percentage of the saturation of the sample of water, it can be done by calculating from a diagram prepared by the Commissioners, for instances of sea and land waters, contained on p. 58 of appendix VI of the *5th Report of the Royal Commission on Sewage Disposal*. This diagram gives the saturation figures at different temperatures for sea water and distilled water. (See Addenda of this book, p. 38 for table of solubilities of oxygen and nitrogen in distilled water and sea water.)

Estimation of dissolved oxygen in the presence of much nitrate and organic matter. Winkler (*Zeit. Angew. Chem.* 1916, XXIX, 44, and *Analyst*, 1916, XLI, 151). The water is placed in a 250 c.c. bottle, which is completely filled, and to it are added, by means of a pipette at the bottom of the bottle, 10 drops of 50 per cent. sulphuric acid and 1 c.c. of a hypochlorite solution (containing 0·5 gram of calcium hypochlorite and 25 grams of sodium sulphate per 100 c.c.). The bottle is stoppered and the contents are well mixed; after standing for 10 minutes, 1 c.c. of manganous chloride solution and 2 c.c. of sodium hydroxide-potassium iodide solution are added, and the resulting mixture is titrated with sodium thiosulphate solution. The same process is again carried out without the addition of manganous chloride and allowance is made in the calculation for the excess of chlorine thus determined.

Typical analyses of various sewage effluents
(in parts per 100,000).

Ammoniacal nitrogen	0·02	0·03	0·26	1·40	0·26	1·66	2·12
Albuminoid nitrogen ..	0·10	0·07	0·27	0·24	0·16	0·27	0·18
Nitrous nitrogen ..	trace	trace	0·02	0·04	nil	0·03	0·02
Nitric nitrogen ..	1·92	3·10	2·28	1·83	0·45	0·61	0·55
Oxygen absorbed in four hours at 80° F.	0·87	0·87	3·41	2·33	1·90	1·91	1·54
Solids in suspension ..	2·00	0·70	8·10	4·40	3·20	2·80	0·90
Oxygen in solution ..	nil	—	—	—	—	—	—
Dissolved oxygen taken up in five days at 65° F.	0·34	0·39	3·10	3·44	3·12	3·77	0·68
Remarks	earthy smell; bright; clear; small amount of fine brown solids	bright; no smell; trace of suspended matter	turbid; considerable brown suspended matter	brownish; opalescent; strong fishy smell	turbid; earthy smell	brownish; opalescent; strong fishy smell	brownish slightly opalescent; fishy smell

See also the 4th *Report of the Royal Commission on Sewage Disposal* (1904), vol. IV, parts 2 and 5, which describes methods of chemical analysis as applied to sewage and sewage effluents, and also contains tables of analyses.

RIVER-WATER AND SEWAGE

The following tables (pp. 67–72) contain the results of the determinations of the amount of oxygen dissolved in, and taken up by, a river, a sewage effluent and mixtures of the effluent with a river during the summer and winter months of 1913. They are extracted from an investigation by Purvis and Black on the oxygen content of the River Cam before and after receiving the Cambridge sewage effluent (*Proc. Camb. Phil. Soc.* vol. XVII, pt V, p. 353). They are typical results on the basis of the standard of the amount of dissolved oxygen which is consumed in five days at 18° C. suggested by the 8th *Report of the Royal Commission on Sewage Disposal* (1912), vol. I.

The more important facts which arise from a comparison of the above analyses are the following: (a) The solids in suspension in the effluent were, on several occasions in the summer months, above the standard of three grams per 100,000; and on these occasions an offensive smell was noticed after five days' incubation. On four occasions during the winter months

The River Cam and the Sewage Effluent of Cambridge.

Tables containing the results of the determinations of the amount of oxygen dissolved and absorbed by the effluent and the river at various times.

Date 1913	Hour of collecting	Location of the sample	Temperature of the water °C.	Barometric pressure in mm.	Dilution	Feet below the surface	Total suspended solids in grams per 100,000	Oxygen dissolved in c.c. per litre at 0° C. and 760 mm.		Oxygen absorbed in five days in grams per 100,000	Putrefaction on incubation at 18° C.
								At the commencement	After five days' incubation at 18° C.		
May 29	1 p.m.	River 150 feet above the effluent outfall	20	760	—	1·5	—	7·183	6·208	0·142	—
,,	,,	Sewage effluent	20	,,	—	—	3·2	0·807	nil	9·903	H₂S present
,,	,,	Mixture of effluent and river water 50 feet below effluent outfall	20	,,	1 to 15	1·5	—	5·557	2·822	0·392	—
,,	,,	River ¼ mile below the effluent outfall	20	,,	—	1·5	—	7·057	5·180	0·338	—
June 12	10.30 a.m.	River 150 feet above the effluent outfall	15	764	—	1·5	—	7·776	7·479	0·041	—
,,	,,	Sewage effluent	15	,,	—	—	2·9	0·230	nil	6·451	H₂S present
,,	,,	Mixture of effluent and river water 50 feet below effluent outfall	15	,,	1 to 16	1·5	—	7·559	3·465	0·586	—
,,	,,	River ¼ mile below the effluent outfall	15	,,	—	1·5	—	8·651	4·934	0·561	—
June 13	10 a.m.	River 150 feet above the effluent outfall	16	767	—	1·5	—	10·086	9·268	0·117	—
,,	,,	Sewage effluent	16	,,	—	—	2·8	2·727	nil	4·3	nil
,,	,,	Mixture of effluent and river water 50 feet below effluent outfall	16	,,	1 to 16	1·5	—	9·796	7·912	0·270	—
,,	,,	River ¼ mile below the effluent outfall	16	,	—	1·5	—	10·057	7·437	0·375	—

The River Cam and the Sewage Effluent of Cambridge (contd.).

Date 1913	Hour of collecting	Location of the sample	Temperature of the water °C.	Barometric pressure in mm.	Dilution	Feet below the surface	Total suspended solids in grams per 100,000	Oxygen dissolved in c.c. per litre at 0° C. and 760 mm.		Oxygen absorbed in five days in grams per 100,000	Putrefaction on incubation at 18° C.
								At the commencement	After five days' incubation at 18° C.		
July 10	10 a.m.	River 150 feet above the effluent outfall	16	758	—	1·5	—	7·793	7·496	0·042	—
,,	,,	Sewage effluent	—		Sample Bottle lost in sewer						—
,,	,,	Mixture of effluent and river water 50 feet below effluent outfall	16	758	1 to 15	1·5	—	7·311	5·849	0·209	—
,,	,,	River ¼ mile below the effluent outfall	16	,,	—	1·5	—	8·542	7·487	0·151	—
July 17	10 a.m.	River 150 feet above the effluent outfall	17	762	—	1·5	—	5·693	5·397	0·041	—
,,	,,	Sewage effluent	17	,,	—	—	3·0	1·098	nil	7·066	nil
,,	,,	Mixture of effluent and river water 50 feet below effluent outfall	17	,,	1 to 15	1·5	—	5·556	2·942	0·377	—
,,	,,	River ¼ mile below the effluent outfall	17	,,	—	1·5	—	6·818	4·428	0·342	—
July 24	1 p.m.	River 150 feet above the effluent outfall	15	765	—	1·5	—	8·364	7·474	0·127	—
,,	,,	Sewage effluent	15	,,	1 to 17	—	3·3	1·386	nil {spoilt	4·547 {spoilt	H₂S present
,,	,,	Mixture of effluent and river water 50 feet below effluent outfall	15	,,		1·5	—	8·188	7·018	0·167	—
,,	,,	River ¼ mile below the effluent outfall	15	,,	—	1·5	—	8·949	6·553	0·342	—

Date 1913	Hour of collecting	Location of the sample	Temperature of the water °C.	Barometric pressure in mm.	Dilution	Feet below the surface	Total suspended solids in grams per 100,000	Oxygen dissolved in c.c. per litre at 0° C and 760 mm.		Oxygen absorbed in five days in grams per 100,000	Putrefaction on incubation at 18°C.
								At the commencement	After five days' incubation at 18°C.		
July 31	10.30 a.m.	River 150 feet above the effluent outfall	17	762	—	1·5	—	7·479	6·886	0·085	—
"	"	Sewage effluent	17	"	—	—	1·7	1·959	nil	2·919	nil
"	"	Mixture of effluent and river water 50 feet below effluent outfall	17	"	1 to 12	1·5	—	7·019	5·557	0·209	—
"	"	River ¼ mile below the effluent outfall	17	"	—	1·5	—	8·120	6·792	0·190	—
Aug. 7	12 m.	River 150 feet above the effluent outfall	16	762	—	3	—	8·661	8·067	0·085	—
"	"	Sewage effluent	16	"	—	—	6·2	2·251	nil	5·220	H₂S present
"	"	Mixture of effluent and river water 50 feet below effluent outfall	16	"	1 to 14	3	—	7·311	0·876	0·922	—
"	"	River ¼ mile below the effluent outfall	16	"	—	3	—	8·942	6·818	0·304	—
Aug. 14	10.30 a.m.	River 150 feet above the effluent outfall	17	763	—	3	—	7·479	6·589	0·127	—
"	"	Sewage effluent	17	"	—	—	2·5	1·959	nil	0·617	nil
"	"	Mixture of effluent and river water 50 feet below effluent outfall	17	"	1 to 17	3	—	6·727	4·972	0·251	—
"	"	River ¼ mile below the effluent outfall	17	"	—	3	—	8·385	7·323	0·152	—

The River Cam and the Sewage Effluent of Cambridge (contd.).

Date 1913	Hour of collecting	Location of the sample	Temperature of the water °C.	Barometric pressure in mm.	Dilution	Feet below the surface	Total suspended solids in grams per 100,000	Oxygen dissolved n c.c. per litre at 0° C. and 760 mm.		Oxygen absorbed in five days in grams per 100,000	Putrefaction on incubation at 18° C.
								At the commencement	After five days' incubation at 18° C.		
Oct. 10	12 m.	River 150 feet above the effluent outfall	12	764	—	3	—	7·179	5·101	0·297	—
,,	,,	Sewage effluent	12	,,	—	—	10·0	1·389	nil	1·804	nil
,,	,,	Mixture of effluent and river water 50 feet below effluent outfall	12	,,	1 to 17	3	—	6·142	3·802	0·335	—
,,	,,	River ¼ mile below the effluent outfall	12	,,	—	3	—	7·379	5·743	0·234	—
Oct. 18	12 m.	River 150 feet above the effluent outfall	12	764	—	3	—	7·852	5·991	0·266	—
,,	,,	Sewage effluent	12	,,	—	—	4·0	3·799	nil	5·680	nil
,,	,,	Mixture of effluent and river water 50 feet below effluent outfall	12	,,	1 to 17	3	—	8·515	5·264	0·466	—
,,	,,	River ¼ mile below the effluent outfall	12	,,	—	3	—	8·306	7·106	0·172	—
Oct. 29	10 a.m.	River 150 feet above the effluent outfall	12	744	—	3	—	6·292	3·649	0·378	—
,,	,,	Sewage effluent	12	,,	—	—	1·0	2·824	nil	3·001	nil
,,	,,	Mixture of effluent and river water 50 feet below effluent outfall	12	,,	1 to 17	3	—	5·263	1·769	0·500	—
,,	,,	River ¼ mile below the effluent outfall	12	,,	—	3	—	6·813	4·042	0·397	—

Date 1913	Hour of collecting	Location of the sample	Temperature of the water °C.	Barometric pressure in mm.	Dilution	Feet below the surface	Total suspended solids in grams per 100,000	Oxygen dissolved in c.c. per litre at 0°C and 760 mm.		Oxygen absorbed in five days in grams per 100,000	Putrefaction on incub at 18°C
								At the commencement	After five days' incubation at 18°C.		
Nov. 5	12 m.	River 150 feet above the effluent outfall	10	752	—	3	—	6·300	4·539	0·252	—
"	"	Sewage effluent	10	"	—	—	6·1	2·238	nil	3·045	nil
"	"	Mixture of effluent and river water 50 feet below effluent outfall	10	"	1 to 17	3	—	4·468	1·184	0·470	—
"	"	River ¼ mile below the effluent outfall	10	"	—	3	—	7·046	4·315	0·391	—
Nov. 12	11 a.m.	River 150 feet above the effluent outfall	9	744	—	3	—	6·913	4·231	0·384	—
"	"	Sewage effluent	9	"	—	—	1·3	1·961	nil	2·484	nil
"	"	Mixture of effluent and river water 50 feet below effluent outfall	9	"	1 to 17	3	—	5·559	nil	0·796	—
"	"	River ¼ mile below the effluent outfall	9	"	—	3	—	6·496	2·371	0·591	—
Nov. 19	10.30 a.m.	River 150 feet above the effluent outfall	8	771	—	3	—	7·776	5·995	0·255	—
"	"	Sewage effluent	8	"	—	—	2·6	2·824	nil	2·752	nil
"	"	Mixture of effluent and river water 50 feet below effluent outfall	8	"	1 to 15	3	—	6·705	1·022	0·814	—
"	"	River ¼ mile below the effluent outfall	8	"	—	5	—	8·176	5·723	0·351	—

The River Cam and the Sewage Effluent of Cambridge (contd.).

Date 1913	Hour of collecting	Location of the sample	Temperature of the water °C.	Barometric pressure in mm.	Dilution	Feet below the surface	Total suspended solids in grams per 100,000	Oxygen dissolved in c.c. per litre at 0° C. and 760 mm.		Oxygen absorbed in five days in grams per 100,000	Putrefaction on incubation at 18° C.
								At the commencement	After five days' incubation at 18° C.		
Nov. 26	11 a.m.	River 150 feet above the effluent outfall	8	769	—	3	—	7·479	5·406	0·297	—
,,	,,	Sewage effluent	8	,,	1 to 20	—	0·292	3·112	nil	2·592	nil
,,	,,	Mixture of effluent and river water 50 feet below effluent outfall	8	,,	—	3	—	7·842	3·002	0·693	—
,,	,,	River ¼ mile below the effluent outfall	8	,,	—	3	—	8·722	6·248	0·354	—
Dec. 3	11.30 a.m.	River 150 feet above the effluent outfall	9	755	—	3	—	8·073	6·297	0·254	—
,,	,,	Sewage effluent	9	,,	—	—	7·0	3·112	nil	2·873	nil
,,	,,	Mixture of effluent and river water 50 feet below effluent outfall	9	,,	1 to 17	3	—	7·544	4·422	0·447	—
,,	,,	River ¼ mile below the effluent outfall	9	,,	—	—	—	8·722	5·702	0·432	—
Dec. 8	11.30 a.m.	River 150 feet above the effluent outfall	5	767	—	3	—	8·373	5·995	0·340	—
,,	,,	Sewage effluent	5	,,	—	—	2·1	2·531	nil	2·334	nil
,,	,,	Mixture of effluent and river water 50 feet below effluent outfall	5	,,	1 to 15	3	—	7·550	3·579	0·596	—
,,	,,	River ¼ mile below the effluent outfall	5	,,	—	3	9·4	8·293	4·359	0·563	—

the suspended solids were also above the standard; but, on the other hand, there was no smell after five days' incubation. On examining these solids microscopically it was found that they chiefly consisted of zoogloea masses of a filamentous bacillus which had developed and grown on the inside of the drain pipes and inspection chambers carrying the effluent to the river. They were not fæcal substances which produced an unpleasant smell like those noticed in the summer. (b) The amount of oxygen absorbed by the river above the outfall was always above the standard of a clean river water (0·2 gram) in the winter months from October to December inclusive, whereas in the summer months, from May to August inclusive, it was always below the standard. It cannot be said, therefore, that the river itself always satisfies the standard of the Royal Commission. (c) Only on two occasions (August 14 and October 10) was the amount of oxygen taken up by the effluent below the standard of the Commissioners. (d) On the other hand, the purification which takes place when the effluent mixes with the river water is fairly rapid; and, although the mixture of the effluent and river at 50 feet below the outfall gives a figure which is sometimes above and sometimes below the standard of 0·4 gram of oxygen absorbed in five days at 18° C., yet the river ¼ mile down as regards its cleanliness compares fairly well with the standards of a diluting water suggested by the Commissioners. For example, five of the analyses would grade the river as "clean," ten as "fairly clean" and three as "doubtful" at ¼ mile below the effluent outfall.

It will be noticed that the differences in the summer and winter months are very striking.

Three factors at least may be suggested to explain these differences and these are: (1) the varying amount of the rainfall, with which is connected a considerable amount of pollution derived mainly from road washings and the surface water from agricultural land, (2) the number of hours of sunshine, with which is connected the purifying power of the oxygen given out by aquatic plants under its influence, and (3) the changes in the temperature of the water (and therefore closely allied to the second factor), with which is connected the varying amounts of oxygen dissolved from the air at different temperatures. As the rainfall increases the amount of oxygen absorbed by the river in five days increases, and this was particularly noticeable in the rainy season in October. In the summer months, the number of hours of sunshine was greater than in the winter months, and the amount of oxygen in the river was increased as a consequence of the response to this influence by the aquatic plants. In the winter months, on the other hand, from November 12 to December 8, there was a distinct rise in the amount of oxygen dissolved, and this was explained by the decrease in the rainfall, and a fall in the temperature of the water, so that there was a kind of balance. In the summer months, the decreased solubility of the oxygen of the air caused by the higher temperature was more than compensated by the increased discharge of the oxygen from the aquatic plants; and the increased solubility of the oxygen of the air caused by the lower winter temperature partly compensated for the disappearance of the oxygen discharged by the aquatic plants.

At the same time, as Letts has indicated (6th appendix (1908), 5th *Report of the Royal Commission on Sewage Disposal*) in his experiments with the sea weed *Ulva latissima*, it is most likely that aquatic plants generally may be of considerable importance in the purification of a polluted stream. They are able to absorb some of the ammonia salts and nitrates, in addition to their ability to give off oxygen under the influence of sunshine.

Besides the above estimations of the amount of oxygen dissolved in, and taken up by, a river, the table on p. 75 contains the results of a series of chemical and bacterial analyses of the River Cam in an investigation by Purvis and Rayner (*Jour. Roy. San. Inst.* 1913, vol. XXXIV (X), p. 478). They show the chemical and bacterial (as regards *Bacillus coli*) variations at different parts beginning at 100 feet above the effluent outfall and extending four miles below it. There is some further pollution at two miles below the outfall. The samples were taken from 18 inches below the surface of the river and in midstream, and were obtained between 6 a.m. and 8 a.m. The numbers are the mean of three analyses on two days in May and one day in June, 1912.

It is clear from the table on p. 75 that the river is polluted

Average Chemical (*in parts per* 100,000) *and* Bacterial (*in* 1 *c.c.*) *Analyses of the Cam Water above and below the Effluent Outfall.*

	100 feet above Outfall	Crude Effluent	8 feet from Outfall	¼ mile below Outfall	½ mile below Outfall	¾ mile below Outfall	1 mile below Outfall	1¼ miles below Outfall	2 miles below Outfall	2½ miles below Outfall	3 miles below Outfall	4 miles below Outfall
Free and saline ammonia	·068	—	·379	·112	·0846	·102	·074	·0712	·0862	—	—	—
Albuminoid ammonia ..	·0336	—	·0846	·032	·0286	·034	·035	·0275	·0412	—	—	—
Oxygen absorbed in 4 hours at 80° F. ..	·3143	—	·678	·2039	·2035	·254	·222	·216	·2213	—	—	—
Nitrogen as nitrates ..	·55	—	·55	·65	·583	·65	·575	·575	·575	—	—	—
Nitrogen as nitrites ..	Only traces were found, but there was a tendency to an increase down the river.											
Chlorine	3·06	—	4·483	3·4	3·4	3·5	3·35	3·35	3·35	—	—	—
B. coli found in 1 c.c. ..	661	102,422	27,522	—	6,670	—	14,443	8,540	6,377	2,349	1,525	30

at a place two miles below the effluent. The bacterial analysis shows marked pollution at about three-quarters of a mile down, and the chemical figures are higher than at half a mile; and, even at two miles, the two ammonia figures are higher than at 100 feet above the effluent.

It is of some importance, however, to note that the figure for the absorbed oxygen goes down very rapidly, so that at a quarter of a mile it is below that at 100 feet above the outfall; it increases at three-quarters of a mile and again rapidly decreases, so that at two miles it is again lower than at 100 feet above the outfall. There is, therefore, definite proof that the dissolved oxygen in the stream comes at once into action, and thereby decreases the amount of easily oxidizable substances in the effluent. The results are quite comparable with those of the oxygen absorbed figures described before, in Purvis and Black's observations.

The river therefore purifies itself chemically from the contaminating effluent quite satisfactorily; for between half a mile and three-quarters of a mile, the albuminoid ammonia and the oxygen absorbed figures are lower than at 100 feet above the effluent outfall.

The dangerous pollution, as indicated by *B. coli*, coming from the discharge of the sewage effluent into the stream, is still well marked at between three and four miles below the effluent outfall. It will be observed, however, that there is a definite amount of purification in this respect at four miles below, as compared with that at 100 feet above, the outfall. If the river were to receive no further pollution after that which is poured into it from the effluent outfall, it is, perhaps, probable that at about three miles below the outfall the water would be comparatively free from *Bacillus coli*.

See also the *8th Report of the Royal Commission on Sewage Disposal*, vol. II, appendix: "On Standards and Tests for sewage and sewage effluents discharging into rivers and streams."

SEA-WATER AND SEWAGE

An analysis of sea-water from the British Channel is given
below. There are variations in such a sample and one taken
from the Irish Sea or the North Sea.

	parts per 1000
Sodium chloride	28·00
Magnesium sulphate	2·30.
Magnesium chloride	3·60
Magnesium bromide	0·03
Calcium sulphate	1·30
Calcium carbonate	0·03
Potassium chloride	0·74
Iodides	traces

Thorp and Morton (*Jahresb. für Chemie*, 1870, p. 1380) state
that the Irish Sea contained 0·002 part of magnesium nitrate
per 1000 of the water. This represents less than 0·04 part of
nitrogen per 100,000 parts of water. It is difficult to realize
that this represents the final product of the nitrification of the
immense amount of organic nitrogenous compounds including
nitrates which must have been poured in the sea, and which is
continually being poured in from rivers of all kinds and all
sizes. The matter is of considerable importance when sewage
and sewage effluents are discharged into the sea or river; for it
is desirable to know the nature and extent of the chemical, as
well as the bacterial purification together with the length of
time such purification may take.

Sea-water usually contains little or no free and saline ammonia, and very small amounts of albuminoid ammonia,
whereas nitrogen as nitrates and nitrites has rarely been found,
and then in very small quantities. The possibilities of pollution
of tidal estuaries, and indeed of the sea itself by the sewage
poured into it from towns situated on the coast, is a serious
matter. The Royal Commission on Sewage Disposal has collected a large amount of evidence from places where sewage
has been deposited in the sea and tidal estuaries. Of great importance is the evidence in vol. VII of the Commissioners' Report given by Dr W. E. Adeney and Professor Letts. These in-
vestigators in a series of laboratory experiments mixed sea-
water with 1 per cent. of sewage, and from time to time they
estimated the two ammonias, and the nitrites and nitrates.

They concluded from their experiments that nitrifying organisms can exist in such mixtures, although it was stated to be very remarkable that a large proportion of free ammonia remained unnitrified even after 11 months' inoculation. And, further, in Adeney and Letts' later experiments they found that the nitrates present at the beginning of the incubation disappeared after an interval of 21 months.

In an investigation by Purvis and Coleman[1] on "The influence of the saline constituents of sea-water on the decomposition of sewage," they give the results of the estimation of the two ammonias and of the nitrates and nitrites when sewage was incubated, not only with sea-water, obtained off the Norfolk coast, both sterilized and unsterilized, but also when it was incubated with several of the principal saline constituents of sea-water. The chief result of Purvis and Coleman's varied experiments was to show that the organic substances of sewage when in sea-water only slowly decomposed; for even after eight weeks' incubation there was a comparatively small decrease in the amounts of the two ammonias; and, what is perhaps of greater importance, neither nitrates nor nitrites were produced. In fact, in two series of experiments where the original sewage contained traces of nitrates and nitrites, even these traces disappeared after three days' incubation.

In a later paper by Purvis and Courtauld[2] two series of experiments were conducted by incubating unfiltered sewage with (a) ammonia-free water made faintly alkaline with soda, and (b) with distilled water, and of such strength that each solution contained 1 per cent. sewage. The general results of these experiments were comparable in some respects with those of Purvis and Coleman in so far as there was a very slow and gradual decrease in the two ammonias. But with regard to the production of nitrates there was some difference, in that both in the alkaline and non-alkaline mixtures very small quantities of nitrates were produced, and in one or two experiments there were also traces of nitrites. In these experiments the zinc-copper couple method as described by Dr McGowan was used to determine nitrates and nitrites. At the same

[1] Jour. Roy. San. Inst. vol. xxvii, No. 8 (1906), p. 433.
[2] Proc. Camb. Phil. Soc. vol. xv, Part iv, p. 354.

time, attention was called to the possibility that this method
might give fictitious results. It was used by Dr McGowan
(*Report of Royal Commission on Sewage Disposal*, vol. IV, pt V,
p. 17), as well as by Adeney and Letts. It was suggested that
such a couple might not only reduce the nitrates and nitrites
to free ammonia, but that nitrogenous compounds, like the
albuminoids, might be partly reduced to simple forms, of
which ammonia would be one; and that, consequently, on distillation the figure obtained for nitrates would be correspond-
ingly high.

In order to substantiate this suggestion, Purvis and Courtauld, some months later (*Proc. Camb. Phil. Soc.* vol. XIV, pt V,
p. 441), showed that such a zinc-copper couple did actually
reduce peptones, blood serum, albumin and sewage containing
no nitrates or nitrites when in solution in strengths varying
from 1 per cent. to 0·001 per cent. of the various organic
substances. The investigation was divided into three parts:
(1) spontaneous decomposition of the dissolved organic nitrogenous substances; (2) the action of a copper-zinc couple upon
such solutions; and (3) the action of the couple on these solutions when a definite amount of potassium nitrate was also
present. The conclusions were that the couple not only reduced
the nitrates to ammonia, but also, partly, the nitrogenous substances as well; and that, therefore, the accuracy of this
method could not be relied upon for estimating nitrates and
nitrites in water charged with organic nitrogenous substances.

Purvis and Coleman used the indigo method described on
p. 11, for nitrates, and the metaphenylene diamine method
for nitrites (p. 13). In the later experiments, the phenol sulphuric acid method was used for estimating nitrates (p. 9).

In an investigation by Purvis, Macalister, and Minnett
(*Proc. 7th Internat. Congress Applied Chemistry*, 1909, Sec.
VIII a, p. 272), the subject was further studied, bacterially as
well as chemically. The series of experiments was undertaken
to see if stronger sewage and stronger mixtures would indicate
the presence of nitrates and nitrites better than in the weaker
sewage and weaker mixtures. The following Table (I) contains
the results, in parts per 100,000, of the analysis of a 10 per
cent. mixture of sewage with sea-water:

TABLE I.

10 per cent. strong afternoon sewage in sea-water; mixed 2.3.09.

Date of analysis	Free NH₃	Albuminoid NH₃	Total NH₂	Nitrites	Nitrates
Filtered—					
2.3.09 ..	0·760	0·144	0·904	not done	not done
10.3.09 ..	0·450	0·024	0·474	,,	,,
20.3.09 ..	0·600	0·048	0·648	,,	,,
Unfiltered—					
2.3.09 ..	1·200	0·200	1·400	0·021	none
3.3.09 ..	not done	not done	—	0·018	,,
4.3.09 ..	,,	,,	—	0·011	,,
5.3.09 ..	,,	,,	—	0·009	,,
6.3.09 ..	,,	,,	—	none	,,
10.3.09 ..	0·500	0·300	0·800	,,	,,
20.3.09 ..	0·640	—	—	not done	not done

The following Table (II) contains the estimations of the nitrites and nitrates in the 5 per cent. and 1 per cent. mixtures of unfiltered sewage and sea-water mixed 2.3.09:

TABLE II.

Date			Nitrites	Nitrates
3.3.09 ..	5 per cent. mixture		0·014	none
4.3.09 ..	,,	,,	0·005	,,
5.3.09 ..	,,	,,	0·004	,,
6.3.09 ..	,,	,,	none	,,
10.3.09 ..	,,	,,	,,	,,
3.3.09 ..	1 per cent. mixture		0·002	,,
4.3.09 ..	,,	,,	none	,,
5.3.09 ..	,,	,,	,,	,,
6.3.09 ..	,,	,,	,,	,,
10.3.09 ..	,,	,,	,,	,,

The chemical results showed: (1) that in all the mixtures of sea-water, with either strong or weak sewage (with variations from 1 to 10 per cent. of sewage), there remained about 70 per cent. of undecomposed and unacted upon nitrogenous organic compounds after 18 days' incubation; (2) that mixtures of 1 per cent. weak sewage and sea-water showed neither nitrates nor nitrites after 18 days; (3) that mixtures of 5 per cent. weak sewage and sea-water showed neither nitrates nor nitrites after 18 days; (4) that mixtures of 10 per cent. *strong* sewage and sea-water gave nitrites for four days and then they disappeared, but that nitrates did not appear; (5) that mixtures of 5 per cent. *strong* sewage and sea-water showed nitrites for three days and then they disappeared, but that no nitrates were produced; and (6) that mixtures of 1 per cent. *strong*

sewage and sea-water showed nitrites at the end of the first
day of incubation and then they disappeared, but that no
nitrates were produced.

The bacterial results of a 10 per cent. mixture of sewage
and sea-water proved that there was a rapid diminution of the
organisms when the sewage was incubated with sea-water
(Tables III, IV, V, pp. 82–83). The rapid disappearance of the
bacteria is very marked, and the growths of organisms, for
example nitrifying organisms, may be inhibited at a very early
stage. In fact the salts in the sea-water act not unlike anti-
septics, and the result is that the organic substances are only
slowly broken down; and even this decomposition is probably
caused by the oxygen dissolved from the air.

TABLE III.

	Intervals between receipt of sample and bacterial analysis					
	2 hours only		4 days		7 days	
	Sewage	Sewage and sea-water	Sewage	Sewage and sea-water	Sewage	Sewage and sea-water
Colonies in 1 c.c. on agar in 48 hours at 37° C.	26,000,000	2,688,000	39,840,000	3,144,000	8,800,000	36,000
Colonies in 1 c.c. on gelatine in four days at 22° C.	1,072,000,000	11,660,000	250,000,000	206,000,000	188,000,000	1,080,000
B. coli communis in 1 c.c.	1,000,000,000	100,000,000	100,000,000	10,000,000	1,000,000	100
B. ent. spor. in 1 c.c.	1,000	100	1,000	100	100	absent
Strept. faecalis in 1 c.c.	10,000	1,000	10,000	100	100	absent

TABLE IV.

The sample was received 3rd February, 1909: a portion was at once diluted in the proportion of sewage 1 part and sea-water 9 parts, i.e. a 10 per cent. mixture. Both the original sewage and the mixture were allowed to stand for 12 hours at the laboratory temperature before analysis. The original sewage was diluted with sterile water immediately before analysis to make the results comparable.

	Intervals between receipt of sample and bacterial analysis					
	12 hours after receipt		4 days		7 days	
	Sewage	Sewage and sea-water	Sewage	Sewage and sea-water	Sewage	Sewage and sea-water
No. of colonies in 1 c.c. capable of developing on agar at 37° C. in 48 hours	98,400,000	1,000,000	Not examined	11,600	Not examined	100
No. of colonies in 1 c.c. capable of developing on gelatine at 22° C. in four days	Not counted	Not counted		40,160,000		1,200
No. of B. coli communis present in 1 c.c.	100,000,000	100,000		10,000		100
No. of B. ent. spor. present in 1 c.c.	100	nil		nil		nil
No. of streptococcus faecalis in 1 c.c.	100	10		nil		nil

The enormous reduction in the number of organisms in seven days is very striking.

TABLE V.

Sewage received 18th February, 1909, and mixed with sea-water in the proportion of 1 to 9, on receipt; they were allowed to stand at the laboratory temperature for 24 hours and used for analysis on 19th February, 1909.

	Intervals between receipt of sample and bacterial analysis					
	24 hours		4 days		7 days	
	Sewage	Sewage and sea-water	Sewage	Sewage and sea-water	Sewage	Sewage and sea-water
Colonies per c.c. on agar in 48 hours at 37° C.	1,480,000	126,800	268,000	15,600	224,000	2,500
Colonies per c.c. on gelatine in four days at 22° C.	69,200,000	6,200,000	1,024,000	75,600	572,000	32,000
B. coli communis in 1 c.c.	1,000,000	100,000	100,000	100	100,000	100
B. ent. spor. in 1 c.c.	absent	absent	absent	absent	absent	absent
Streptococcus faecalis in 1 c.c.	100	10	100	10	absent	absent

The decrease in the number of organisms at the end of seven days is again very striking; and the decrease in the number of organisms in the mixture of sea-water and sewage is much greater than the decrease in the sewage. The presence of considerable quantities of *B. coli* is noticeable in the three series of experiments even after seven days.

Purvis, McHattie, and Fisher (*Jour. Roy. San. Inst.* 1911, vol. XXXII, p. 442), continued these experiments and during the incubation, dry air, free from carbon dioxide, was slowly and continuously bubbled through mixtures of sea-water and sewage, and of sea-water and distilled water. The original figures are not inserted here but the results of the observations were: (1) that after 70 days' incubation of 10 per cent. sewage in sea-water, with every facility for complete æration, there was no production of nitrates or nitrites; (2) that there were some nitrates produced when the sewage was incubated with distilled water in 42 days; (3) that the free-ammonia figure was increased in the sewage and sea-water at the end of 42 days, but it decreased in the sewage and distilled water at the end of the same period of time.

The authors suggested that the most obvious explanation of these facts was to assume that the sea-water destroyed the useful nitrifying organisms, as indicated by the bacterial and chemical investigations of Purvis, Macalister, and Minnett (*loc. cit.*). At the same time, some explanation was necessary with regard to the increase in the free ammonia of the sewage and sea-water, as well as the decrease in the ammonia of the sewage and distilled water and the presence of nitrates in the latter. It was suggested that the free and continuous æration oxidized the nitrogenous compounds of the sewage, and slowly decomposed them to less complex compounds, one of which was ammonia, and that this oxidation was continued a stage further in the sewage and distilled water, so that the presence of the nitrates was accompanied by a corresponding decrease in the free ammonia.

With regard to the continuous presence of free ammonia even after 52 days' incubation, it was remarked that it supported the suggestion of Kenwood and Kay-Menzies (*Internat. Congress Applied Chemistry*, 1909, Sec. VIII a, p. 259) as affording a valuable clue to the contamination of sea-water by sewage.

Letts and Richards (*7th Report Royal Commission on Sewage Disposal*, vol. XI, appendices, part I, pp. 104–113) also showed that nitrates were only produced in mixtures of sewage and sea-water after about 70 days' incubation.

Purvis and Walker completed another series of experiments both chemically and bacterially and mixed the afternoon unfiltered sewage from the Cambridge Sewage Farm with sea-water obtained from off the Norfolk coast near Lowestoft, as in the previous investigations (*Jour. Roy. San. Inst.* 1912, vol. XXXIII (9), p. 368; 1913, vol. XXXIV (1), p. 71).

The mixtures, and the sea-water itself, were placed in three large unstoppered Winchester bottles. The air, freed from carbon dioxide, and washed by passing through ammonia-free water, was aspirated through each bottle by connection with a water pump, and the aspiration of the air went on day and night. The average temperature was between 14°–15° C. The following tables contain the results of the analyses under the conditions of this constant temperature and continuous and thorough æration, and they give the number of days after the mixtures had been made. The numbers represent parts per 100,000.

TABLE E.—*Analyses of the sea-water* alone.

	1st May (9 days)	7th May (16 days)	20th May (29 days)	3rd June (42 days)	10th June (49 days)
Free and saline NH_3	not done	not done	not done	not done	0·025
Albuminoid NH_3 ..	„	„	„	„	0·005
Total NH_3	„	„	„	„	0·030
N as nitrites ..	nil	nil	nil	·020	trace
N as nitrates ..	nil	nil	nil	nil	nil

TABLE F.—5 *per cent. mixture of sewage in sea-water.* Mixed 22nd April, 1912.

	1st May (9 days)	7th May (16 days)	20th May (29 days)	28th May (37 days)	3rd June (42 days)	10th June (49 days)
Free and saline NH_3 ..	·68	·15	·30	·05	·15	·325
Albuminoid NH_3	·11	·08	·08	·05	·085	·045
Total NH_3	·79	·23	·38	·10	·235	·370
N as nitrites	·0037	nil	·006	? trace	nil	nil
N as nitrates	nil	nil	nil	nil	nil	·02

TABLE G.—10 *per cent. mixture of sewage in sea-water. Mixed 22nd April, 1912. There were no nitrates or nitrites in the sewage.*

	1st May (9 days)	7th May (16 days)	20th May (29 days)	28th May (37 days)	3rd June (42 days)	10th June (49 days)
Free and saline NH_3	1·02	1·40	·52	·18	·28	·425
Albuminoid NH_3	·15	·17	·17	·15	·15	·145
Total NH_3 ..	1·17	1·57	·69	·33	·43	·570
N as nitrites ..	·0044	trace	·0118	·0059	·0059	nil
N as nitrates ..	nil	nil	nil	? trace	nil	·05

The chief results of the above analyses are (1) the very slow decomposition and decrease in the two ammonias, even after 49 days' incubation. (2) The appearance of nitrites in the sea-water alone in about 42 days, and their appearance in nine days in the two mixtures; their disappearance, and their reappearance, in about 29 days and their decrease in the 10 per cent. mixtures in 42 days; and their disappearance in the 5 per cent. mixture in the same time. (3) The appearance of nitrates after 49 days in the two mixtures.

It is to be noted also that the changes in each mixture are proportionately the same. For example, the total ammonia in both mixtures at the end of 49 days is about one-half that at the end of nine days; and the nitrites in the 5 per cent. mixture are about one-half those in the 10 per cent. mixture at the end of 29 days; and the nitrates in the 5 per cent. mixture at the end of 49 days are about one-half those in the 10 per cent. mixture. The numbers indicate that the conditions of the experiments were very similar.

Letts and Richards (*loc. cit.*) found oxidized nitrogen after 21 days and 27 days in a 5 per cent. mixture, but they did not differentiate it into nitrites and nitrates. They also found both nitrites and nitrates after 73 and 103 days: "the nitrites gradually disappearing and the nitrates becoming stronger, so that after five and a half months every trace of nitrous nitrogen had disappeared while nitric nitrogen had largely replaced it."

The bacterial investigations were limited to the number of organisms which appeared on agar at 37° C., and on gelatine at 22° C. The following (Table D_2) contains the bacterial results of the sea-water and the mixtures, of which the chemical results are contained in Tables E, F and G (p. 85). The dates represent the days of the month when the incubations on agar and gelatine were commenced.

TABLE D_2.

The sea-water and the two mixtures were analysed at once on the 22nd April, 1912, and then at the intervals which are noted. The numbers represent bacteria per c.c. E = sea-water alone. F = 5 per cent. sewage and sea-water. G = 10 per cent. sewage and sea-water.

			Number of organisms in 1 c.c. capable of developing on agar at 37° C. in 2 days	Number of organisms in 1 c.c. capable of developing on gelatine at 22° C. in 3 days
22nd April, 1912	..	E	6,000	400,000
		F	1,200,000	4,820,000
		G	2,500,000	10,200,000
26th April, 1912	..	E	6,400	550,000
(4 days)		F	1,840,000	11,200,000
		G	3,350,000	27,650,000
30th April, 1912	..	E	740	86,000
(8 days)		F	17,800	1,050,000
		G	29,750	2,850,000
5th May, 1912	..	E	254	2,550
(13 days)		F	11,400	72,000
		G	20,800	114,000
13th May, 1912	..	E	84	480
(21 days)		F	942	674
		G	1,380	820
20th May, 1912	..	E	3	82
(29 days)		F	109	82
		G	220	90
28th May, 1912	..	E	2	42
(37 days)		F	74	55
		G	93	63
3rd June, 1912	..	E	53	14
(42 days)		F	87	102
		G	83	276
10th June, 1912	..	E	71	31
(49 days)		F	94	346
		G	78	1,000

The results of the bacterial investigation are: (1) In the first place they show that a certain number of organisms were in the sea-water itself, although, of course, very considerably fewer than in the mixtures. (2) There was an enormous reduction of the organisms by the 21st day. (3) This reduction steadily went on until the 37th day, and the number growing on agar at 37° was greater than on gelatine at 22° C., whereas it was the reverse of this at the commencement. (4) That by the 42nd and 49th day there was a gradual increase in the number of organisms.

The experiments were continued for some time after the

49th day, and the effect of the oxidation of *sterilized* sewage and of sterilized sewage mixed with small quantities of the incubations just described was also investigated.

The results showed (1) that the trace of nitrites found in the sea-water alone on the 42nd day remained practically the same on the 61st, the 89th, and the 106th day; and that by the 115th day a trace of nitrates appeared, and also on the 176th day: (2) that there was an alternate slow disappearance and reappearance of both nitrites and nitrates in the two mixtures between the 42nd day and the 115th day; and that by the 176th day both mixtures contained no nitrites, but definite amounts of nitrates: (3) that the sea-water and mixtures contained definite amounts of both ammonias at the end of the 176th day.

The following table contains the results of the bacterial analyses, which, as in the earlier experiments, were limited to the number of organisms which appeared on agar at 37° C. and on gelatine at 22° C.

E^1 = sea-water alone.
F^1 = 5 per cent. mixture of sewage and sea-water.
G^1 = 10 per cent. mixture of sewage and sea-water.

		Number of organisms in 1 c.c. capable of developing on agar at 37° C. in 2 days	Number of organisms in 1 c.c. capable of developing on gelatine at 22° C. in 3 days
22 June, 1912 (61 days)	E^1	62	17
	F^1	87	287
	G^1	65	760
9 July, 1912 (78 days)	E^1	43	22
	F^1	75	159
	G^1	67	423
22 July, 1912 (89 days)	E^1	31	7
	F^1	39	129
	G^1	58	317
6 August, 1912 (106 days)	E^1	19	2
	F^1	33	81
	G^1	47	208
15 October, 1912 (176 days)	E^1	A few moulds only	A few moulds only
	F^1	A few moulds	A few moulds
	G^1	A few moulds	A few moulds and 7 colonies

The outstanding results of the bacterial analyses were the steady decrease in the number of organisms from the slight increase on the 42nd and on the 49th days; and the final disappearance of all the bacteria by the 176th day, with the exception of seven colonies developed in gelatine in the 10 per cent. mixture. There was nothing but moulds left. A comparison of the corresponding chemical results shows that nitrates were present in the mixture by this time.

Sterilized sewage. Another part of the investigation was to incubate definite portions of sterilized sewage and of sterilized sewage mixed with definite amounts of the 5 per cent. and 10 per cent. mixtures, in order to ascertain how far the decomposition and nitrification are affected in the richer sterilized sewage.

About one litre of fresh sewage was sterilized in an autoclave at 120° C. and 126 lbs. pressure for one hour. Definite volumes of this sterilized sewage were then mixed in the following proportions:

1. 500 c.c. of sterilized sewage were mixed with 500 c.c. sterilized distilled water. This is referred to in H in the table below.

2. 50 c.c. of the sterilized sewage were mixed with 50 c.c. of the 5 per cent. mixture of sewage and sea-water of the earlier incubations, and also with 900 c.c. of sterilized distilled water. This is referred to in J in the table (p. 90).

3. 100 c.c. of sterilized sewage were mixed with 100 c.c. of the 10 per cent. mixture of sewage and sea-water of the earlier incubations, and also with 800 c.c. sterilized distilled water. This is referred to in K in the table (p. 90).

These mixtures were made on the 27th September, 1912, and allowed to incubate as in the earlier incubations. That is to say, pure filtered air was aspirated regularly and continuously through them at a definite temperature of 14°–18° C., and they were analysed from time to time chemically and bacterially.

TABLE H.—*Chemical Analysis of the sterilized sewage (see above) in parts per* 100,000.

	28th Sept.	4th Oct. (5 days)	10th Oct. (11 days)	15th Oct. (16 days)	20th Oct. (21 days)	5th Nov. (36 days)
Free and saline NH₃	1·95	1·95	1·80	not done	·30	·30
Albuminoid NH₃ ..	·20	·20	·25	,,	·20	·25
Total NH₃	2·15	2·15	2·05	,,	·50	·55
N as nitrites ..	nil	·059	·09	·147	·251	·225
N as nitrates ..	nil	nil	? trace	·150	·450	·900

TABLE J.—*Chemical Analysis of the sterilized sewage to which a portion of the old 5 per cent. mixture had been added (see above).*

	28th Sept.	4th Oct. (5 days)	10th Oct. (11 days)	15th Oct. (16 days)	20th Oct. (21 days)	4th Nov. (36 days)
Free and saline NH₃	3·0	1·8	1·4	not done	·15	·08
Albuminoid NH₃ ..	1·0	1·0	1·0	,,	·08	nil
Total NH₃	4·0	2·8	2·4	,,	·23	·98
N as nitrites ..	small trace	·004	·06	·009	? trace	·0001
N as nitrates ..	? trace	nil	? trace	·002	·05	·09

TABLE K.—*Chemical Analysis of the sterilized sewage to which a portion of the old 10 per cent. mixture had been added (see p. 89).*

	28th Sept.	4th Oct. (5 days)	10th Oct. (11 days)	15th Oct. (16 days)	20th Oct. (21 days)	4th Nov. (36 days)
Free and saline NH₃	5·5	6·0	5·4	not done	·2	·13
Albuminoid NH₃ ..	1·0	1·5	2·2	,,	·15	·05
Total NH₃	6·5	7·5	7·7	,,	·35	·18
N as nitrites ..	trace	·0118	·13	·005	? trace	·0003
N as nitrates ..	? trace	? trace	·10	·200	·45	·75

The results contained in the above tables H, J and K clearly show that nitrites were first produced slowly in all three solutions, and that this was followed by the production of nitrates. At the same time the total ammonia figure is also reduced. That is to say, the oxidation of sterilized sewage resulted in the production of nitrites and nitrates (without the assistance of bacteria), as shown by Table H.

The following table contains the results of the bacterial analyses of which the chemical analyses are in Tables H, J, K (above).

		No. of organisms in 1 c.c. capable of developing on agar at 37° C. in 2 days	No. of organisms in 1 c.c. capable of developing on gelatine at 22° C. in 3 days
29 Sept. 1912	H	No bacterial colonies; 2 colonies of proteus	No bacterial colonies; 1 mould
	J	1 colony	No colonies; 3 moulds
	K	7 colonies	11 ,, no moulds — No colonies; 1 proteus
7 Oct. 1912	H	1 colony	224 ,,
	J	11 colonies	368 ,,
	K	35 ,,	1 colony
10 Oct. 1912	H	No colonies	218 colonies
	J	11 colonies	320 ,,
	K	19 ,,	No colonies
15 Oct. 1912	H	No colonies	93 colonies
	J	2 colonies	215 ,,
	K	8 ,,	No colonies
22 Oct. 1912	H	No colonies	27 colonies
	J	1 colony	148 ,,
	K	11 colonies	No colonies
4 Nov. 1912	H	No colonies	18 colonies
	J	1 colony	107 ,,
	K	3 colonies	No colonies

The most striking result of the above table is to show that no bacterial colonies appeared in the sterilized sewage; and that in the sterilized sewage which had been inoculated with small quantities of the old 5 per cent. and 10 per cent. incubations the number of colonies slightly increased between the date of the inoculation (28th September) and nine days afterwards, and gradually decreased after that date.

If these numbers are compared with the chemical analyses of the 5th November (Table H, p. 89) it will be seen that there were considerable amounts of nitrites and nitrates in the sterilized sewage, and *that not a single bacterial colony was found.*

Results. To sum up the results of these investigations, it is clear that while nitrites and nitrates were produced there was also a reduction in the number of bacteria. The first series of experiments with unsterilized sewage indicated that, although the number of organisms decreased, the oxidation of the nitrogenous compounds was not diminished. In the second series of experiments with sterilized sewage, it was proved that nitrites and nitrates were produced even when no bacteria were present; and although there was a slight increase in the number of organisms in the 5 per cent. and 10 per cent. incubations, no doubt caused by the fresh food which had been added, the numbers gradually decreased, and yet nitrites and nitrates were present in considerable amounts.

The whole series of experiments proves that where thorough æration goes on in mixtures of sewage and sea-water, the production of nitrites and nitrates need not be brought about by the action of the nitrifying organisms. It is a reasonable explanation to suggest that the dissolved oxygen slowly breaks down the complex compounds in sewage; and that, in course of time, nitrites and nitrates are among the final products of this slow oxidation. The salts in the sea-water are antagonistic to the growth of bacteria, the latter gradually die out, and amongst them, it may be, are the useful nitrifying organisms. The result is that a rapid oxidation of the complex chemical compounds is impossible; and it is only slowly brought about partly by the dissolved oxygen obtained from the air which is gradually used up in the process, and is replenished by the systematic solution of more oxygen from the atmosphere, and partly obtained from aquatic plants which, under the influence of sunshine, give out considerable quantities of oxygen.

The effect of the high temperature and pressure in the sterilized sewage experiments would be to break down the organic compounds to a considerable extent, and thereby the oxidation would proceed more rapidly than in the unsterilized sewage.

The application of these results to the disposal of sewage in the sea or in estuaries or lakes or rivers is direct. The growth and development of useful nitrifying organisms are retarded; and the decomposition and breakdown of the complex organic compounds are slowly accomplished by the oxygen dissolved in the larger body of water. This oxygen is soon used up by the first lot of sewage; and it is only by the continuous solution of more oxygen that the decomposition can proceed. Consequently, the final production of nitrates in this way is a very slow process. An important point to bear in mind is, therefore, the necessity of a thorough and rapid dilution of the sewage or effluent when these are poured into the water of the sea or an estuary or a river, even after they have undergone some preliminary treatment. A more rapid and efficient oxidation is thereby assured, quite apart from the further purification which proceeds from the ability of aquatic plants to absorb ammonia salts, as well as nitrates. And, of course, a moving water, like the sea, or a river, will also assist the purification. (See Royal Commission on Sewage Disposal, 8th Report, vol. II, appendix: "On Standards and Tests for sewage and sewage effluents discharging into rivers and streams.")

REFERENCES TO INVESTIGATIONS ON THE DECOMPOSITION OF
SEWAGE IN SEA-WATER.

1. Royal Commission on Sewage Disposal, vol. VII. Evidence of Dr Adeney and Prof. Letts.
2. Royal Commission on Sewage Disposal. 5th Report. Appendix VI. Report by Prof. Letts and Dr Adeney; and the same report and appendix, experiments by Dr Fowler.
3. Purvis and Coleman. Journ. Roy. Sany. Inst. vol. XXVII, No. 8 (1906), p. 433.
4. Purvis and Courtauld. Proc. Camb. Phil. Soc. vol. XIV, p. 441, and vol. XV, p. 354.

5. Purvis, Macalister and Minnett. *Proc. 7th Int. Congress.* Applied Chemistry (1909), Sec. VIII a, p. 272.

6. Purvis, McHattie and Fisher. *Journ. Roy. Sany. Inst.* vol. XXXII, No. 9 (1911), p. 442.

7. Royal Commission on Sewage Disposal. *7th Report,* vol. II. Appendices, Part I. Experiments by Prof. Letts and Mr Richards.

8. Letts. *Journ. Roy. Sany. Inst.* vol. XXXIII, No. I, p. II.

9. Purvis and Walker. *Journ. Roy. Sany. Inst.* vol. XXXIII, No. 9 (1912), p. 368; and vol. XXXIV, No. I (1913), p. 71.

The whole subject of "The principles and practice of the dilution method of Sewage Disposal" will be discussed by Dr W. E. Adeney in one of the volumes of The Cambridge Public Health Series.

WORKS EFFLUENTS

Very serious contamination of streams and brooks often occurs in the neighbourhood of works in which manufacturing processes are carried out. This contamination is due to the waste waters from the processes used which frequently contain large quantities of highly oxidisable material, together with suspended matter, both volatile and non-volatile, and ingredients such as fats, tar oils, acid, etc. It is essential in the interests of the public health that as far as possible all offensive and poisonous material should be removed from such effluents before they are permitted to enter any brook or stream.

Methods of analysis. The determination of free and saline ammonia, albuminoid ammonia, solids in suspension and oxygen absorbed are carried out in accordance with the directions for sewage analysis (pp. 55–65); estimations of total solids, chlorine, sulphates, nitrates and nitrites and the physical characters are made as directed under water analysis (pp. 2–23).

Putrescibility. A stoppered bottle is completely filled with the effluent and kept at a temperature of 27° C.; the time taken for blackening or for the smell of sulphuretted hydrogen to appear is noted.

Determination of fat. 100 c.c. of the effluent are made acid with sulphuric acid and extracted with ether; the ethereal layer is separated and the ether is evaporated off in a weighed flask; the residue is dried in a water oven and weighed; the

final weight, less the weight of the flask, represents the amount
of fat in 100 c.c. of the effluent.

The following methods of analysis are due to Linder (*Reports
of the Chief Inspector of Alkali Works*, 1905, *et seq.*).

Determination of total sulphur. 50 c.c. of the effluent
are slowly dropped into a flask containing excess of pure
bromine covered by water which has been moderately acidified
with hydrochloric acid; the resulting liquid is evaporated to
dryness on a water bath; the residue extracted with water and
filtered; the filtrate is cooled and made up to 250 c.c. and the
sulphate is precipitated in 100 c.c. with barium chloride solution in the usual way; the result will be:

sulphur in grams per 100 c.c.
    $= 5 \times 0\cdot1373 \times$ grams of barium sulphate obtained.

Determination of sulphur as sulphates. 250 c.c. of the
effluent are concentrated to about 10 c.c. on a water bath;
2 c.c. of concentrated hydrochloric acid are then added and
the evaporation is continued to dryness; the residue is extracted with water and filtered; the filtrate is made up to
250 c.c. and the sulphate is precipitated with barium chloride
solution in the usual way.

Sulphur as sulphates in grams per 100 c.c.
    $= 0\cdot1373 \times$ grams of barium sulphate obtained.

Determination of sulphur as sulphide. 10 c.c. of the
effluent are diluted to 500 c.c.; acidified with hydrochloric
acid and titrated with N/10 iodine solution, the flask being
closed and well shaken at the end of the titration in order to
reabsorb the sulphuretted hydrogen above the solution; the
volume of iodine solution used determines the volume of the
effluent taken.

10 c.c. (or more if necessary) of the effluent are run into
excess of N/5 ammoniacal zinc chloride solution; diluted to
about 80 c.c.; the resulting liquid is warmed in order to coagulate the sulphide, and filtered; the precipitate is washed
with water at 40–50° C., and is then washed into excess of
N/10 iodine solution with hydrochloric acid; the mixture is
well shaken in order to complete the solution of the sulphide

(this is very important and essential) and the excess of iodine is determined with N/10 sodium thiosulphate solution.

Sulphur as sulphide in grams per 100 c.c.
$$= 10 \times 0.0016 \times \text{c.c. of iodine solution used.}$$

Sulphuretted hydrogen in grams per 100 c.c.
$$= 10 \times 0.0017 \times \text{c.c. of iodine solution used.}$$

$$\text{H.E. (Hydrogen equivalent)} = \frac{\text{Sulphuretted hydrogen in grams}}{0.017}.$$

Determination of sulphur as thiocyanate (sulphocyanide).

(1) *Ferrocyanides absent.* 50 to 100 c.c. of the effluent are boiled to expel volatile salts; excess of sodium acid sulphite solution is then added, followed by excess of 10 per cent. copper sulphate solution; the liquid is then set aside in a closed flask for $1\frac{1}{2}$ to 2 hours at 25–30° C., in order to deposit the cuprous salt, and then filtered; the precipitated cuprous thiocyanate is washed with hot water until the washings give no colour with potassium ferrocyanide or ammonium sulphide; the precipitate is then washed back into the flask, digested at 30–40° C. with 25 c.c. of a 4 per cent. solution of sodium hydroxide (free from chlorine) and filtered; to the filtrate 5 c.c. of nitric acid (free from oxides of nitrogen and 50 per cent. strength) and 1 c.c. of a saturated solution of iron alum are added; the solution is filtered, if necessary, and titrated with N/10 silver nitrate solution; or the precipitated cuprous thiocyanate may be washed into a platinum dish, 1 c.c. of concentrated nitric acid added and the whole evaporated to dryness on the water bath; the residue is gently ignited, moistened with nitric acid and again cautiously ignited to expel oxides of nitrogen; the residue is then dissolved in N. sulphuric acid; a slight excess of sodium carbonate added and the separated carbonate dissolved in acetic acid; to the clear green solution thus obtained, excess of potassium iodide is added and the liberated iodine titrated with N/10 sodium thiosulphate solution. For technical purposes, the evaporation of the cuprous thiocyanate with nitric acid may be omitted. The salt should be washed back into the flask and oxidized therein for 15–20 minutes with 2 c.c. of concentrated nitric acid; the free acid

is neutralized with sodium carbonate and the solution is prepared for titration as before.

Sulphur as thiocyanate in grams per 100 c.c.
= 2 × 0·0032 × c.c. of N/10 silver nitrate solution used.

Hydrocyanic acid in grams per 100 c.c.
= 2 × 0·0027 × c.c. of N/10 silver nitrate solution used.

(2) *Ferrocyanides present.* In order to remove the ferrocyanides, a sufficient excess of ferric chloride solution is added to the slightly acidified and boiled effluent to produce a decided red colour; the liquid is then warmed gently (40–50° C.) and filtered; to the cooled filtrate excess of sodium acid sulphite solution is added and the determination carried out as described above.

Estimation of sulphur as thiosulphate and sulphite. The sulphur present as sulphate, thiocyanate and sulphide is deducted from the total sulphur, giving the sulphur present as thiosulphate and sulphite.

Determination of free ammonia. (*a*) *By direct titration.* 10 c.c. of the effluent are diluted to 100 c.c. and titrated with N/2 sulphuric acid, using methyl orange as an indicator.

(*b*) *By distillation.* 10 c.c. of the effluent are diluted to 300 c.c. and distilled, 150 c.c. of distillate are collected in N/2 sulphuric acid, the excess of acid is then titrated with N/2 sodium carbonate solution.

Determination of fixed ammonia. To the residual liquor obtained above, 100 c.c. of N/2 sodium hydroxide solution are added and the distillation continued as before.

Grams of ammonia per 100 c.c.
= 10 × 0·0085 × c.c. of N/2 acid used.

$$\text{H.E.} = \frac{\text{Ammonia in grams}}{0·017}.$$

Determination of CO_2. 10 c.c. of the effluent are diluted to 400 c.c. in a suitable flask, fitted with a Bunsen rubber valve; 10 c.c. of ammoniacal calcium chloride solution (1 c.c. = 0·044 gram CO_2) are added and the whole is heated on a water bath for $1\frac{1}{2}$ to 2 hours; the liquid is filtered, the precipitated calcium carbonate is washed back into the flask, dissolved in N/2 hydrochloric acid and the excess of acid is titrated with N/2 sodium carbonate solution.

CO_2 in grams per 100 c.c. = 10 × 0·011 × c.c. of N/2 acid used.

$$H.E. = \frac{CO_2 \text{ in grams}}{0·022}.$$

Determination of chlorine in the presence of thiocyanate. To 10 c.c. of the effluent, diluted to 50 c.c., 25–50 c.c. of hydrogen peroxide solution (10 volumes; free from chlorine) are added, and the liquid is boiled for 15 minutes; 6 drops of a 10 per cent. solution of potassium chromate are then added and the boiling is continued for 1 minute; the resulting liquid is filtered, cooled and made up to 250 c.c. and an aliquot part is titrated with N/10 silver nitrate solution, after bringing back to the neutral point with very dilute nitric acid. A blank experiment should be made at the same time, using 10 c.c. of N/10 sodium chloride solution and the same volume of water, hydrogen peroxide solution and potassium chromate solution.

Determination of hydrocyanic acid. 50 c.c. of the effluent are distilled with excess (50–100 c.c.) of a 20 per cent. solution of lead carbonate; the distillate is collected in 25 c.c. of N/2 sodium hydroxide solution and diluted to 400 c.c.; 0·2 gram of potassium iodide is then added and the liquid is titrated with N/10 silver nitrate solution. The distillation is carried out in the ammonia distillation apparatus and the heating must be cautiously done in order to avoid frothing; the distillation is complete when 100 c.c. have passed over; at the end of the distillation a current of air should be drawn through the apparatus as a precaution; during the distillation, the end of the delivery tube must dip into the sodium hydroxide solution.

1 c.c. of silver nitrate solution
$$= 0·0054 \text{ gram of hydrocyanic acid.}$$

Hydrocyanic acid in grams per 100 c.c.
$$= 2 × 0·0054 × \text{ c.c. of N/10 silver nitrate solution used.}$$

$$H.E. = \frac{\text{Hydrocyanic acid in grams}}{0·027}.$$

Determination of ferrocyanides. 250 c.c. of the effluent are boiled to expel volatile salts; 10 to 15 c.c. of 6N sodium hydroxide solution are added, and the liquid is boiled for 15 minutes in order to remove fixed ammonia and also to dissolve the ammonium ferrous ferrocyanide; the resulting liquid is cooled and made up to 250 c.c.; 50 c.c. are diluted to 100–150 c.c. and raised to the boiling point; 5 c.c. of 6N sodium hydroxide solution and 30 c.c. of 3N magnesium chloride solution (606 grams of $MgCl_26H_2O$ per litre) are added, the latter slowly and with constant shaking in order to avoid clots; the liquid is then boiled for 5 minutes and 25–50 c.c. of boiling N/10 mercuric chloride solution (27·1 grams of mercuric chloride per litre) are added, and the solution is boiled for not more than 10 minutes and then distilled for 20 minutes with 30 c.c. of 6N sulphuric acid; the distillate is collected in 25 c.c. of N/2 sodium hydroxide solution; to the distillate a pinch of lead carbonate is added and the liquid is filtered and diluted to 400 c.c., a crystal of potassium iodide is then added and the solution is titrated with N/10 silver nitrate solution.

1 c.c. of N/10 silver nitrate solution

> $= 0·0054$ gram of hydrocyanic acid
>
> $= 0·00947$ gram of ammonium ferrocyanide.

Determination of phenol. 100 c.c. of the effluent are treated with 1 c.c. of ammonium polysulphide in order to convert any cyanide into thiocyanate; the mixture is allowed to stand for some time and is then made up to 200 c.c.; sufficient solid lead carbonate to precipitate the sulphide is then added and the mixture is well shaken and filtered. To 100 c.c. of the filtrate, 25 c.c. of 50 per cent. sodium hydroxide solution are added and the liquid is evaporated until the salts begin to crystallize out; the residue is washed into a litre flask with 150 c.c. of water, and, when cold, is acidified with dilute sulphuric acid and distilled until the salts begin to separate out; 100 c.c. of water are then added to the distillation flask and a second distillate is obtained; a third distillate is also similarly obtained; each of the distillates is then neutralized with 1 gram of calcium carbonate and a small quantity of lead carbonate; the first distillate is then redistilled, followed by the second and then the third. The final distillates are united and made up to 500 c.c.; 100 c.c. of the mixed distillates are made alka-

line with 4 c.c. of N/10 sodium hydroxide solution and warmed
to 60° C.; an excess of N/10 iodine solution is then run into
the flask, which is immediately stoppered and allowed to cool
with frequent shaking; the contents of the flask are then
acidified with N/10 sulphuric acid and the excess of iodine is
titrated with N/10 sodium thiosulphate solution. The end
point is marked by a transition from blue to rose pink.

After the distillation, Wilkie (*J.S.C.I.* 1911, xxx, 398)
makes up the final distillates to 500 c.c. and to 100 c.c. of the
mixed distillates, adds equal volumes of N/10 sodium carbonate solution and N/10 iodine solution; and, after standing
for 5 minutes, neutralizes the sodium carbonate with N/10
sulphuric acid and then titrates with N/10 sodium thiosulphate
solution as before. The amount of iodine absorbed multiplied
by 0·1235 gives the phenol. A few pieces of pumice should be
added to the distillation flask, which should be placed on a
sand bath, otherwise violent bumping will occur.

Standards

The Royal Commission on Sewage Disposal (*9th Report*,
1915) recommended that the following standards should be
enforced for Trade Waste Waters:

(1) The effluent from distilleries should not contain more
than 3 parts of suspended matter per 100,000.

(2) The effluent from coal washing, paper mills (wood pulp
only), breweries and maltings, shale oil distilleries, woollen
dyeing works, cotton dyeing and printing works, tanneries
and dairies should not contain more than 4 parts of suspended
matter per 100,000.

(3) The effluent from tin, lead and zinc mines, china clay
works, stone quarries, tin plating and galvanising works,
paper works (other than wood pulp), wool scouring effluent,
and bleaching effluent should not contain more than 6 parts
of suspended matter per 100,000.

(4) The effluent from distilleries should not absorb more
than 2 parts of dissolved oxygen in 5 days.

(5) The effluent from breweries and maltings, shale oil distilleries and tanneries should not absorb more than 4 parts of
dissolved oxygen per 100,000 in 5 days.

CHAPTER II

MILK—CREAM—DRIED MILK—CONDENSED MILK

MILK

MILK is the fluid secreted by the mammary glands of all female mammals for the purpose of nourishing their young. It is a perfect food and is composed of fat, proteids, mineral salts and sugar. Milk varies slightly in composition, and the milk of the cow, is, of course, of the greatest importance as a food.

Genuine cow's milk of good average quality has a specific gravity of about 1032 and is slightly yellow in colour, due to the suspended fat. The proteids of milk consist of casein, albumin, globulin, fibrin, and other nitrogenous substances; the mineral matter consisting of the chlorides and phosphates of potassium, sodium, calcium and magnesium, with traces of iron and sulphates. When drawn from the cow it is amphoteric in reaction, *i.e.* it turns red litmus blue, and blue litmus red; but it soon becomes faintly acid owing to the formation of small quantities of lactic acid. This is produced by a micro-organism, *Bacillus acidi lactici*, which gradually decomposes the lactose in milk with the formation of lactic acid. The acid causes the milk to curdle or become "sour," and the length of time required to produce this curdling of milk is chiefly dependent on the temperature. It is well known that milk becomes sour more quickly in summer than in winter. The average yield of milk from a good cow is from two to two and a half gallons per day.

Milk is undoubtedly the most adulterated of all articles of food. The chief methods of adulteration are :

(*a*) The removal of a portion of the fat or cream,
(*b*) The addition of water,
(*c*) The addition of skimmed or separated milk,
(*d*) The incomplete emptying of the udder, the last drawn fluid being always the richest in fat.

The composition of milk, as sold in this country, is controlled by the Sale of Milk Regulations (1901), issued by the Board of Agriculture, in which it is directed that "Where a sample of milk (not being sold as skimmed or separated or condensed milk) contains less than 3 per cent. of fat, it shall be presumed ...that the milk is not genuine by reason of the abstraction therefrom of milk fat or the addition thereto of water" and that "Where a sample of milk (not being sold as skimmed, separated or condensed milk) contains less than 8·5 per cent. of milk solids other than milk fat, it shall be presumed...that the milk is not genuine by reason of the abstraction therefrom of milk solids other than milk fat or the addition thereto of water." This standard must be regarded as unduly lenient, as regards the fat content of genuine milk. It is a fact that few healthy, properly-fed cows will produce milk containing as little as 3 per cent. of fat. This is recognized in other countries; as, for example, in the United States of America, where the fat standard is 3·25 per cent.; in the State of Western Australia, where the standard is 3·2 per cent.; in Paris, where the standard is 4·0 per cent.; in Berne, where the standard is 3·5 per cent.; in New Zealand, where the standard is 3·25 per cent.; and in Victoria and Saskatchewan, where the standard is 3·5 per cent.

Greatly increased powers are taken by the Ministry of Health under the Milk and Dairies Act, 1914, and under the Milk and Dairies (Consolidation) Act, 1915, for the regulation of the milk supply. Under these Acts, the Ministry is authorized to issue Milk and Dairies Orders for providing standards for milk. Further, under section 5, sub-sections 3 and 4, the medical officer of health of one authority may direct the medical officer of health of another authority to take and forward to him, samples of milk forwarded from a dairy outside his authority, and, for the purposes of the Sale of Food and Drugs Acts, such samples are deemed to have been taken within the area of the first-named medical officer of health. And the third schedule to the Act makes regulations for dealing with the "warranty" defence. Under this schedule "Within sixty hours after the sample of milk was procured from the purveyor, he may serve on the Local Authority a

notice stating the name and address of the seller, from whom
he received the milk and the time and place of delivery to the
purveyor by the seller or consignor of the milk from a corresponding milking and requesting them to take immediate steps
to procure, as soon as practicable, a sample of the milk in
course of transit or delivery from the seller or consignor to the
purveyor, unless a sample has been so taken since the sample
was procured from the purveyor, and where a purveyor has
not served such a notice as aforesaid, he shall not be entitled
to plead a warranty as a defence in any such proceedings."

Richmond has given in the *Analyst*, vols. XXVIII to XLI, the
average fat in the samples of milk examined in the Laboratory
of the Aylesbury Dairy Company, and his results in percentages for the fourteen successive years are given below.

	1903	1904	1905	1906	1907	1908	1909	1910	1911	1912	1913	1914	1915	1916
Fat	3·83	3·74	3·73	3·71	3·75	3·75	3·74	3·73	3·71	3·68	3·67	3·72	3·76	3·82
Solids, not fat	8·95	8·94	8·97	8·93	8·94	8·88	8·92	8·89	8·80	8·86	8·81	8·80	8·86	8·85

These numbers represent the results of the analyses of many
thousands of milks annually.

Determination of the Specific Gravity. The sample is
first carefully shaken or stirred thoroughly to mix any cream
which may have risen to the top, and great care should be
taken to avoid the inclosure of air, as milk retains air bubbles
rather tenaciously.

The specific gravity of the milk is taken at 60° F. (16° C.)
and the sample should be brought to this temperature by
allowing it to stand in water. The specific gravity may be
determined either with a delicate hydrometer, a Westphal
balance or with a specific gravity bottle. The two former read
the specific gravity directly, but the specific gravity bottle
method is the most accurate, although it is not the most ex-
peditious. The specific gravity of normal milk, which is about
1032, is lowered by the addition of water and raised by skim-
ming.

Example: the weight of water contained in a specific gravity
bottle was 49·987 grams.

The weight of a sample of milk contained in the same bottle
was 51·051 grams.

The specific gravity of the sample therefore was

$$\frac{51 \cdot 051}{49 \cdot 987} = 1030 \cdot 56.$$

Estimation of total solid matter. 5 grams of the sample are weighed out into a flat-bottomed platinum dish, evaporated on the water bath to dryness, and, when dry, placed in a water oven (at 100° C.). It is allowed to cool in a desiccator and weighed from time to time until the weight is constant. From two to three hours in the water oven may be required.

For the rapid estimation of total solid matter, Revis (*Analyst*, 1907, XXXII, 284) weighs out 2·5 grams of milk, and adds 1 c.c. of acetone and places the mixture on a water bath for 12 minutes, finally drying to constant weight in a water oven.

Example: The residue from 5 grams of milk was 0·613; therefore the total solids in the milk were

$$0 \cdot 613 \times 20 = 12 \cdot 26 \text{ per cent.}$$

Ash. The residue from the determination of the total solids is carefully incinerated over a Bunsen flame until a white ash remains. Great care should be taken that the temperature does not rise too high otherwise the result will be low owing to the volatilization of some of the sodium chloride. The ash of milk averages about 0·75 per cent., and it is slightly alkaline. If the alkalinity is marked it would probably indicate the addition of carbonate in the form, perhaps, of calcium carbonate or chalk.

Fat. There are many methods for the determination of fat in milk; but for all practical purposes the following will suffice:

The Leffman-Beam process. This well-known method is the most accurate and the most convenient of all centrifugal methods. The results obtained with it, by a skilled worker, never vary more than 0·1 per cent. from the most accurate of the other methods.

The process depends upon the liberation of the fat by the addition of concentrated sulphuric acid, and its separation by the application of centrifugal force. Before the liberation of the fat a mixture of fusel oil and hydrochloric acid is added which produces a greater difference in the surface tension between the fat and acid liquid and this causes a readier separation of the fat.

The bottles used in the process are flat bottomed and hold about 30 c.c.; they are graduated on the neck into 80 divisions, each division representing 0·1 per cent. of fat by weight.

15 c.c. of the milk are measured into the bottle, 3 c.c. of a mixture of equal parts of amyl alcohol and concentrated hydrochloric acid are added and the liquids well mixed; 9 c.c. of concentrated sulphuric acid are then added slowly with constant agitation, and then the bottle is filled almost to the zero mark with a hot mixture of equal parts of sulphuric acid and water. It is then placed in the centrifugal machine (if one test only is being made, the machine must be balanced with a bottle filled with equal parts of sulphuric acid and water) and rotated for two minutes. After the rotation, the fat will have risen to the top of the bottle, and the percentage is read off directly. The reading must be made from the extreme top to the extreme bottom of the column of fat.

The Werner-Schmidt process. This method is particularly suitable for sour milks. 10 grams of the sample are placed in a special tube (which is graduated from 20 to 50 c.c.), and the tube is filled to the 20 c.c. mark with concentrated hydrochloric acid. The contents of the tube are well mixed and the tube is put in a beaker of water, which is heated to boiling, until the contents turn dark brown. The tube is allowed to stand for about five minutes and afterwards cooled in water; pure ether is then added to the 50 c.c. mark, the tube corked and shaken for one minute. After shaking, let the tube stand until the acid and ether layers have completely separated. The volume of the ether layer is read off and 20 c.c. are transferred into a weighed fat flask, by means of a pipette. The ether is evaporated and the fat dried in the water oven for 45 minutes and weighed.

Example: 10 grams of milk were taken for the estimation; the volume of the ethereal layer was 25·5 c.c., the weight of fat obtained from 20 c.c. was 0·253 gram, then

$$\frac{0·253 \times 25·5 \times 10}{20} = 3·225 \text{ per cent. of fat.}$$

Many analysts prefer to extract the fat completely from

5 grams of the milk instead of taking an aliquot part of the ether extract. This is done by transferring the ethereal layer to a beaker, and repeating the process of washing the water residue with several quantities of ether, and then evaporating the mixed ethereal extracts to dryness.

The Adams' process. This is a general method of extraction and a Soxhlet apparatus is used. With regard to the extraction of the fat in milk, 5 c.c. are run over one of the long strips of fat-free paper specially manufactured for the process. The paper is then rolled into a coil and dried in a water oven. When it is completely dried, place it in the Soxhlet apparatus attached to a weighed dry flask. Pure ether is then run in from the top of the inverted condenser in sufficient amount to fill the Soxhlet tube about one and a half times. Place the flask on a water bath and heat with a small flame. The ether should be allowed to siphon over about a dozen times when it will have dissolved the whole of the fat. The ether is distilled over at the end of the siphonings; the flask detached and dried in the water oven until the weight is constant. This weight, less the weight of the flask, represents the weight of fat in 5 c.c. of the milk, from which the percentage can be calculated.

Example: 5 c.c. of milk gave 0·165 gram of fat: the specific gravity of the milk was 1031, therefore the 5 c.c. weighs 5·155 grams: hence

$$\frac{100 \times 0·165}{5·155} = 3·2 \text{ per cent. of fat.}$$

The fat-free papers used in this process usually contain small quantities of substances which are soluble in ether. It is desirable, therefore, that the papers should be extracted with ether first, and then dried, otherwise the results will be too high.

The Gottlieb-Rose method (*Analyst*, 1898, XXIII, 259). Place 5 grams of milk in a 50 c.c. stoppered cylinder; add 0·5 c.c. of ammonia (specific gravity 0·880), and thoroughly mix the contents of the tube; then add 5 c.c. of alcohol (97 per cent.) to the mixture and again mix the contents of the tube; to the mixture add 12·5 c.c. of ether and mix the liquid, followed by 12·5 c.c. of petroleum ether and again thoroughly mix; allow the liquids to separate and, by means of a wash-bottle tube, blow off the clear liquid containing the fat into a weighed fat flask; the liquid remaining in the cylinder is again shaken up twice with 25 c.c., and once with 20 c.c. of the mixed solvents, and the washings are each in turn blown over into the same flask. The solvents are evaporated; the flask dried in a water oven and weighed; the weight of fat obtained multiplied by 20 gives the percentage of fat.

Calculation method. Several formulæ have been proposed by which the third factor may be calculated when any two are known. Richmond's formula has been found to be the most satisfactory and is in almost universal use:

$$T = 0 \cdot 25G + 1 \cdot 2F + 0 \cdot 14,$$

where T = total solids, G = the excess specific gravity over 1000, and F = the percentage of fat.

Upon this formula, Richmond's slide rule has been based, by which the fat may be read off when the specific gravity and total solids are known, or the total solids when the fat and specific gravity are known.

Schoore (*Pharm. Weekblad.* 1918, LVI, 1645) suggests the formula:

$$T = \frac{G + 5F}{4}.$$

Total Proteids. These are best determined by calculation from the total nitrogen obtained by the Kjeldahl method.

Solutions required: Concentrated sulphuric acid.

Strong sodium hydroxide solution. 50 grams of sodium hydroxide are dissolved in 50 c.c. of water and the solution is allowed to stand until it is clear; the clear liquid is poured off and kept in a rubber stoppered bottle.

$N/10$ sulphuric acid solution.

$N/10$ sodium hydroxide solution.

Weigh out 5 grams of milk into a Kjeldahl flask and evaporate to dryness on a water bath; to the dry residue add 5 grams of powdered potassium sulphate, and 20 c.c. of concentrated sulphuric acid; the flask is then placed in an inclined position and heated gently with a naked flame until all the frothing ceases; the flame is then raised until the acid boils briskly. As soon as the liquid is colourless it is allowed to cool, and is then rinsed out into a distilling flask, about 200 c.c. of water being used for this purpose. Strong sodium hydroxide solution is added in sufficient quantity to make the liquid alkaline and also a few pieces of pumice; the flask is at once connected to the condenser. Into the receiving flask, place 50 c.c. of the N/10 sulphuric acid solution, which is to absorb the ammonia as it distils over. The distillation is continued until about 200 c.c. have passed over; the excess of sulphuric acid in the receiver is then titrated with the N/10 sodium hydroxide solution. Each c.c. of N/10 sulphuric acid solution used = 0·0014 gram of nitrogen.

The total proteids are obtained by multiplying the amount of nitrogen by 6·38.

A blank experiment should be conducted with the materials used.

In this method organic nitrogen is converted into ammonia, and the ammonia combines with the sulphuric acid to form ammonium sulphate. This is decomposed by the sodium hydroxide solution, and the liberated ammonia is distilled over and collected in the N/10 sulphuric acid solution in the receiver.

Example: In a determination of the total proteids, 5 grams of milk were used and 21·4 c.c. of the N/10 sulphuric acid solution were neutralized by the ammonia formed.

Then 21·4 × 0·0014 × 20 × 6·38 = 3·823 per cent. of total proteid.

The total proteid may also be determined approximately by calculation from Richmond's formula:

$$P = 2\cdot8T + 2\cdot5A - 3\cdot33F - 0\cdot7\frac{G}{D}.$$

P = the percentage of proteid.
T = the percentage of total solids.
A = the percentage of ash.
F = the percentage of fat.
D = the specific gravity (water being 1).
G = the excess gravity over 1000.

Olson (*Journ. Ind. and Eng. Chem.* 1909, I, 256) calculates the proteins from the formula:

$$P = TS - \frac{TS}{1\cdot34},$$

where P = proteins,
TS = total solids.

Lythgoe (*Journ. Ind. and Eng. Chem.* 1914, VI, 899) makes use of the following formula, for calculating the proteins from the fat:

$$P = 0\cdot4\,(F - 3) + 2\cdot8,$$

where P = proteins,
F = fat.

Determination of aldehyde value. Richmond (*Analyst,* 1911, XXXVI, 9).

Solutions required:

N/10 solution of strontium hydroxide (this solution requires standardizing every time it is used), or N/10 solution of sodium hydroxide. A 40 per cent. solution of formaldehyde.

The process. The number of c.c. of the N/10 strontium hydroxide solution or sodium hydroxide solution, required to neutralize 2 c.c. of the formaldehyde solution, is first determined; 10 c.c. of the sample of milk are then neutralized with the N/10 strontium or sodium hydroxide solution, a few drops of phenol phthalein solution being added as an indicator; 2 c.c. of the formaldehyde solution are then added and the mixture is again titrated with the N/10 strontium or sodium hydroxide solution until the same pink tint reappears; the number of c.c. used, less the number of c.c. due to the acidity of the formaldehyde solution, gives the aldehyde figure; this is usually returned as the number of c.c. of normal alkali required per litre of milk; the aldehyde value of normal milk is usually from 18 to 20. The aldehyde value multiplied by 0·17 (when strontium hydroxide solution is used) or by 0·19 (when sodium hydroxide solution is used) gives a close approximation to the total proteids.

Milk Sugar (Lactose). Milk sugar may be determined with sufficient accuracy by calculation. The fat, proteids and ash subtracted from the total solids will give the lactose. A slight error is introduced owing to the fact that the ash is not the same as the salts existing in the milk; and that it is assumed that everything besides fat, ash and proteid is lactose, a supposition which is not strictly accurate.

A fairly accurate determination of lactose can be made by Fehling's method.

Solution required: Weigh out 34·6 grams of pure crystallized copper sulphate, which has been crushed and dried between blotting paper; dissolve in distilled water and make up to 500 c.c. Also weigh out 173 grams of rochelle salt and 65 grams of sodium hydroxide; dissolve each separately in distilled water; mix the two solutions and dilute to 500 c.c.

The process. Weigh out 10 grams of milk and dilute to 100 c.c. with distilled water; add a few drops of acetic acid and shake thoroughly well to coagulate the proteids. Neutralize the acetic acid with soda solution, filter from the precipitated proteids; take 10 c.c. of the filtrate and dilute to 100 c.c. with distilled water, so that a 1 per cent. solution of the milk is thus obtained. Place 25 c.c. of the copper solution and 25 c.c. of the rochelle salt and soda solution in a dish; add about 100 to 150 c.c. of water; mix well; raise the temperature so that the solution first simmers (not boils) and run in the 1 per cent. milk solution from a burette, stirring well all the time. The blue colour of the Fehling's solution will gradually disappear; but it is not easy to see the exact point when all the copper is precipitated as cuprous oxide. In order to do this a series of drops of ferrocyanide of potassium, made very slightly acid with a drop of acetic acid, are placed on a porcelain dish. Towards the end of the experiment a drop of the solution in the dish, taken out at the end of a stirring rod, is brought in contact with the drop of ferrocyanide of potassium. If the copper has not been completely precipitated by the lactose, a chocolate coloured precipitate will be noticed. When this disappears, all the copper in the Fehling's solution has been precipitated. It is then easy to calculate the percentage of sugar, for 50 c.c. of Fehling's solution are equivalent to 0·3380 gram lactose or milk sugar.

The percentage of lactose is also accurately determined by means of the polarimeter after removing the fat and proteids.

The specific rotatory power of a substance means the amount of rotation in angular degrees of the plane of polarization produced when a ray of polarized light passes through a solution of the substance containing 1 gram of the substance in 1 c.c. in a tube 1 decimetre long; and it is usually expressed for the monochromatic light of a sodium flame as:

$$[a]_D = \frac{100\,a}{l \times c},$$

where a = the observed angle of rotation,

$\quad\quad l$ = the length of the observation tube in decimetres,

$\quad\quad c$ = the concentration per 100 c.c.,

and $[a]_D$ = the angular rotation for lactose and is equal to $52.5°$.

Solution required: Acid mercuric nitrate solution. Dissolve a small quantity of metallic mercury in twice its weight of nitric acid (specific gravity 1·42) and when dissolved, add an equal volume of water.

For the estimation, place 60 c.c. of the milk in a 100 c.c. flask; add 1 c.c. of the acid mercuric nitrate solution and fill the flask to the mark with distilled water; shake the solution well and filter through a dry filter paper; place the filtrate in a polarimeter tube and take several readings of the angular rotation.

In calculating the results, correction must be made for the volume of the precipitated fat and proteids; the weight of the fat multiplied by 1·075 gives its volume; and the volume of the proteids is obtained by multiplying the weight by 0·8; the sum of these two is the volume in c.c. of the precipitate.

Example: The specific gravity of a sample of milk was 1031·0; the percentage of fat 3·5; and the percentage of proteids 3·55.

The weight of milk was 60 c.c. × 1·031 = 61·86 grams.

The weight of the fat was $\dfrac{3 \cdot 5 \times 61 \cdot 86}{100}$ = 2·165 grams.

The volume of fat was then 2·165 × 1·075 = 2·33 c.c.

The weight of proteids in the milk was

$$\frac{3 \cdot 55 \times 61 \cdot 86}{100} = 2 \cdot 30 \text{ grams.}$$

The volume of proteid was 2·30 × 0·8 = 1·84 c.c.

The volume of the solution taken for the determination of the lactose was therefore $100 - (2 \cdot 30 + 1 \cdot 84) = 95 \cdot 86$ c.c.

The angle of rotation in a 200 mm. tube was $2 \cdot 5°$; substituting these values in the above equation we get:

$$52 \cdot 5 = \frac{95 \cdot 86 \times 2 \cdot 5}{c \times 2}$$

or $$c = 2 \cdot 28,$$

that is, there are $2 \cdot 28$ grams of lactose in $61 \cdot 86$ grams of milk or $3 \cdot 69$ per cent. of lactose.

Determination of total soluble matter. To 20 grams of the milk, 80 c.c. of water and 1 c.c. of 10 per cent. acetic acid solution are added, and the resultant liquid is filtered through a dried and weighed filter paper; the precipitate is well washed with water, dried and weighed; this percentage deducted from the total solids gives the total soluble matter. Ledent (*Ann. Fals.* 1919, XII, 219) states that when the percentage of total soluble matter is divided by the ratio of casein to fat, the resulting figure is never less than 6 in the case of a genuine milk; if a figure of less than 6 is obtained, fat has been abstracted from the sample.

Detection of cane sugar. Elsdon (*Analyst*, 1918, XLIII, 292).

Molybdate test. To 10 c.c. of milk, 2 c.c. of a saturated solution of ammonium molybdate and 8 c.c. of hydrochloric acid (1 in 8) are added; the temperature of the mixture is gradually raised to 80° C. and maintained at that temperature for 5 minutes; in the presence of cane sugar, a blue colour is obtained.

Resorcinol test. 1 c.c. of 3N-hydrochloric acid solution and 0·5 gram of resorcinol are added to 15 c.c. of milk; five drops of the mixture are placed on a white tile and evaporated to dryness on a water bath; in the presence of cane sugar, a red colour is obtained.

Non-fatty solids. The non-fatty solids are obtained by subtracting the percentage of fat from the percentage of total solids; or by calculation from the fat and specific gravity. The formula for the latter is

$$SNF = \frac{S + F}{4},$$

where SNF = the percentage of non-fatty solids,

      S = the specific gravity less 1000,

      F = the percentage of fat.

Calculation of adulteration. The calculation of the percentage of added water in a sample of milk is made from the percentage of non-fatty solids. The non-fatty solids in a sample of genuine milk should not fall below 8·5 per cent. For example, V parts of non-fatty solids correspond to $\dfrac{V \times 100}{8\cdot5}$ parts of genuine milk, and the percentage of added water in the sample is found from the formula

$$100 - \frac{V \times 100}{8\cdot5}.$$

Example: A sample of milk gave 8·00 per cent. of non-fatty solids, then $100 - \dfrac{8\cdot00 \times 100}{8\cdot5} = 5\cdot88$ per cent. of added water.

Since the minimum percentage of fat in a genuine milk is 3·0, the deficiency in a sample is calculated from the formula

$$100 - \frac{F \times 100}{3}.$$

Example: A sample of milk contains 2·7 per cent. of fat, then

$$100 - \frac{2\cdot7 \times 100}{3} = 10$$

and the sample is deficient of 10 per cent. of its fat.

Where a sample has been deprived of a portion of its fat and also watered, an allowance must be made in the percentage deficiency in fat for the deficiency caused by the addition of the water.

Example: The results of an analysis of a sample of milk were 2·40 per cent. of fat and 7·65 per cent. of solids not fat; and, calculating on the formula, the sample contains 10 per cent. of added water. The original milk before the water was added contained $\dfrac{100 \times 2\cdot4}{90} = 2\cdot66$ per cent. of fat,

and $100 - \dfrac{2\cdot66 \times 100}{3\cdot0} = 11\cdot33.$

The sample, therefore, contained 10 per cent. of added water, and, in addition, was deficient of 11·33 per cent. of its fat.

L. J. Harris (*Analyst*, 1918, XLIII, 345) prefers to calculate the amount of added water from the formula

$$W = 100 - \frac{10,000N}{3N + 8\cdot5\,(100 - F)},$$

where N = the percentage of solids-not-fat,
  F = the percentage of fat,
  W = the percentage of added water.

Formulæ for calculating both the percentage of skimmed milk and the percentage of added water in a sample. Liverseege (*J.S.C.I.* 1908, XXVII, 604). Both the percentage of skimmed milk and the percentage of added water in a sample of milk may be calculated from the following simultaneous equations:

  (1) $0\cdot085m - 0\cdot09s$ = solids-not-fat found,
  (2) $0\cdot035m + 0\cdot002s$ = fat found,
  (3) $m + s + w = 100$,

where m = percentage of average milk (fat 3·5, solids-not-fat 8·5) in the sample,
  s = percentage of separated milk (fat 0·2, total solids 9·0) in the sample,
  w = percentage of added water in the sample.

Analysis of a sour milk. It is often necessary, especially in summer, to undertake the analysis of a sour milk; but, with care, the results should not differ materially from the analysis of the milk before it has gone sour. The greatest difficulty is to obtain an even mixture of the sample; but it is generally possible to obtain this if the whole of the sample is poured into a beaker and mixed with a wire egg beater.

The fat is estimated by the Werner-Schmidt or the Gottlieb-Rose method.

Determination of the total solids. Approximately 5 grams of the well-mixed sample are weighed into a platinum dish; one drop of phenol phthalein is added, and then N/10 sodium hydroxide solution drop by drop until a pink colour is just permanent; the sample is then evaporated on a water bath;

dried in a water oven and weighed; from the weight is subtracted 0·0022 gram for each c.c. of N/10 sodium hydroxide
solution added.

Example: 5·30 grams of a sour milk required 4·5 c.c. of N/10
sodium hydroxide solution to produce a permanent pink
colour; and, after drying, the residue weighed 0·587 gram;
4·5 × 0·0022 = 0·0099; and therefore,

$$\frac{(0·587 - 0·0099) \times 100}{5·30} = 11·06 \text{ per cent. of total solids.}$$

Determination of the specific gravity of a sour milk.
Richmond (*Analyst*, 1900, xxv, 116) adds 5 c.c. of strong ammonia solution to each 100 c.c. of the milk, and, to the specific
gravity of the mixture, applies a constant correction which he
has deduced from the change in specific gravity when 5 c.c. of
strong ammonia solution are added to 100 c.c. of fresh milk;
the correction has varied from 0·0065 to 0·0070 with different
samples of ammonia solution.

Government laboratory method of analysis. Thorpe
(*Jour. Chem. Soc.* 1905, LXXVII, 206). The contents of the bottle
are transferred to a suitable vessel and thoroughly mixed with
a wire whisk; 10 grams are weighed out into a flat-bottomed
platinum capsule which has been weighed together with a
short glass rod with a flattened end; a few drops of phenol
phthalein solution are added, and N/10 strontium hydroxide
solution is run in until the mixture is neutral; the whole is
then evaporated on a water bath until the residue is of the
consistency of dry cheese; 20 c.c. of dehydrated ether are added
and the whole carefully triturated with the glass rod; the
ethereal solution is passed through a filter paper which has
been dried and weighed in a weighing bottle, and the extraction
is repeated eight times; the ethereal solution is evaporated and
the weight of the dried fat is ascertained.

Before becoming quite dry, the solids, after extraction, are
transferred as far as possible to the weighing bottle; the filter
paper is replaced in the bottle and the whole (including the
platinum capsule) is dried at 100° C. for three hours and
weighed; dried again for two hours and reweighed, and finally
weighed after a further period of one hour. 0·00428 gram is

deducted for each c.c. of N/10 strontium hydroxide solution used; the result gives the amount of solids-not-fat actually present in the quantity taken.

100 grams of the milk are distilled; the distillate is neutralized with N/10 sodium hydroxide solution and redistilled; the specific gravity of the distillate is then determined in a 50 c.c. pycnometer; the alcohol corresponding to the specific gravity is obtained from a table, and this, deducted from 1000 and multiplied by 0·977, gives the anhydrous milk sugar lost.

10 grams of the milk, in a platinum capsule, are neutralized with N/10 sodium hydroxide solution to the extent of half the total acidity, and then evaporated to dryness on a water bath with frequent stirring; 20 c.c. of boiling water are added and the whole titrated with N/10 sodium hydroxide solution; phenol phthalein solution being used as an indicator. The difference between the volume of N/10 sodium hydroxide solution used for the original acidity and that used after evaporation multiplied by 0·0255 gives the loss in percentage of milk sugar, due to conversion into volatile acids.

2 grams of the milk are made up to 100 c.c. with ammonia-free distilled water and filtered; 10 c.c. of the filtrate are diluted to 50 c.c. and the ammonia is determined with Nessler's reagent (p. 2). Each part of ammonia so obtained represents 5·2 parts of casein lost.

The three corrections, thus obtained, are added to the solids-not-fat found, giving the solids-not-fat in the original milk.

Detection of added water. Monier Williams (*L.G.B. Food Reports*, No. 22) has shown that the freezing point of genuine milk varies from − 0·558 to − 0·514° C. and that the percentage of added water may be calculated from the formula

$$W = 100 - \frac{100\Delta}{0.535},$$

where Δ = the observed freezing point depression and W = the probable percentage of added water.

In his conclusions, Monier Williams states: "The freezing point appears to be the most constant of any of the properties exhibited by genuine milk. Although unaffected by the removal of fat from, or the addition of separated milk to genuine milk, it is raised by the addition of water to the milk. The method may, in certain circumstances, be applied with advantage as a confirmatory test to the detection of added water and to the approximate estimation of the amount present."

Estimation of dirt in milk by Lowe's Method (*Chemical News*, 1912, vol. CIV, p. 61). The apparatus required is a conical settling tube to which is attached, by a rubber band, a small tube graduated in 0·01 c.c.; 500 c.c. of the milk are placed in the settling tube and allowed to stand overnight; a few drops of formalin being added to prevent curdling; the volume of the sediment is read off in the morning and is reported as parts per 100,000 by volume; or, the sediment may be collected, dried at 100° C. and weighed, in which case the dry residue should be multiplied by eight, as it has been proved that only ⅛th part by weight of cow dung can be recovered from the milk. The sediment should be carefully examined under the microscope after washing. A clean milk should not contain more than 2 parts of dirt per 100,000 of milk.

Fendler and Kuhn's method (*Zeit. Unt. Nahr. Gen.* 1909, XVII, 513). 100 c.c. of the milk are subjected to centrifugal force in a vessel with a narrow graduated stem; the sediment is separated and shaken with 15 c.c. of a 10 per cent. ammonia solution; after standing for one hour, the mixture is diluted with 15 c.c. of water and again subjected to centrifugal force; the sediment is transferred to a platinum crucible, washed with alcohol and ether, and dried at 100° C. to constant weight. The sediment so obtained in a clean milk should not exceed 0·001 gram per 100 c.c.

Test for cow dung. The sediment is treated with a strong solution of sugar in a watch glass; the sugar solution is poured off, and the sediment dried at 100° C.; one drop of concentrated sulphuric acid is now added, and the particles of dung will become a reddish purple colour, which is readily seen with a hand glass.

The sediment should also be examined microscopically for any moulds or bacteria and for any vegetable parenchyma and cells and other dirt.

Colouring Matter

The addition of colouring matter to milk is very common; and, as it is added for the purpose of producing in a poor milk the high colour usually associated with a high fat content, it should be looked upon as a fraudulent addition. Annatto is usually employed for this purpose and is detected by allowing a small strip of white filter paper to stand overnight in contact with a portion of the milk to which a small quantity of sodium bicarbonate has been added; in the presence of annatto, a brown stain is produced on the filter paper.

Occasionally milk is coloured with coal-tar dyes; these may be detected by Lythgoe's method (*J. Amer. Chem. Soc.* 1900, XXII, 813) in which 10 c.c. of the sample of milk are treated with 10 c.c. of concentrated hydrochloric acid; when, on mixing, a pink colour is produced in the presence of coal-tar dyes.

Skimmed milk

Skimmed milk is the residue left after the removal of a large proportion of the fat from a milk by hand or by centrifugal means. The removal of the fat causes a slight increase in the proportion of non-fatty solids, and also an increase in the specific gravity.

The sale of skimmed milk in this country is controlled by the Sale of Milk Regulations, 1912, issued by the Board of Agriculture, by which it is directed that "Where a sample of skimmed or separated milk (not being condensed milk) contains less than 8·7 per cent. of milk solids other than milk fat it shall be presumed...until the contrary is proved, that the milk is not genuine, by reason of either the addition thereto of water or the abstraction therefrom of milk solids other than milk fat."

The analysis of a skimmed milk is carried out exactly as if it were a full cream milk.

Buttermilk

Buttermilk is the residue left in the churn after the removal of the butter. Its composition varies considerably owing to the fact that a certain amount of water is added to facilitate the separation of the butter, and the amount varies with the temperature. Nevertheless, the addition of 25 per cent. of water should be regarded as exceptional, and anything above 25 per cent. as fraudulent. The analysis of buttermilk is carried out as if it were a sour milk.

Preservatives in Milk

The presence of any preservative substance in milk is prohibited under the Public Health (Milk and Cream) Regulations, 1912, formulated by the Local Government Board under the provisions of the Public Health (Regulations as to Food) Act, 1907. But preservative substances are to a certain extent still used; those most commonly employed being compounds of boron and formaldehyde.

Detection of boric acid and borax. Place about 5 c.c. of the milk in a porcelain crucible; add six drops of tincture of turmeric and three drops of dilute hydrochloric acid (1 in 3); the mixture is then gently evaporated on the top of a water oven. In the presence of either boric acid or borax, a pink colour is developed at the edges; this colour is characteristic, and the reaction is very delicate.

Estimation of boric acid by Thompson's Method (*Analyst,* 1893, XVIII, p. 184). 50 c.c. of the milk are evaporated to dryness with 1 gram of sodium hydroxide; the residue is incinerated at a low temperature and the ash dissolved in dilute hydrochloric acid; the contents of the dish are washed into a 100 c.c. flask, the volume must not exceed 50 to 55 c.c.; 0·5 gram of dry calcium chloride is added and one drop of phenol phthalein solution; sodium hydroxide solution is then run in until the solution is alkaline, and, finally, 20 c.c. of lime water are added and the solution is made up to 100 c.c. In this way, all the phosphates are precipitated as calcium phosphate. The solution is now well mixed and filtered through a dry filter paper; 50 c.c. of the filtrate (= 25 c.c. of milk) are taken for the estimation, and normal sulphuric acid is added until the pink colour is discharged; a few drops of methyl orange are then added, and the addition of sulphuric acid is continued until the yellow colour becomes pink; N/10 sodium hydroxide solution is now added until the pink colour just becomes yellow. All the acids, except boric acid and carbonic acid, now exist as salts neutral to phenol phthalein; the carbonic acid is expelled by boiling, the solution is cooled, and 30 grams of glycerine or 2 grams mannitol are added; N/10 sodium hydroxide solution is then run in until a permanent pink colour is produced. 1 c.c. N/10 sodium hydroxide=0·0062 gram of boric acid. This method of estimating boric acid is now rarely used.

Example: A sample of milk treated in this way required 7·9 c.c. of N/10 sodium hydroxide after the addition of glycerine to produce a permanent pink colour; therefore

$$7·9 \times 0·0062 \times 4 \times 700 = 137·14$$

grains of boric acid per gallon of milk.

Richmond's method (*Analyst*, 1907, XXXII, 152). To 10 c.c. of the sample of milk, 5 c.c. of phenol phthalein solution (0·5 per cent.) are added, and the solution is titrated with N/10 sodium hydroxide solution until a permanent pink colour is obtained; the mixture is then boiled and titrated, while still boiling, with N/10 sulphuric acid solution, until the pink colour is just discharged; N/10 sodium hydroxide solution is then added until the pink colour reappears; 30 per cent. of glycerine is added and the titration is continued with N/10 sodium hydroxide solution until the permanent pink colour is again obtained. Each c.c. of N/10 sodium hydroxide solution used in the final titration represents 0·0062 gram of boric acid.

Detection of formaldehyde. One of the best tests is that of Jorissons; take about 10 c.c. of the milk and add several drops of an aqueous solution of phloro-glucinol; shake well; and then add a few drops of sodium hydroxide, a pink colour is produced in the presence of formalin.

Hehner's test. Take 5 c.c. of milk and dilute with about 25 c.c. of water; add a drop of carbolic acid and then carefully run some strong sulphuric acid down the side of the test-tube; a red ring at the junction of the two solutions indicates the presence of formaldehyde.

On the whole, if formalin is suspected, it is better to distil about two-thirds of 10 c.c. of the milk, and use the distillate for the tests.

Schiff's test. A very dilute solution of magenta is decolorized with sulphurous acid; add one c.c. of the distillate to this and allow to stand for a few minutes; the colour will be reproduced by traces of formaldehyde.

Estimation of formaldehyde. Solutions required: Acid silver nitrate solution; to 30 c.c. of N/10 silver nitrate add 15 drops of concentrated nitric acid;

N/10 solution of potassium sulphocyanide;

N/1 solution of potassium cyanide containing 6·5 grams per 1000 c.c.

The method is based on the fact that when solutions of silver and an alkaline thiocyanide are mixed in the presence of a ferric salt, so long as silver is in excess, the thiocyanate of that metal is precipitated, and any brown ferric thiocyanate which may form is at once decomposed. When, however, the thiocyanate is added in the slightest excess, brown ferric thiocyanate is formed and a colour produced.

Place 100 c.c. of milk in a distilling flask with 1 c.c. of dilute sulphuric acid (1 in 3), and distil the mixture carefully until 20 c.c. of the distillate have been collected; these 20 c.c. contain approximately one-third of the formaldehyde present in the original 100 c.c. To the distillate add 5 c.c. of the N/1 potassium cyanide solution, and then 10 c.c. of the acid silver nitrate solution, add a few drops of ferric sulphate solution; shake the mixture; make it up to 50 c.c.; filter; take out 25 c.c. with a pipette for the estimation; and titrate with the N/10 potassium sulphocyanide solution (Volhard's method).

10 c.c. of the acid silver nitrate solution are then added to 5 c.c. of the N/1 potassium cyanide solution; add a few drops of ferric sulphate solution; make up to 50 c.c., well mix and filter; 25 c.c. are taken out and titrated with the N/10 potassium sulphocyanide solution till a red colour is produced.

The difference in the two titrations is owing to the fact that some of the potassium cyanide forms a double compound with the formaldehyde. Each c.c. of potassium sulphocyanide = 0·006 gram of formaldehyde.

Example: In a milk containing formaldehyde, 2·3 c.c. of potassium sulphocyanide solution were used for 25 c.c. without formaldehyde, and 3·3 c.c. for the 25 c.c. with formaldehyde;

the difference being 1·0 c.c. Therefore 1·0 × 2 × 0·006 × 3 =
0·036 gram of formaldehyde in 100 c.c. of milk.

Jones' method (*Chemical News*, 1908, xcvii, p. 247). *Solutions required: Acid reagent.* Dissolve 0·25 gram of pure iron
wire in hydrochloric acid; oxidize the solution with nitric acid
and precipitate the iron with ammonia; wash the precipitate and dissolve it in 500 c.c. of concentrated hydrochloric
acid.

Dilute formalin solution. 1 c.c. of formalin (40 per cent.
formaldehyde) is diluted to 1000 c.c. 0·1 c.c. of this solution
added to 10 c.c. of milk gives a product containing one part of
formalin per 100,000 parts of milk, or one part of formaldehyde
per 250,000 parts of milk.

The process; 10 c.c. of the suspected milk in a large test-tube
(one inch by six inches) are treated with 10 c.c. of the acid
reagent. Into each of two similar tubes, 10 c.c. of pure milk
are placed; and, to one of these 0·1 c.c. and to the other 0·2
c.c. of the standard formalin solution is added and also 10 c.c.
of the acid reagent to each; the contents of the tubes are well
mixed; the tubes are placed simultaneously in a water bath at
90° C., and subsequently kept at 80° to 85° C. for 20 to 25
minutes; to each tube 30 c.c. of cold water are added and the
mixture is well shaken; cooled; filtered; each filter washed with
10 c.c. of water and the filtrates made up to 100 c.c. in each
case.

The blue colours which are obtained are compared in Nessler
cylinders; if the colour shown in the sample filtrate be darker
than that given by the 0·1 c.c. of the standard filtrate, it is
better to dilute the 0·2 c.c. standard filtrate. The sample and
standards must be submitted to exactly the same conditions
side by side.

Shrewsbury and Knapp's process (*Analyst*, 1909, xxxiv,
12). *Solution required:* To 10 c.c. of concentrated hydrochloric
acid, 0·1 c.c. of pure nitric acid is added; this reagent must
always be freshly prepared.

The process; Place 5 c.c. of the sample of milk in a test-tube,
add 10 c.c. of the reagent and shake the mixture violently;
place the test-tube in a water bath at 50° C. and allow it to
stand for 10 minutes; the contents of the tube are then quickly

cooled to 15° C., when, in the presence of formaldehyde, a violet colour is produced; the depth of the colour is proportionate to the amount of formaldehyde present, and is determined by comparison of the colour with that obtained in tubes containing known proportions of formaldehyde. If the colour is very deep, the original milk should be diluted with milk free from formaldehyde; the best colour is obtained when the sample contains less than 6 parts of formaldehyde per million of milk.

Detection of mystin. A proprietary article called mystin has been used as a preservative with the intention of defeating the usual tests for preservatives. This substance consists of a solution of formaldehyde and sodium nitrite in water; the sodium nitrite is added to prevent the colouration for formaldehyde being obtained in the Hehner test.

Dr Monier Williams (*Local Government Board Food Report*, No. 17, 1912) has shown that if 5 c.c. of a sample of milk containing mystin are treated with 0·05 gram of urea and 1 c.c. of N/1 sulphuric acid in a boiling water bath for two minutes and then cooled, the resulting liquid will give a well defined Hehner colouration.

Stokes' method (*Analyst*, 1912, XXXVII, 178). A portion of the milk is coagulated with dilute sulphuric acid and filtered; a 2 per cent. solution of diphenylamine in sulphuric acid is added to the filtrate, when, in the presence of mystin, a deep blue colour is obtained; this colour is due to the presence of nitrites or nitrates in the mystin.

Detection of benzoates. Sodium benzoate has been used as a preservative of milk. It may be identified by adding a drop or two of acetic acid to the milk; shake well; filter from the coagulated proteids; neutralize the filtrate carefully with sodium hydroxide and add ferric chloride when a buff coloured precipitate will be produced insoluble in acetic acid if a benzoate is present.

Detection of nitrates. Elsdon and Sutcliffe (*Analyst*, 1913, XXXVIII, 450). *Preparation of the serum. Reagent required.* A solution containing 2·5 grams of mercuric chloride and 5 grams of hydrochloric acid in 100 c.c.

Add 25 c.c. of the reagent to 25 c.c. of the milk, shake

the mixture and filter; 25 c.c. of the filtrate are collected for the test.

The test. Reagent required: To 0·085 gram of diphenylamine sulphate in a large flask add 50 c.c. of water, followed by the gradual addition of 450 c.c. of concentrated sulphuric acid.

The process. To 1 c.c. of serum in a test-tube add 4 c.c. of the reagent, thoroughly mix and cool the contents of the tube; in the presence of even minute traces of nitrate a blue colour is obtained. As nitrites interfere with this reaction, a test for them should always be first performed.

Estimation of nitrates. Reagent required: Dissolve 0·2 gram of brucine in 75 c.c. of sulphuric acid (specific gravity 1·82), and add the solution to 25 c.c. of water. This reagent gives a red colour in the presence of nitrites, which gradually fades to a straw colour in three hours in the absence of nitrates.

The process. (1) In the absence of nitrites;

To 5 c.c. of serum in a test-tube add 10 c.c. of the reagent, mix the contents of the tube thoroughly, and pour them into a Nessler cylinder; allow the contents of the cylinder to stand for 30 minutes; then compare the colour with that obtained from standards similarly prepared and containing known quantities of nitrate.

(2) In the presence of nitrites;

To 5 c.c. of serum in a test-tube add 10 c.c. of the reagent, and, at the same time, prepare standards containing known quantities of nitrate, and, also, in each standard 10 parts per 100,000 of sodium nitrite; after standing for 3 hours, the colours obtained are matched against those of the standards.

In view of the fact that milk contains no nitrates and that the majority of natural waters do contain a small trace of nitrate, the above method may be used (in the absence of added nitrate) to confirm the addition of water.

Detection of salicylic acid. A portion of the milk is treated with one or two drops of acetic acid; shake well; add a few drops of mercuric nitrate; filter off the precipitated proteids; shake the filtrate with ether, repeating the extraction several times; and evaporate the extractions to small bulk; add one or two drops of ferric chloride when a violet colour will be produced in the presence of salicylic acid.

Detection of hydrogen peroxide. Adam (*J. Pharm. Chim.* 1906, XXIII, 273). *Reagent required*; Schardinger's reagent, prepared by adding 5 c.c. of formalin and 5 c.c. of a concentrated alcoholic solution of methylene blue to 190 c.c. of distilled water.

The test. To 10 c.c. of milk an equal volume of the reagent is added, when, if the sample has never contained hydrogen peroxide, the reagent is decolorized; whereas milk, which has been treated with hydrogen peroxide, loses its power of decolorizing the reagent for about 5 days. Untreated milk also gives a red colour with tincture of guiacol after the addition of a few drops of hydrogen peroxide, and also a blue colour with para-phenylene-diamine and a few drops of hydrogen peroxide; sour milk does not give either the red colour with tincture of guiacol or the blue colour with para-phenylene-diamine, but it does decolorize the reagent.

Milk which has been treated with hydrogen peroxide, gives the red colour with tincture of guiacol and the blue colour with para-phenylene-diamine without the addition of hydrogen peroxide.

Milk which has been treated with hydrogen peroxide and from which the preservative has disappeared, gives the red colour with tincture of guiacol, and the blue colour with para-phenylene-diamine without further addition of hydrogen peroxide, but will not decolorize the reagent. Boiled milk does not give any of these reactions.

Wilkinson and Peter's method (Zeit. Unter. Nahr. Gen. 1908, XVI, 51). To 10 c.c. of the sample of milk, 3 c.c. of a 4 per cent. alcoholic solution of benzidine (*p*-diamidophenyl) acetate, and two or three drops of acetic acid are added, when, in the presence of hydrogen peroxide, a blue colour is obtained.

Detection of Abrastol. Leffman (*Chem. Zeit.* 1905, XXIX, 1086). *Solution required:* Acid mercuric nitrate solution (p. 110). 0·5 c.c. of the acid mercuric nitrate solution is added to 10 c.c. of the milk; when, in the presence of abrastol (*a*-naphtol sulphonate), a yellow colour is obtained. A control test with 10 c.c. of milk, free from abrastol, should always be made.

(Also see Chap. XII for the detection and estimation of preservatives in foods.)

Typical Analyses of Milk (in percentages).

	(1)	(2)	(3)	(4)	(5)	(6)	(7)
Fat	3·53	2·85	3·20	2·23	7·27	0·60	0·53
Solids, not fat ..	8·91	8·70	8·02	7·52	7·40	7·15	3·68

	(8)	(9)	(10)
Fat	0·20	1·12	5·81
Solids, not fat ..	8·90	8·56	10·25

No. (1) is a genuine milk of good quality.

No. (2) is a milk deficient of 5 per cent. of its fat.

No. (3) is a milk containing 5·5 per cent. of added water.

No. (4) is a milk containing 11·5 per cent. of added water, and deficient in 16 per cent. of its fat.

No. (5) is a sample of milk improperly taken; it was taken from the top of a churn without first mixing the contents.

No. (6) is a genuine sample of buttermilk containing 15·5 per cent. of added water.

No. (7) is a sample of buttermilk containing 56·7 per cent. of added water, an excess of 31·7 per cent.

No. (8) is a genuine sample of skimmed milk.

No. (9) is a typical analysis of fore milk.

No. (10) is a typical analysis of strippings.

The following analyses of milk (in percentages) have been kindly supplied by Dr Laird, the Medical Officer of Health for Cambridge. The samples were analysed by Mr J. West Knights, Public Analyst for Cambridge.

	(11)	(12)	(13)	(14)	(15)	(16)	(17)	(18)
Total solids ..	11·70	10·92	10·68	11·74	11·74	7·82	11·60	9·94
Solids, not fat ..	8·75	7·90	7·98	9·01	8·86	5·47	8·90	6·59
Milk fat.. ..	2·95	3·02	2·70	2·73	2·88	2·35	2·70	3·35
Ash	0·74	0·72	0·60	0·76	0·70	0·48	0·72	0·58

(11) deficient in 2 per cent. of its fat; (12) 7 per cent. added water; (13) 6 per cent. added water; (14) deficient in 9 per cent. of its fat; (15) deficient in 4 per cent. of its fat; (16) adulterated with 35 per cent. water; (17) deficient in 10 per cent. of its fat; (18) deficient in 22 per cent. non-fatty solids.

The following series of analyses show that the various samples of milk are of a higher quality.

	(19)	(20)	(21)	(22)	(23)	(24)	(25)	(26)
Total solids ..	11·88	11·82	13·24	13·96	11·84	13·60	13·90	12·68
Solids, not fat ..	8·58	8·17	9·44	9·26	8·54	9·10	9·80	8·18
Milk fat	3·30	3·65	3·80	4·70	3·30	4·50	4·10	4·50
Ash	0·72	0·70	0·78	0·74	0·68	0·68	0·80	0·68

The chemical changes produced in boiled and sterilized milk have been investigated by Purvis, Brehaut and McHattie (*Jour. Roy. San. Inst.* 1912, vol. XXXIII, p. 154) who showed that definite amounts of proteids, phosphates and fat are thrown out of solution and form the well-known scum. In round numbers the loss in phosphorus in boiled milk was found to be 11 per cent. and in sterilized milk 4 per cent.; the loss in proteids in the boiled milk was about 14 per cent. and in the sterilized milk about 6 per cent.; and the loss in fat in the boiled milk was about 6 per cent. Besides these losses, it means that definite chemical changes take place in milk when it is either boiled or sterilized. In connection with boiled milk, the *Reports to the Local Government Board* (New Series, 63 and 76) by Dr T. E. Lane-Claypon should be consulted. These discuss the value of boiled milk and the "biological properties" in relation to the feeding of infants. See also Dr Lane-Claypon's *Milk*.

A full discussion of the natural variations in the composition of cows' milk is contained in the *Departmental Committee's Report on Milk and Cream Regulations*, 1901 (Cd. 491); and a considerable number of analyses are quoted.

The final *Report of the Irish Milk Commission*, 1911 (Cd. 7129), is also of great importance as regards the milk supply and its purity.

CREAM

Cream is obtained either by allowing milk to stand, when it rises to the top and is skimmed off, or by the separation of the cream from the milk in a centrifugal separator.

The chief adulterations of cream are deficiency in fat and the addition of thickening substances and preservatives.

The fat content of a good cream varies from 40 to 60 per cent.

The addition of preservatives to cream is now controlled by the Public Health (Milk and Cream) Regulations, 1912, issued under the Public Health Act, 1907. Under these regulations, the addition of thickening substances to any cream, and the addition of preservative substances to cream containing less than 35 per cent. of fat; or the addition to cream containing more than 35 per cent. of fat of any preservative substance other than boric acid or hydrogen peroxide is prohibited. Further, any cream containing preservative must be described as "Preserved Cream" and the amount of the preservative present must be stated on a label of specified form and size.

The Public Health (Milk and Cream) Regulations (1912) Amendment Order, 1917, amends the above order by providing that boric acid may not be added to cream in excess of 0·4 per cent. and the product must be sold as preserved cream; and also the preserved cream, whether containing boric acid or hydrogen peroxide, shall be labelled "not suitable for infants or invalids."

Estimation of fat. This can be done by any of the methods used for milk; but in the Werner-Schmidt process a definite weight of the cream should be diluted with a definite volume of distilled water. In Adams' process the cream can be easily plastered over the long strip of fat-free paper and then dried in the hot water oven.

A fairly accurate determination of the fat in cream may be made by means of the modified Leffman-Beam process for milk. Two grams of the sample are weighed in a flat porcelain dish, and about 5 c.c. of water are added; the mixture is warmed gently and thoroughly stirred, and poured into one of the Leffman-Beam bottles; the dish is washed twice with about 4 c.c. of water; the washings are added to the rest of the liquid in the bottle; amyl alcohol and hydrochloric acid are then added followed by sulphuric acid as described under milk (pp. 103–104). The Leffman-Beam bottles are graduated for 15·55 grams of milk so that the percentage of fat read off is multiplied by 7·775.

For a more accurate determination, the Werner-Schmidt method is used; 2 grams of cream are taken for the estimation and diluted with about 8 c.c. of water.

The total solids, ash, sugar and proteids are determined by the methods described under milk (pp. 103, 106, 108).

Test for gelatine. *Solution required:* Acid mercuric nitrate solution which is prepared by dissolving one part of mercury in two parts of concentrated nitric acid; when all the mercury is dissolved the liquid is cooled and diluted with an equal volume of water. 10 c.c. of the milk are placed in a test-tube, diluted with 20 c.c. of water and thoroughly shaken; 10 c.c. of the acid mercuric nitrate solution are added and the mixture is thoroughly shaken for several minutes; the tube is set aside for the proteids to settle; the contents are filtered; an equal volume of saturated picric acid solution is added to the filtrate when, in the presence of gelatine, a heavy flocculent precipitate is formed.

Detection of gelatine in sour cream (A. Seidenberg, *Jour. Ind. Eng. Chem.* 1913, 927). In the detection of gelatine by the above method in sour cream, some soluble decomposition products may produce a precipitate; but this is insoluble in hot water whereas the gelatine precipitate is soluble. In such cases the mixture is shaken vigorously and filtered; the precipitate is washed first with ammonia water until the washings are alkaline to litmus, and then with water; the washed precipitate is heated to boiling with 10 to 20 c.c. of water; filtered and cooled; and the filtrate is treated with an equal volume of picric acid solution; in the presence of gelatine a precipitate is formed. By this method it is possible to detect as little as 0·5 per cent. of gelatine.

Test for starch. A few c.c. of the cream are diluted with water in a porcelain dish and a few drops of iodine solution added; a blue colour is obtained when starch is present.

Viscogen in cream. Viscogen is a solution of cane sugar in lime, a very small quantity of which has a remarkable effect in thickening either milk or cream. Its presence may be detected either by the determination of the relative proportion of lime in the ash or by the determination of the alkalinity of the ash. A small proportion of viscogen increases the alkalinity of the ash very materially.

Test for viscogen. Mix 1 c.c. of sesamé oil; 1 c.c. of hydrochloric acid and 0·5 gram of the suspected cream; shake the mixture thoroughly for one minute and allow it to stand for 30 minutes; in the presence of viscogen a crimson colour is produced. As little as 1 per cent. of cane sugar can be detected by this method; but for so small a quantity it is necessary to allow the mixture to stand for a somewhat longer period.

Baier and Neumann's method (*Zeit. Unt. Nahr. Gen.* 1908, XVI, 51). To 25 c.c. of the cream, 10 c.c. of a 5 per cent. solution of uranium acetate are added; the mixture is then filtered and 2 c.c. of a saturated solution of ammonium molybdate and 8 c.c. of hydrochloric acid (1 : 7) are added to 10 c.c. of the filtrate; the mixture is heated on the water bath for 5 minutes; in the presence of calcium sucrate, a blue colour is obtained.

Preservatives in cream

Boric acid. The most convenient method for the estimation of boric acid in milk and cream is that devised by Richardson (*Analyst*, 1913, vol. XXXVIII, p. 140).

Solution required: Copper sulphate solution containing 5 grams of copper sulphate per 100 c.c. 10 grams of cream are mixed with 40 c.c. of water, and 5 c.c. of the copper sulphate solution are added, the mixture is well stirred and heated to boiling point for a few seconds; about 0·5 gram of zinc dust is added to remove the excess of copper; the mixture is filtered through a dry filter paper and the contents of the paper are well washed; to the cold filtrate add a few drops of phenol phthalein solution and N/10 sodium hydroxide until a permanent pink colour just appears; glycerine is now added to the extent of one-third of the total volume or 2 grams of mannitol are added and the mixture is again titrated with N/10 sodium hydroxide until the pink colour becomes permanent. Each c.c. of N/10 sodium hydroxide solution used after the addition of glycerine or mannitol = 0·0062 gram of boric acid.

Many analysts prefer to dispense with the use of copper sulphate and to use Richmond's method described under milk (p. 119).

Fluorides. For the detection of fluorides, 100 grams of the cream are made alkaline with ammonium carbonate and boiled; a few c.c. of calcium chloride solution are added and the boiling continued for five minutes; the precipitate is collected on a filter paper; washed, dried, and ignited in a platinum dish; a few drops of concentrated sulphuric acid are added to the residue in the dish, which is then covered with a watch glass, partly protected by means of vaseline; the dish is kept at 75° to 85° C. for an hour, when in the presence of fluorides the watch glass will be found to have been etched.

Detection of hydrogen peroxide in cream. Solution required:
Schardinger's reagent. Mix together 5 c.c. of a concentrated
alcoholic solution of methylene blue, 5 c.c. of formaldehyde
and 190 c.c. of water.

Adam (*Jour. Pharm. Chim.* 1906, vol. 273) has shown that
Schardinger's reagent is invariably decolorized by a cream
which has never contained H_2O_2, whatever its age may be;
but a cream, which has once been treated with H_2O_2, loses its
power of decolorizing the reagent and only regains it after
about five days, when bacterial decomposition has set in.

Another method for the detection of hydrogen peroxide in
milk and cream is described by Wilkinson and Peters (*Zeit.
Nahr. Genuss.* 1908, vol. XVI, p. 172). It consists in adding
ten drops of a 2 per cent. solution of benzidine to 10 c.c. of
the sample, and then a few drops of dilute acetic acid; a blue
colour is produced in the presence of hydrogen peroxide.

Typical analyses of cream.

		Raw Cream	Thick Cream	Devonshire Cream
Water	..	67·93	37·62	33·76
Fat	..	24·44	58·77	59·79
Lactose	..	2·96	1·46	1·01
Proteid	..	4·04	1·83	4·97
Ash	..	0·63	0·32	0·47
		100·00	100·00	100·00

The following analyses of various creams (in percentages)
were kindly supplied by Mr J. West Knights.

			(1)	(2)	(3)	(4)	(5)	(6)
Total solids	..	..	59·46	57·44	39·72	34·24	53·46	58·00
Non-fatty solids..		..	6·99	5·06	9·60	6·47	6·75	5·00
Fat	..	..	52·47	52·38	33·12	27·77	46·71	53·00
Ash	..	..	·50	·48	·54	·50	·50	·30
Boric acid	..	..	·42	·40	none	none	·38	none

Nos. (3) and (4) are poor in fat.

The following typical analysis of a cream adulterated with
condensed milk is given by Richmond (*Analyst*, 1909, XXXIV,
210).

Total solids	..	..	37·89 per cent.
Fat	..	..	27·42 ,,
Ash	..	..	1·23 ,,
Solids-not-fat	..	..	10·47 ,,

Richmond states that a genuine cream with this percentage
of fat would contain only 6·5 per cent. of solids-not-fat.

DRIED MILK

There are a number of products on the market obtained by
the almost total removal of water from milk; and, it is piob-
able, that in the future the number of these will be considerably increased, owing to the very great reduction in bulk and
the consequent saving in the cost of transport as compared
with new or condensed milk. Also the keeping qualities are
greatly improved, and the product only requires the addition
of water to reproduce to some extent the original milk. The
composition of dried milk varies considerably and should be
proportionate to the composition of the original milk. A dried
milk made from a sample of milk which exactly complied with
the requirements of the Board of Agriculture, would contain
26·09 per cent. of fat and 73·91 per cent. of solids-not-fat.

Dr Coutts (*Local Government Board Food Reports*, No. 24)
states that dried milk made from other than full-cream milk
should be labelled "machine skimmed milk" or "separated
milk"; and also that the expression "milk" in the Public
Health (Milk and Cream) Regulations, 1912, includes dried
milk and that, therefore, the addition of preservatives to
dried milk is prohibited, such preservatives including sodium
carbonate as well as the ordinary chemical preservatives.

Methods of analysis. Richmond (*Analyst*, 1906, XXXI, 219).
The sample should first be ground in a mortar and well mixed.

Determination of moisture. 1 gram of the ground and
mixed sample is dried on a water bath to constant weight, the
loss in weight represents moisture.

Determination of fat. The fat in a dried milk cannot be
estimated by direct extraction; it should be determined either
by the Werner-Schmidt method (p. 104) or by the Gottlieb-
Rose method (p. 105). In the presence of sugar other than
milk sugar, the ethereal solution should be mixed with an
equal bulk of petroleum ether and shaken with water, made
slightly alkaline with ammonia, before the ethereal solution is
evaporated.

Determination of milk sugar. 10 grams of the dried milk are ground in a mortar with sufficient hot water to make a paste; this is gradually thinned with hot water and the solution is made up to 100 c.c.; a few drops of ammonia are added if all the powder does not go into solution; unless this method is followed incomplete extraction of the sugar results; the lactose is then estimated by the method described under milk (p. 108).

Determination of the proteids. The proteids in a dried milk are estimated by Kjeldahl's method, described under milk (p. 106), the nitrogen being multiplied by 6·87.

Determination of fat. Richmond (*Analyst*, 1908, XXXIII, 389) prefers to use the Gottlieb-Rose method, carried out as follows: 0·5 to 0·7 gram of the sample is weighed into a narrow 50 c.c. stoppered cylinder; sufficient water is added to make up to 5·15 grams; 0·5 c.c. of ammonia solution (0·88 ammonia diluted with an equal volume of water) is also added and the dried milk is dissolved by shaking, and, if necessary, by warming; 5 c.c. of 97 per cent. alcohol are then added and the whole is well shaken until it is homogeneous; 12·5 c.c. of ether (specific gravity 720) are then poured into the cylinder and the whole is well mixed by thorough shaking, 12·5 c.c. of petroleum ether (B.P. below 60° C.) are then added, and the contents of the cylinder are again thoroughly mixed; after separation, the upper layer is drawn off, further quantities of a mixture of equal parts of ether and petroleum ether are added in order to extract the whole of the fat; the mixed solvents are then evaporated and the fat is dried and weighed. The fat obtained is redissolved in petroleum ether and the solution is decanted from the minute residue; after three or four washings with petroleum the residue is dried and weighed and the weight obtained is deducted from the original weight of fat. This method can be used and is the most accurate and rapid for the analysis of all milk and milk products, and it is also applicable to the estimation of fat in eggs, egg yolk and dried egg preparations.

Detection of cane sugar. Dobbie (*Local Government Board Food Reports*, No. 24). The method used is that of Rothenfuser (*Zeit. Nahr. Gen.* 1906, XVI, 51).

Solutions required:

Di-phenylamine solution. Mix 25 c.c. of a 5 per cent. alcoholic (95 per cent. by volume) solution of di-phenylamine
with 60 c.c. of glacial acetic acid and 120 c.c. of dilute hydrochloric acid (equal parts of water and hydrochloric acid). This
reagent should be freshly prepared.

Ammoniacal lead acetate solution. 430 grams of neutral lead
acetate and 130 grams of litharge are boiled with 560 grams of
water for half an hour; the liquid is allowed to cool and the
clear solution is decanted and diluted with cold, recently
boiled, distilled water until the specific gravity is 1·15. Immediately before use, two volumes of the solution are mixed
with one volume of ammonia.

The process. Warm 1 gram of the powder with 10 c.c. of
water and 10 c.c. of freshly-made ammoniacal lead solution;
thoroughly shake the mixture and filter at once; to 4 c.c. of
the filtrate, add 8 c.c. of di-phenylamine reagent and place
the liquid in a boiling water bath for 10 minutes; in the presence of cane sugar, a blue colour is formed.

Estimation of lactose. Dobbie (*Local Government Board
Food Reports*, No. 24). 2·5 grams of the sample are ground to
a thin paste with hot water and then neutralized with N/10
sodium hydroxide solution, using phenol phthalein solution as
an indicator. The liquid is then washed into a 250 c.c. flask
with 200 c.c. of water and a volume of N/10 sulphuric acid
equal to the volume of N/10 sodium hydroxide solution used,
is added. Fehling's copper solution, in sufficient quantity to
precipitate the proteids, is then added; the volume is made
up to 250 c.c. and the copper reducing power is taken on 50
c.c. The amount of hydrated lactose is obtained from the
following table:

Hydrated lactose, $C_{12}H_{22}O_{11}H_2O$ from CuO.

CuO in grams	·000	·001	·002	·003	·004	·005	·006	·007	·008	·009
·02	—	—	—	—	—	—	·151	·0156	·0161	·0166
·03	·0172	·0177	·0182	·0188	·0194	·0200	·0206	·0212	·0218	·0224
·04	·0230	·0236	·0242	·0248	·0254	·0260	·0266	·0272	·0278	·0284
·05	·0290	·0296	·0302	·0308	·0314	·0320	·0326	·0332	·0338	·0344
·06	·0350	·0356	·0362	·0368	·0374	·0380	·0386	·0392	·0399	·0405
·07	·0411	·0417	·0423	·0429	·0435	·0441	·0447	·0453	·0459	·0465
·08	·0471	·0478	·0484	·0490	·0496	·0502	·0508	·0514	·0520	·0526
·09	·0532	·0538	·0544	·0550	·0556	·0562	·0568	·0574	·0580	·0586
·10	·0592	·0598	·0604	·0610	·0616	·0622	·0628	·0634	·0640	·0646
·11	·0652	·0658	·0664	·0670	·0676	·0682	·0688	·0694	·0700	·0706
·12	·0712	·0718	·0724	·0730	·0736	·0742	·0748	·0754	·0760	·0766
·13	·0772	·0778	·0784	·0790	·0796	·0802	·0808	·0814	·0820	·0826
·14	·0832	·0838	·0844	·0850	·0856	·0862	·0869	·0875	·0881	·0887
·15	·0893	·0900	·0906	·0912	·0918	·0924	·0930	·0936	·0942	·0948
·16	·0954	·0960	·0966	·0972	·0978	·0984	·0990	·0996	·1002	·1008
·17	·1014	·1020	·1026	·1032	·1038	·1044	·1050	·1056	·1062	·1068
·18	·1074	·1080	·1086	·1092	·1098	·1104	·1110	·1116	·1122	·1128
·19	·1135	·1141	·1147	·1154	·1160	·1166	·1172	·1178	·1184	·1191
·20	·1197	·1203	·1210	·1216	·1222	·1228	·1234	·1241	·1247	·1254
·21	·1260	·1266	·1272	·1278	·1285	·1291	·1297	·1303	·1309	·1316
·22	·1322	·1328	·1334	·1340	·1347	·1353	·1359	·1365	·1372	·1378
·23	·1384	·1390	·1396	·1402	·1409	·1415	·1421	·1427	·1433	·1440
·24	·1446	·1452	·1458	·1464	·1470	·1476	·1482	·1489	·1495	·1501
·25	·1507	·1514	·1520	·1526	·1532	·1538	·1544	·1550	·1557	·1564
·26	·1570	·1576	·1582	·1588	·1594	·1600	·1606	·1612	·1618	·1624
·27	·1630	·1637	·1644	·1650	·1656	·1662	·1668	·1674	·1680	·1686
·28	·1692	·1699	·1705	·1711	·1717	·1723	·1730	·1736	·1742	·1748
·29	·1755	·1761	·1767	·1776	·1784	·1790	·1798	·1804	·1810	·1817
·30	·1823	·1830	·1836	·1843	·1850	·1856	·1862	·1869	·1876	·1882
·31	·1889	·1896	·1902	·1908	·1914	·1922	·1928	·1934	·1941	·1948
·32	·1954	·1960	·1967	·1974	·1980	·1987	·1993	·2000	·2007	·2014
·33	·2020	·2027	·2034	·2040	·2047	·2054	·2060	·2067	·2074	·2080
·34	·2087	·2094	·2100	·2107	·2113	·2120	·2126	·2133	·2140	·2146
·35	·2153	·2160	·2166	·2173	·2180	·2187	·2194	·2200	·2207	·2213
·36	·2220	·2226	·2234	·2240	·2246	·2253	·2260	·2266	·2273	·2280
·37	·2286	·2293	·2300	·2306	·2313	·2320	·2326	·2332	·2340	·2346
·38	·2352	·2359	·2366	·2372	·2379	·2386	·2392	·2399	·2406	·2412
·39	·2419	·2426	·2432	·2439	·2446	·2452	·2459	·2466	·2472	·2478
·40	·2486	·2492	·2498	·2505	·2511	·2517	·2523	·2529	·2535	·2541
·41	·2547	·2554	·2560	·2566	·2572	·2578	·2584	·2590	·2596	·2602
·42	·2609	·2615	·2621	·2628	·2634	·2640	·2646	·2654	·2660	·2666
·43	·2672	·2679	·2686	·2692	·2699	·2705	·2712	·2718	·2724	·2731
·44	·2738	·2744	·2751	·2758	·2764	·2770	·2777	·2784	·2790	·2797
·45	·2804	·2810	·2817	·2824	·2830	·2837	·2844	·2851	·2858	·2865

Detection of preservatives. Dobbie (*Local Government Board Food Reports*, No. 24).

Boric acid. A few drops of 10 per cent. sodium hydroxide solution are added to 1 gram of the sample, the mixture is dried and extracted with ether to remove the fat; the ethereal solution is filtered, the filter paper is returned to the dish and the residue is re-extracted with ether, and finally incinerated at a low temperature; the ash is dissolved in dilute hydrochloric acid and tested with turmeric paper.

Fluorides. 5 grams of the sample are treated with sodium hydroxide solution, dried, and ashed, and the etching test is carried out on the residue.

Sulphites. Boil 2 grams of the sample with dilute hydrochloric acid, and test the vapour with potassium iodate and starch paper; a blue colour will be produced by the action of the vapour of sulphur dioxide.

Salicylic acid. A little of the sample is tested directly with neutral ferric chloride solution; and, if present, the salicylic acid is estimated colorimetrically on 5 grams of the sample.

Benzoic acid. Use is made of the method of Jonescu (*J. Pharm. Chim.* 1909, XXIX, 523) in which 5 grams of the sample are placed in a 300 c.c. flask with 30 c.c. of water, 2 grams of potassium bi-sulphate and a little pumice powder are added, and the mixture is distilled, as far as possible without charring the residue; the distillate is collected in a Nessler tube, and 2 drops of a 1 per cent. neutral solution of ferric chloride are added to it; in the absence of a violet coloration, 2 drops of hydrogen peroxide (one volume) are added, and the mixture is allowed to stand for some time; in the presence of benzoic acid, a violet colour slowly develops. If a violet colour appears immediately on the addition of the ferric chloride solution, the distillate is heated on a water bath for 15 minutes with 1 c.c. of potassium permanganate solution (2 grams of potassium permanganate and 4 grams of potassium hydroxide in 100 c.c.), care being taken that excess of potassium permanganate is present all the time; after heating, the excess of potassium permanganate is removed by the addition of dilute sulphuric acid and oxalic acid and the solution is again distilled; the distillate is then again tested with ferric chloride solution.

The following typical analyses of dried milks are given by Richmond (*Analyst*, 1906, XXXI, 220):

	(1)	(2)	(3)	(4)	(5)	(6)	(7)
Moisture ..	6·39	4·92	3·30	3·55	4·74	5·15	6·03
Fat	27·35	27·98	23·97	2·55	29·16	19·90	25·60
Milk sugar ..	31·42	34·16	37·32	45·60	32·24	34·96	32·83
Cane sugar ..	—	1·25	1·53	2·80	—	—	2·00
Proteids ..	27·48	24·59	26·38	35·45	26·66	31·10	23·84
Ash	6·00	6·24	6·19	7·89	5·63	7·11	6·44

Richmond states that No. (4) is made from a separated milk and that No. (6) is deprived of a portion of its fat. Nos. (2), (3), (4) and (7) contain added cane sugar.

The following typical analyses of dried milk are taken from Dr Coutts' report on dried milk (*Local Government Board Food Reports*, No. 24):

	(8)	(9)	(10)	(11)
Moisture	5·30	4·20	8·60	6·00
Fat	22·58	31·28	0·67	21·92
Proteids	26·51	22·88	32·25	25·01
Lactose	35·83	35·72	49·59	39·28
Ash	6·40	5·75	7·54	6·40
Cane sugar	Trace	Nil	Nil	1·84

	(12)	(13)	(14)	(15)
Insoluble in water	4·20	3·61	4·85	4·20
Soluble in water	2·20	2·14	2·69	2·20
Alkalinity (as Na_2CO_3) ..	0·24	0·29	0·11	0·16
Chlorides (as NaCl) ..	1·15	0·94	1·44	1·15
Lime (as CaO)	1·34	1·23	1·76	1·62
Phosphates (as P_2O_5) ..	1·73	1·46	2·19	1·61

Nos. (8) and (9) are prepared from whole milks; Nos. (10) and (11) from impoverished and skimmed milks; No. (12) is the ash of No. (8), No. (13) is the ash of No. (9); No. (14) is the ash of No. (10), and No. (15) is the ash of No. (11).

CONDENSED MILK

The sale of condensed milk has increased considerably of late years and it is now an article of food of considerable importance. It is usually prepared by evaporating milk under diminished pressure to about one-third of its original volume, and this is sometimes followed by the addition of cane sugar. The percentage of fat in a condensed milk prepared from whole milk should not be less than ten. The actual adulteration of condensed milk is very rare, but misrepresentation is very common. For example, condensed milk made from separated milk, and containing 1·0 per cent. of fat or less, is frequently sold as condensed milk whereas the purchaser expects to obtain condensed whole milk. There is, of course, no objection to the sale of condensed milk made from skimmed milk, provided that the fact is disclosed on the label as required by section XI of the Sale of Food and Drugs Act, 1899. There is also considerable misrepresentation as regards the proportion of water necessary to dilute the sample in order to obtain a liquid comparable with new milk.

Methods of Analysis. Weigh out 10 grams of the condensed milk; dissolve it in water and make it up to 100 c.c.

Total solids. 10 c.c. of the 10 per cent. solution are placed in a platinum dish and the mixture is evaporated to dryness; the residue is dried in a water oven and weighed; the increase in weight represents the solids in 1 gram of the condensed milk.

Ash. The residue from the total solid determination is carefully incinerated over a Bunsen flame; cooled and weighed; the residue multiplied by 100 gives the percentage of ash.

Fat. The fat can be determined by any of the methods described under milk; but, as in the analysis of cream, a definite weight of the condensed milk should be diluted with a definite amount of distilled water.

Leach's method. 5 grams of the condensed milk are weighed into a small beaker; dissolved in 15 c.c. of water and carefully washed into a Leffman-Beam bottle; the bottle is filled nearly to the neck with water and 4 c.c. of copper sulphate solution (containing 7 grams of copper sulphate in 100 c.c.) are added; the contents of the bottle are thoroughly mixed and rotated in the centrifuge; the proteids and fat sink to the bottom; the supernatant liquid contains the sugar; this liquid is drawn off with a long-drawn-out pipette; the precipitated fat and proteids are washed twice with water and finally sufficient water is added to bring the contents of the bottle to 15 c.c.; the test is then continued as in the ordinary Leffman-Beam method for the estimation of fat in milk. The reading on the bottle multiplied by 3·11 gives the percentage of fat.

Proteids. For this determination 20 c.c. of the diluted milk are used; and the amount of proteids is estimated by the Kjeldahl method as described for milk (p. 106), or the following method may be used.

5 grams of the sample are dissolved in water and made up to 100 c.c.; to 50 c.c. of this solution, a solution of copper sulphate (as described under fat above, or copper Fehling's solution, p. 109) is added drop by drop until no further precipitate is obtained; the mixture is then filtered through a dried and tared filter paper; the precipitate is well washed, dried and weighed; the filter paper and the precipitate are then incinerated and the residue weighed; the weight of precipitate obtained, less the weight of the ash and the weight of fat, multiplied by 40, gives the percentage of proteid in the sample.

Milk sugar. Weigh out 10 grams of the condensed milk; dissolve it in water; add a few drops of citric acid and make up to 250 c.c.; filter through a dry filter paper. Place 25 c.c. of copper Fehling's solution, 25 c.c. of alkaline Fehling's solution (prepared before, p. 109) and 25 c.c. of distilled water in a beaker of 250 c.c. capacity; place it in a boiling water bath; after the beaker has stood in the water bath for five minutes, run in from a pipette 25 c.c. of the filtrate obtained above; allow the beaker to remain in the water bath for exactly 12 minutes; quickly filter the solution through a good filter paper; wash the precipitate with hot water until the filtrate gives no alkaline reaction; dry the precipitate in a water oven; incinerate in a platinum dish and weigh as CuO; from the weight of CuO thus obtained subtract the weight of ash in a blank experiment. The weight of CuO multiplied by 0.5758 = the weight in grams of anhydrous lactose in the 25 c.c. taken for the experiment.

Example: In an experiment carried out as described 0.253 gram of CuO was obtained, therefore

$$0.253 \times 0.5758 \times 100 = 14.57 \text{ per cent. of lactose.}$$

Cane sugar. A rough approximation of the cane sugar may be obtained by subtracting the sum of the percentages of the fat, ash, proteid and milk sugar from the total solids.

The cane sugar is accurately determined by Fehling's method. To 50 c.c. of the filtrate obtained as described in the determination of milk sugar, add one gram of citric acid and boil for 15 minutes; allow the solution to cool; just neutralize it with caustic soda and make it up to 200 c.c.; the copper reduction is then determined as described above.

From the weight of CuO obtained subtract the weight of CuO due to lactose, and the remainder, multiplied by 0·4091, gives the cane sugar.

Revis and Payne's method for determination of cane sugar and lactose (*Analyst*, 1914, XXXIX, 476). 65·085 grams of the condensed milk are washed into a 250 c.c. graduated flask with sufficient water to make the solution up to 220 c.c.; the solution is heated in boiling water for 5 to 10 minutes, and then made up to the mark and well mixed; 100 c.c. are measured into a stoppered cylinder, 10 c.c. of acid mercuric nitrate solution are added and the mixture is violently shaken for 30 seconds; after standing for 5 minutes the mixture is filtered through a dry filter paper, the temperature of the filtrate is raised to 20° C., and the angle of rotation noted in the polarimeter. A further quantity of 25 c.c. of the filtrate is placed in a 50 c.c. flask which is counterpoised; this is heated in boiling water for 8 minutes and then cooled and the weight is adjusted by the addition of distilled water; the solution is filtered, if necessary, and the angle of rotation at 20° C. is again noted; the correction for fat and proteids is obtained from the following formula:

$$C = 10 - \left\{ \frac{(F \times 1\cdot11) + (P \times 0\cdot82)}{100} \right\} \times 26\cdot034 \text{ c.c.,}$$

where F = percentage of fat,
   P = percentage of proteid,
   C = correction.

The polarimetric readings are multiplied by $(100 + c)$ to give correct readings for normal weight, then:

$$\text{Percentage of cane sugar} = \frac{(D - I) \times 100}{\left(R_c - \dfrac{I}{2}\right)} = S,$$

$$\text{Percentage of lactose} = (D - S) \times \frac{R_l}{26\cdot034} \times 100,$$

where D = corrected direct reading,
    I = corrected invert reading,
    T = temperature of invert reading,
   $\left.\begin{array}{l} R_c \\ R_l \end{array}\right\}$ = inversion and lactose factors.

Revis and Payne, from careful calculation, arrive at the following values for R_c and R_l:

$$R_c = 141\cdot71,$$
$$R_l = 0\cdot3086.$$

The acid mercuric nitrate solution required in the above process is obtained by dissolving pure mercuric oxide in twice its weight of nitric acid (specific gravity $1\cdot42$), the resulting solution being diluted to five times its volume with water.

Some analyses of Condensed Milk in percentages.

	Sweetened	Unsweetened	Skimmed
Total solid matter..	76·5	36·3	67·4
Fat	10·0	11·3	0·7
Ash	1·9	1·5	1·9
Proteid	8·3	9·0	10·0
Lactose	15·6	14·5	15·4
Cane sugar	40·7	—	39·4

Dr Coutts' Report to the Local Government Board on condensed milks (*Food Reports*, No. 15, 1911) contains a considerable number of analyses of various brands of condensed milk, and it gives a very complete bibliography of the literature of the subject. The Reports to the Local Government Board by Dr Coutts and Mr J. L. Baker (*Food Reports*, No. 20) in relation to proprietary foods used for infant feeding should be consulted; also the Reports to the L.G.B. by Dr Coutts and Mr G. Winfield (*Food Reports*, No. 24) on dried milks are of importance; and Prof. Delepine's Report (*Food Reports*, No. 21) in which the bacterial content is discussed.

CHAPTER III

BUTTER, MARGARINE—LARD, DRIPPING, SUET— CHEESE, CREAM CHEESE—EDIBLE OILS

BUTTER AND MARGARINE

DURING the churning of milk, the fat corpuscles and part of the casein are made to adhere together and are removed as butter; the water, the remainder of the casein and the mineral salts are left behind as buttermilk. Butter fat consists of the glycerides of butyric, caproic, capric, caprylic, myristic, palmitic, stearic and oleic acids. After milk, butter is probably the most adulterated of all articles of food; the usual adulterations practised are complete or partial substitution of margarine and excess of water.

The amount of water in butter is controlled by the Sale of Butter Regulations, 1902, and by the Butter and Margarine Act, 1907, under which the maximum amount of water in butter may not exceed 16 per cent. Butter containing more than 16 per cent. of water may be legally sold, provided that it is sold under a fancy name approved by the Board of Agriculture.

Margarine is the product obtained by churning together animal or vegetable fats or both and milk. When carefully prepared it is very similar to butter in appearance; the percentage of water in margarine is limited, as in butter, to 16 per cent. by the Butter and Margarine Act, 1907. The Sale of Food and Drugs Act, 1899, section VIII, permits the presence of 10 per cent. of butter fat in margarine fat; the Butter and Margarine Act, 1907, permits 10 per cent. of butter in margarine; section XIII of the Butter and Margarine Act, 1907, defines margarine as "Any article of food, whether mixed with butter or not, which resembles butter and is not milk-blended butter." Owing to the recent developments in the hydrogenization of oils and the production of solid fats from liquid vegetable and fish oils by comparatively simple methods on a commercial scale, the substitution or the addition of these fats to butter or margarine may be looked for in the near future.

Analysis of butter. Determination of water. Weigh out 5 grams of the sample in a flat-bottomed platinum dish and place it in an air oven at 105° C. until, on imparting a circular motion to the dish, no "crackling" is heard; the water will then have been driven off; the dish is allowed to cool in a desiccator and reweighed; the loss in weight multiplied by 20 gives per cent. of water.

Example: The loss in weight on 5 grams of a sample of butter was 0·631 gram, then 0·631 × 20 = 12·62 per cent. of water.

Salt. The residue from the water determination is incinerated over a Bunsen flame or in a small furnace at as low a temperature as possible, until a white or nearly white ash is obtained; this ash may for all practical purposes be regarded as salt. While there is no fixed standard for salt in butter, yet good salted butter contains from 0·5 to 6 per cent. of salt, and anything above 6 per cent. can only be regarded as an adulteration.

Curd. Weigh out 5 grams of the butter into a small beaker; dissolve the fat in petroleum ether and filter through a dried and weighed filter paper; well wash the residue on the paper with petroleum ether to remove all fat; dry the paper in a water oven and reweigh; the increase in weight represents curd and ash; incinerate the filter paper and residue in a platinum dish; subtract the weight of the filter ash and deduct the remainder from the weight of the curd and ash, thereby giving the weight of curd.

Fat. The filtrate from the curd determination is placed in a weighed fat-flask and the petroleum ether is evaporated off; the flask is then dried in a water oven to constant weight; the increase in weight of the flask multiplied by 20 gives the percentage of fat.

Sorting test for butter samples. A rough method of sorting butter samples containing excess of water from those which have a water content within the above-mentioned limits has been proposed by Russell (*Jour. Roy. San. Inst.* 1906, vol.

XXVII, p. 561). A glass cylinder graduated in c.c. and having a capacity of about 50 c.c. is filled with the butter sample and placed in a water oven until the butter is completely melted; the cylinder is then placed in a centrifugal machine and rotated for two minutes; after the rotation the curd and water will have settled to the bottom leaving a clear column of fat; the volume of the fat column is read off and reduced to a percentage of the total volume. Should the volume of the fat be less than 82 per cent., the percentage of water is estimated by the method given above. This method is exceedingly useful where a large number of butters have to be examined, as the saving of time is very large and the butter samples passed by the method invariably fall within the limits for water.

Examination of the fat. A portion of the sample is placed in a small beaker, in a water oven until melted; the fat rises to the top and is carefully decanted through a dry filter paper; the fat will pass through quite clear and bright.

Preliminary examination. A few years ago the Valenta Acetic-acid Number and the Zeiss Butyro-refractometer Number were sufficiently good sorting tests to indicate the presence of margarine in butter; but, since the introduction of cocoanut oil, most margarines give numbers closely corresponding to those for pure butter fat, thereby rendering these determinations useless.

Heat of bromination. For this determination, weigh out exactly 1 gram of butter fat into a vacuum jacketed test-tube; add 10 c.c. of chloroform from a pipette; mix well with a thermometer (graduated in $\frac{1}{2}$° C.); note the initial temperature of the mixture and surround the tube with cotton wool; now from a pipette allow 1 c.c. of bromine to run down the side of the tube, without stirring; and note the maximum temperature reached; the increase in temperature is the heat of bromination.

The heat of bromination of a genuine butter should be from 4 to 7; of an old fashioned margarine from 9 to 10; of a cocoanut oil from 1·5 to 1·7. The heat of bromination multiplied by 5·5 gives the iodine absorption number.

Determination of the Reichert-Wollny number. The Reichert-Wollny number is a measure of the volatile fatty acids in the sample in terms of N/10 alkali. It is most conveniently determined by Leffman and Beam's modification with glycerol-soda solution; this method has a great advantage over the older and more tedious alcoholic method.

Solutions required: Glycerol-soda solution. Weigh out 100 grams of sodium hydroxide; dissolve it in 100 c.c. of distilled water and allow the solution to stand until clear.

Measure out 20 c.c. of the clear solution and 100 c.c. of pure glycerine; mix the two; keep the mixture in a capped bottle fitted with a rubber bung.

Sulphuric acid solution containing 20 c.c. of concentrated sulphuric acid in 100 c.c.

N/10 sodium hydroxide solution.

The process. Weigh out into a 300 c.c. Jena flask, 5 grams of the clear butter fat; add 20 c.c. of the glycerol-soda solution; carefully heat the flask over a Bunsen burner; the mixture may froth considerably at first, but this ceases as soon as all the water has been driven off; the heating is continued until the mixture becomes clear, when complete saponification will have taken place; 135 c.c. of hot water are now carefully added at first drop by drop, the flask being shaken to avoid frothing; the soap formed dissolves in the water, and, as soon as the solution is complete, sulphuric acid solution is added till just acid, and a few pieces of pumice to prevent bumping; the flask is then connected to a special condenser and heated with a naked flame until 110 c.c. have been distilled; this operation should occupy about 30 minutes. The distillate is well mixed and filtered through a dry filter paper; 100 c.c. of the filtrate are placed in a conical flask; two or three drops of phenol phthalein solution are added, and then N/10 sodium hydroxide run in from a burette until a permanent pink colour is obtained; the number of c.c. of N/10 sodium hydroxide solution used multiplied by 1·1 gives the Reichert-Wollny number.

Genuine butter fat should not give a Reichert-Wollny number of less than 24; the Reichert-Wollny number of margarine is from 0·5 to 1; and of cocoanut oil from 7 to 8.

The Shrewsbury and Knapp number (*Analyst*, 1910, vol. xxxv, p. 385). The Reichert-Wollny process is not capable of detecting small quantities of cocoanut oil; and Shrewsbury and Knapp have devised a process by which they claim to be able to detect as little as 5 per cent. of cocoanut oil in butter fat.

Solutions required: Glycerol-soda solution. Approximately 10N. sodium hydroxide solution is prepared, and 100 c.c. of this solution are mixed with 500 c.c. of glycerine.

Dilute sulphuric acid solution; 100 c.c. of concentrated sulphuric acid are mixed with 400 c.c. of distilled water.

Alcohol; industrial methylated spirit containing 90 per cent. of absolute alcohol by weight.

The process. 5 grams of the filtered fat are weighed into a 300 c.c. Jena flask and saponified with 200 c.c. of the glycerol-soda solution; the soap obtained is at once carefully diluted with boiling water and washed into a separator; the total quantity of boiling water used is exactly 200 c.c.; 5 c.c. of the dilute sulphuric acid solution are at once added and the mixture is vigorously shaken for one minute and allowed to stand for five minutes; the water is then run off from the insoluble fatty acids. The fatty acids in the separator are now dissolved in 50 c.c. of the alcohol, and the solution is poured into a flask and heated, with a piece of pumice to prevent bumping; 30 c.c. of cold water are run into the separator; and immediately the alcohol solution in the flask boils, it is poured into the water in the separator; the mixture is poured back into the flask, which is rotated, and then back into the separator; it is then shaken for 30 seconds and allowed to stand for three minutes so that the insoluble fatty acids may separate; 70 c.c. of the alcoholic solution are run off and titrated with N/10 sodium hydroxide solution using phenol phthalein solution as an indicator.

Average numbers obtained are:

Butter	28 c.c.
Margarine (free from cocoanut oil) ..	20 c.c.
Cocoanut oil	163 c.c.

Detection of cocoanut oil. Hinks (*Analyst*, 1907, XXXII, 160). 5 c.c. of the fat are dissolved in 10 c.c. of ether in a tube, which is then packed with ice; after 30 minutes' cooling, the ethereal layer is rapidly filtered; the filtrate is evaporated on a water bath and the residue is boiled with four times its volume of 96 per cent. (by volume) alcohol; the solution is allowed to cool to the temperature of the room and is then placed in water at 5° C. for 15 minutes; the alcohol layer is rapidly filtered into a tube and kept at 0° C.; a flocculent deposit soon separates, and this deposit is kept at 0° C. for 2 to 3 hours and then examined microscopically; under these conditions, butter gives crystals in round granular masses, cocoanut oil gives needle-shaped crystals, and mixtures of butter and cocoanut oil give granular butter spheres and small very fine, feathery crystals.

Estimation of the percentage of butter fat and cocoanut oil in margarine. Revis and Bolton's modification of the Reichert-Meissl-Polenske-Kirschner process (*Analyst*, 1911, XXXVI, 335). 5 grams of the fat and 20 grams of glycerine are weighed into a 300 c.c. flask, 2 c.c. of 50 per cent. sodium hydroxide solution are added, and the flask and contents are carefully heated over a flame, with constant shaking, until the mixture clears suddenly; the contents of the flask are then cooled and 100 c.c. of recently boiled distilled water are added until complete solution is effected; 0·1 gram of powdered pumice is then added, followed by 40 c.c. of dilute sulphuric acid (25 c.c. of concentrated sulphuric acid diluted to 1000 c.c. and adjusted so that 35 c.c. neutralize 2 c.c. of the 50 per cent. sodium hydroxide solution); the flask is at once connected with the condenser and heated with a small flame until all the insoluble acids are completely melted; the flame is then increased and 110 c.c. are distilled in 19 to 21 minutes, the temperature of the condenser water should be 18° to 21° C. and the apparatus must be the special one devised by Polenske (*Analyst*, 1904, XXIX, 154) and must agree with the specification in all dimensions. When 110 c.c. have distilled, the flame is removed and a 25 c.c. cylinder is placed under the condenser to catch any drops. The 110 c.c. flask and contents are allowed to stand in water at 10° to 15° C. for 15 minutes; the contents of the flask are then well mixed and filtered; 100 c.c. of the filtrate are titrated with N/10 solution of barium hydroxide, using phenol phthalein as an indicator, the number of c.c. used, less the number of c.c. used for the blank and plus 1/10th, is the Reichert-Meissl value. The condenser, cylinder, and 110 c.c. flask are washed with 18 c.c. of cold water, which is then poured over the filter, and the filtrate is rejected; the condenser is washed out with four successive portions of 10 c.c. of neutral alcohol, which are received into the 110 c.c. flask; the mixed alcoholic solutions are titrated with N/10 solution of barium hydroxide, using phenol phthalein as an indicator; the number of c.c. of barium hydroxide solution so used, less the number of c.c. used for the blank, is the Polenske "new butter value" and these, for the corresponding Reichert-Meissl values, are as follows:

Reichert-Meissl values	Polenske "New butter values"
32	3·5
31	3·2
30	3·0
29	2·9
28	2·7
27	2·4
26	2·0
25	1·8
24	1·7
23	1·6

A "new butter value" exceeding by 0·5 c.c. the above corresponding figure for the Reichert-Meissl value indicates the presence of cocoanut oil or palm kernel oil.

Kirschner value. To the 100 c.c. of the 110 c.c. distilled in the Reichert-Meissl determination and titrated with barium hydroxide solution (care being taken not to exceed the neutral point) is added 0·5 gram of finely powdered silver sulphate and the mixture is allowed to stand for 1 hour, with occasional shaking, and is then filtered; to 100 c.c. of the filtrate 35 c.c. of water and 10 c.c. of dilute sulphuric acid (as previously employed) are added, together with a long piece of aluminium wire and 110 c.c. are again distilled off in the standard Polenske apparatus in 20 minutes; 100 c.c. of the distillate are titrated as before with N/10 barium hydroxide solution, and the number of c.c. of barium hydroxide solution so used, less the number of c.c. used for the blank, is calculated to the Kirschner value by means of the following formula:

$$K = X \times \frac{121 \times (100 + y)}{10,000},$$

where X = the corrected Kirschner titration,
     y = the number of c.c. of N/10 barium hydroxide solution used to neutralize 100 c.c. of the Reichert-Meissl distillate.

Bolton and Revis (*Analyst*, 1912, XXXVII, 183) calculate the percentage of butter fat from the following formula:

$$\text{Percentage of butter fat} = \frac{K - (0 \cdot 1P + 0 \cdot 24)}{0 \cdot 244},$$

where K = the Kirschner value found,
    P = the Polenske value found.

Arnaud and Hawley (*Analyst*, 1912, XXXVII, 122) calculate the percentage of cocoanut oil and butter fat from the following formulæ:

Cocoanut oil.

$$P = (P' - P'') - \frac{R}{10} + T,$$

where P = corrected Polenske figure,
    P' = Polenske figure found,
    P'' = Polenske figure of margarine fat, free from cocoanut oil and butter fat (about 0·4),
    T = a correction ascertained from a curve,

then the percentage of cocoanut oil $= \dfrac{100P}{17 \cdot 6}$.

Butter fat.

$$R = (R' - R'') - \text{Reichert due to cocoanut oil found} + T,$$

where R = corrected Reichert-Meissl figure,
    R' = Reichert-Meissl figure found,
    R'' = Reichert-Meissl figure for margarine fat, free from cocoanut oil and butter fat (about 0·6),
    T = a correction ascertained from a curve,

then the percentage of butter fat $= \dfrac{100R}{25}$.

The value of T varies from 0, in the case of a Polenske value of 0·5, to 2 in the case of a Polenske value of 2·5.

The percentage of butter fat is confirmed from the Kirschner value by use of the following formula:

$$K = (K' - 0\cdot5) - \frac{P}{10},$$

where K = corrected Kirschner value,

K' = Kirschner value found,

0·5 = Kirschner value of margarine fat free from butter fat,

P = Polenske value found,

then the percentage of butter fat $= \dfrac{100K}{3}$.

Cranfield (*Analyst*, 1915, XL, 439) gives the following relations between the Kirschner value and Polenske value.

Kirschner value	Polenske value	Limits of Polenske value
19–20	1·46	1·4–1·7
20–21	1·65	1·4–2·2
21–22	2·05	1·7–2·7
22–23	2·43	1·8–2·9
23–24	2·41	2·2–2·6

Richmond (*Analyst*, 1919, XLIV, 166) makes use of the following formula for calculating the percentage of cocoanut oil present, where the Polenske figure exceeds that given in the table:

$$C = \frac{P - P'}{14\cdot4} \times 100,$$

where C = percentage of cocoanut oil,

P = Polenske figure found,

P' = Polenske figure for corresponding Reichert-Meissl figure plus half the Polenske figure.

Richmond also shows that the Polenske figure may be calculated from the Kirschner figure by means of the formula

$$P = (K - 14) \times 0\cdot26,$$

and that if the Polenske figure exceeds $(K - 10) \times 0\cdot26$, the presence of cocoanut oil is certain. In the presence of fats other than cocoanut oil, Richmond expresses the relation between the Reichert-Meissl and Polenske figures by the formula

$$R \times 0\cdot033 - 0\cdot6155 = \log 10 \, (P - 0\cdot48).$$

Elsdon's method (*Analyst*, 1917, XLII, 75 and 295). This is a combination of the Reichert-Meissl-Polenske and Shrewsbury and Knapp processes. The contents of the flask, after the distillation of 110 c.c. in the Reichert-Meissl-Polenske process, are cooled down in water until the fatty acids become caked; this cake is broken up and strained through a wire sieve; the flask and acids being washed with 50 c.c. of cold water; after draining, the fatty acids are returned to the flask and the flask and contents are dried in a steam oven. 100 c.c. of alcohol (which must be exactly of specific gravity 0·9200 at 60° F.) are then added; the flask is corked and heated until the fatty acids completely dissolve; the contents of the flask are cooled below 15·5° C., thoroughly shaken and allowed to stand in water at 15·5° C. for 30 minutes. The liquid is then filtered and 50 c.c. of the filtrate are titrated with N/10 sodium hydroxide solution, using phenol phthalein solution as an indicator. With this process, Elsdon finds that the figures for the alcohol soluble acids in butter always fall within the limits 9·0 to 14·0.

Gilmour's method (*Analyst*, 1920, XLV, 2). This is a modification of the method proposed by Blichfeldt (*J.S.C.I.* 1919, XXXVIII, 150); 20 grams of the clear filtered fat are weighed into a 300 c.c. conical flask and saponified with 30 grams of glycerine and 8 c.c. of potassium hydroxide solution (50 per cent.), and the resulting soap solution is diluted with water to 200 c.c.; to 50 c.c. of this soap solution, 100 c.c. of sulphuric acid (1·25 per cent.) and 0·1 gram of powdered pumice are added and the whole is then distilled in the special Blichfeldt apparatus, which is calibrated to hold 100 grams of water at 65° C.; when the distillate has been collected, the apparatus is disconnected and 0·5 c.c. of phenol phthalein solution (1 per cent.) and N/10 sodium hydroxide solution, slightly in excess of the amount required to neutralize the distillate, are added through the condenser tube; the openings are now closed with corks and the contents are well shaken and then removed to a 200 c.c. measuring flask and cooled to about 15° C.; the excess of sodium hydroxide is then determined with N/10 sulphuric acid and the number of c.c. of N/10 sodium hydroxide solution required to neutralize the volatile acids obtained;

from this figure is deducted 0·4, to allow for the blank, and the corrected figure is represented by T. To the measuring flask is now added a volume of N/10 sulphuric acid equal to $T + 0.4$, followed by 61 grams of pure dry sodium chloride, and the contents of the flask are well shaken, the volume being made up to 200 c.c.; the contents of the flask are now filtered and 190 c.c. of the filtrate are titrated with N/10 sodium hydroxide solution, the number of c.c. required being increased by 1/19th and reduced by 0·4 (to correct for the blank); the number so obtained represents the soluble volatile acids (S) and $T - S$ gives I, the insoluble volatile acids.

The following variations are obtained with the pure fats:

	T	S	I
Butter fat	26·0–33·0	20·0–23·5	5·0– 9·5
Cocoanut oil	19·5–22·5	1·3– 1·8	18·0–20·7
Palm kernel oil	12·0–14·0	1·0– 1·3	11·0–12·7

and the amount of adulteration can be determined from the following equations, which have been calculated from the average figures for pure butter fat, cocoanut oil and palm kernel oil:

Percentage of butter fat $= 4.67S - 0.35I = x$

Percentage of cocoanut oil $= 5I - 0.38x$

Percentage of palm kernel oil $= 7.69I - 0.59x$

Detection of hydrogenized oils. Knapp (*Analyst*, 1913, XXXVIII, 103). 50 grams of the fat are heated in a flask with 20 c.c. of hydrochloric acid with continuous and vigorous shaking; the mixture is allowed to separate while hot; a portion of the acid solution is evaporated to dryness and the residue is dissolved in a drop of water on a white tile, and a drop of ammonium sulphide solution then added; in the presence of nickel (used as a catalyst in the hydrogenization), a black precipitate or coloration is obtained.

Detection of hydrogenized fish oils. Klimont and Meyer (*Zeit. Angew. Chem.* 1914, XXVII, 645). 3 grams of the oil or fat are dissolved in 50 c.c. of acetone; the solution is allowed to stand for 12 hours; the deposited crystals are collected and weighed; if the weight of the crystals exceed 16 per cent., hydrogenized fish oils are certainly present.

Determination of fat in butter. A. Hesse (*Zeit. Nahr. Genuss.* 1904, LIX, 673). 2 grams of the sample are weighed into a stoppered cylinder and melted by the addition of 8 c.c. of boiling water; 1 c.c. of ammonia and 10 c.c. of alcohol are added and the cylinder is shaken until the proteids are dissolved; allow the mixture to cool; add 25 c.c. of ether, followed by 25 c.c. of petroleum ether; the whole is then well shaken and allowed to separate; the ether layer is then pipetted off and the residue again shaken with 25 c.c. of ether, which is again pipetted off; and finally with 25 c.c. of ether and 25 c.c. of petroleum ether. The mixed washings are evaporated and the residue dried in a water oven and weighed; the weight of residue obtained multiplied by 50 gives the percentage of fat.

Preservatives in butter. The most common preservatives used in butter are borax and boric acid or a mixture of these two. About 20 per cent. of the butter sold in this country contains this preservative.

The Report of the Departmental Committee on the use of preservatives and colouring matters of foods (1901, Cd. 833) recommended that the only preservatives to be allowed in butter should be boric acid or borax, or mixtures of these two in proportions not exceeding 0·5 per cent. calculated as boric acid. At the same time it is very doubtful whether the use of this substance is necessary and certainly 0·5 per cent. is excessive.

Determination of the boric acid in butter. Weigh out 10 grams of the well-mixed sample into a 300 c.c. flask and add 200 c.c. of water; warm the mixture over a Bunsen burner until the fat is melted; shake the mixture well and allow it to stand until the fat rises to the surface; siphon off the liquid into a measuring cylinder and note the volume. Place the liquid in a conical flask; add a few drops of methyl orange and dilute sulphuric acid until a pink colour is obtained; boil the solution for two or three minutes; cool in water; and, when cold, add a few drops of phenol phthalein solution, followed by N/10 sodium hydroxide solution until a faint pink colour appears; to the mixture is then added one-third of its volume of glycerine and N/10 sodium hydroxide solution until a permanent pink colour is obtained. The number of c.c. of N/10 sodium hydroxide solution used after the addition of glycerine multiplied by 0·0062 gives the amount of boron compounds calculated as boric acid in 10 grams of the butter.

Hawley's method (*Analyst*, 1915, XL, 150).

Reagents required:

An alcoholic solution of turmeric. 5 grams of powdered turmeric root and 5 grams of tartaric acid are digested with three successive quantities of 150 c.c. of warm alcohol (industrial spirit) for at least 1 hour with each portion; the liquid is filtered and the volume of the mixed filtrates is made up to 500 c.c. with alcohol. This solution should be kept in the dark.

Dilute hydrochloric acid. 20 c.c. of concentrated hydrochloric acid are diluted with water to 100 c.c.

Standard boric acid solution. 1 gram of boric acid is dissolved in 1000 c.c. of dilute hydrochloric acid.

The process. 20 grams of the sample are placed in a small beaker, melted on the water oven and kept warm until the curd and aqueous layer have separated; the fat is poured off, and, to the aqueous layer, 18 c.c. of the dilute hydrochloric acid are added; the contents of the beaker are then stirred and kept warm for a few minutes; 10 c.c. of the fat free liquid are removed from the beaker with a pipette, which is dipped to the bottom of the liquid; while the liquid is held in the pipette, the residue in the beaker is rejected; the liquid in the pipette is then returned to the beaker and allowed to cool, 5 c.c. of the turmeric reagent are then added; in the presence of boric acid, a reddish brown colour is slowly developed, the intensity of which varies with the boric acid content. Standard solutions containing 0·0, 0·1, 0·3 and 0·5 c.c. of the boric acid solution and 0·5 c.c. of milk are made up to 10 c.c. with the dilute hydrochloric acid and the amount of boric acid present in the sample is determined by comparison with the standards.

Detection of colouring matter. Sprinkmeyer and Wagner (*Zeit. Unter. Nahr. Gen.* 1905, LX, 598). 10 c.c. of the clear fat are poured into a separating funnel and 10 c.c. of petroleum ether, followed by 15 c.c. of glacial acetic acid, are added; the mixture is then well shaken and allowed to separate; in the presence of artificial colouring matter the lower layer becomes yellow or red.

Cornelison's method (*J. Amer. Chem. Soc.* 1908, XXX, 1478). 15 grams of glacial acetic acid are added to 10 grams of the fat; the temperature of the mixture is brought to 35° C. and the whole is well shaken and then allowed to separate into two layers; the acid layer is drawn off, its colour is noted, and portions are treated with nitric acid, concentrated sulphuric acid, and sulphuric acid with ether to a clear solution and the following colours are obtained:

	Colour of acid layer	Nitric acid	Concentrated sulphuric acid	Sulphuric acid and ether
Pure butter ..	—	—	Faint pink	—
Soudan I ..	Pink	Pink	Pink	Pink
Annatto ..	Yellow	—	Faint pink	Faint yellow
Turmeric ..	Greenish yellow	Ochre yellow	Pink	Yellow
Carrot ..	Greenish yellow	Yellow	Pink	Yellowish

Detection of coal-tar dyes in butter and margarine. Gilmour (*Analyst*, 1920, XLV, 173). About 1 c.c. of the clear filtered fat, which has been separated at a temperature not exceeding 100° C., is placed in a test-tube and immersed in an oil bath, which is raised to about 185° C.; the test-tube is removed occasionally, shaken and replaced. In the absence of coal-tar dye, the fat will become colourless within 10 minutes; if the fat remains coloured, then coal-tar dyes are present. This method depends on the fact that vegetable butter-dyes and the natural colouring matter of butter are less stable to heat than coal-tar dyes. Butter fat, which has been separated at a temperature exceeding 100° C., does not become colourless on heating.

Typical Analyses of Butter (in percentages).

	Irish	English	"Milk Blended"
Fat	81·7	91·5	74·2
Curd	2·3	1·7	1·1
Salt	1·8	—	2·6
Water	14·2	6·8	22·1

The following analyses of butters have been kindly supplied by J. West Knights.

	(1)	(2)	(3)	(4)	(5)	(6)
Water (per cent.) ..	9·27	12·97	14·57	10·23	15·67	9·43
Reichert-Wollny number in c.c. of N/10 NaHO ..	30·2	24·0	4·00	28·0	3·8	2·0
Boric acid (per cent.) ..	none	·28	·12	none	·25	·20

Nos. (1), (2) and (4) are genuine butters; Nos. (3), (5) and (6) consist entirely of margarine sold as butter.

Margarine must not contain more than 10 per cent. of added butter, 16 per cent. of water, or 0·5 per cent. of boric acid.

LARD

Lard consists of the mixed fats obtained from various parts of the hog; the best lard being obtained from the membranes surrounding the kidneys and from the back.

The chief adulterants of lard are cottonseed oil, beef stearine, paraffin wax and cocoanut oil.

The presence of cocoanut oil is detected, and its amount estimated by Shrewsbury and Knapp's method as described under butter (p. 144).

Lard is graded as follows:

(1) Neutral lard No. 1. This is obtained by rendering the "leaf" or fat from the kidney and bowels at 40° to 50° C.

(2) Neutral lard No. 2. This is obtained by rendering the fat from the back.

(3) Leaf lard. This is obtained by rendering the residue from (1) and (2) with steam under pressure.

(4) Kettle lard, obtained from neutral lard by rendering in steam-jacketed vessels.

(5) Prime steam lard, obtained by rendering, with direct steam, the fat from any part of the animal.

Detection of cottonseed oil. The presence of cottonseed oil in lard is detected by Halphen's test.

Solution required: A solution of sulphur in carbon disulphide, containing 1 gram of sulphur in 100 c.c. of carbon disulphide; this solution is mixed with an equal volume of fusel oil.

Equal volumes of the oil and reagent, about 5 c.c., are placed in a test-tube, loosely stoppered with cotton wool, and heated in a boiling brine bath for 15 minutes. In the presence of cottonseed oil a deep orange to red colour is obtained. Should a very faint colour be obtained it does not necessarily indicate the presence of added cottonseed oil, as the fat obtained from hogs fed on cottonseed meal or cake may give a faint reaction.

Gastaldi's modification (*Analyst*, 1913, XXXVIII, 36).

One drop of pyridin is used in place of amyl alcohol, with which cottonseed oil gives a yellowish rose coloration, and is more delicate than Halphen's test.

Determination of the iodine absorption. *Solutions required:* Wij's iodine solution (*Ber. Chem. Ges.* 1898, vol. XXXI, p. 750). Weigh out 13 grams of pure iodine and dissolve it in 1000 c.c. of glacial acetic acid (99 per cent.); determine the strength of the iodine solution with a standard solution of sodium thiosulphate; a slow stream of chlorine gas, free from hydrochloric acid, is now passed through the solution until the volume of the standard solution of sodium thiosulphate used for the titration is doubled; this occurs when the original dark brown of the solution is changed to light yellow;

A solution of potassium iodide containing 10 grams of the salt in 100 c.c. of water;

N/10 sodium thiosulphate solution.

The process. Weigh out 1 gram of the oil or fat; dissolve it in chloroform, and make the solution up to 100 c.c. with chloroform. Into a wide-mouthed stoppered glass bottle, measure out 20 c.c. of the chloroform solution of the fat; add 20 c.c. of the Wij's iodine solution and set aside for 20 minutes. At the end of 20 minutes, 25 c.c. of the potassium iodide solution are added; the whole is then diluted with 300 c.c. of water and the N/10 sodium thiosulphate solution is run in from a burette, with vigorous agitation of the bottle, until the colour is nearly discharged; a few c.c. of dilute starch solution are then added and the titration continued until the blue colour is discharged. A blank experiment should be performed upon the materials used.

The iodine absorption is obtained from the formula

$$\frac{T \times 0\cdot0127 \times 100}{W},$$

where T = the difference in c.c. in the volume of sodium thiosulphate solution used for the blank experiment and for the oil; W = the weight of oil taken.

The iodine absorption number for lard is from 50 to 63; for beef stearine from 34 to 47; and for cottonseed oil from 101 to 116.

Example: In an experiment with lard 1 gram of the fat was dissolved in 100 c.c. of chloroform and 20 c.c. of the solution used for the experiment.

The volume of sodium thiosulphate solution used for the blank experiment was 39·7 and for the lard 30·3. Then the iodine number of the sample of lard was

$$\frac{9 \cdot 4 \times 0 \cdot 0127 \times 100}{0 \cdot 2} = 59 \cdot 69.$$

Test for paraffin wax (Holde's method, *Jour. Soc. Chem. Ind.* 1892, p. 637). Ten drops of the melted lard are saponified in a test-tube with 5 c.c. of approximately N/2 alcoholic potash; to the clear soap solution, water is added in quantities of 1 c.c. at a time, the solution being observed after each addition. Pure lard gives a clear solution after dilution with 5 c.c. of water, and as little as 0·5 per cent. of paraffin wax gives a characteristic turbidity. This method will detect as little as 0·3 per cent. of paraffin wax in lard or margarine fat.

Shrewsbury's method (*Analyst*, 1909, XXXIV, 348): 5 grams of the melted lard are placed in a 200 c.c. Reichert flask and saponified with 20 c.c. of glycerine soda solution; the hot mixture is dissolved in industrial (non-mineralized) spirits, which is added drop by drop from a pipette, and allowed to cool; if, when the mixture is cold, the solution is clear, no paraffin wax is present; in the presence of 2 per cent. of paraffin wax, the solution is cloudy with opaque flocculi; when the solution has set to a jelly, it is again examined; pure lard gives a slightly opalescent but homogeneous jelly, but as little as 2 per cent. of paraffin wax gives a characteristic cloudy jelly.

Detection of beef stearine. The detection of beef stearine in lard is exceedingly difficult. In the absence of other adulterants, it may be detected by the iodine absorption but it is possible by judiciously mixing cottonseed oil and beef stearine to prepare a product giving an iodine number within the limits for pure lard.

Belfield (*Analyst*, 1898, vol. XIII, p. 70) proposed a microscopical method in which 3 grams of the sample are dissolved in 15 c.c. of warm ether in a test-tube loosely plugged with cotton wool; the solution is cooled to 13° C. and allowed to stand at that temperature overnight; the crystals obtained are examined microscopically. Lard crystallizes in flat rhomboidal plates; while in the presence of beef stearine the characteristic tufts of cylindrical needles are obtained.

Water. Lard is occasionally, though not frequently, adulterated by the addition of water. Pure lard should be absolutely free from water, and also from ash.

DRIPPING AND SUET

Dripping and suet are the rendered fats from various animals, chiefly cows, sheep and hogs. They often contain water as an adulterant, from which they should naturally be free. The addition of starch (in the form of oatmeal or cornflour) to suet to prevent greasy particles from adhering and coalescing together is becoming common; but this addition must be regarded as an adulteration if the sample is sold without adequate declaration.

The fat should be examined by the Shrewsbury and Knapp process (p. 144) and the iodine absorption (p. 156) in order to detect the presence of vegetable oil.

Beef and Mutton Fats

These fats are obtained from the ox and sheep respectively and are so very much alike in composition that any attempt to differentiate between them is very difficult. They should be examined by the Shrewsbury and Knapp process (p. 144), the iodine absorption (p. 156), the Reichert-Meissl-Polenske-Kirschner process (p. 146), and the acidity (p. 163) and saponification value (p. 163) should also be determined. The analyst who has to deal frequently with samples of both of these fats, relies chiefly upon the appearance, the smell, and the taste of the sample; these are materially different, and will serve at least to differentiate between the two fats, but are not capable of detecting mixtures.

CHEESE

Cheese is the compressed and "ripened" product obtained
from milk which has been either naturally or artificially soured.
The "ripening" process is essentially putrefactive and requires
several months to develop the characteristic flavour. Cheese
consists principally of fat, nitrogenous bodies, water, lactose
and mineral matter. It is a noteworthy fact that there is no
standard for cheese in this country, and, as a result, cheese is
sold made from either whole or skimmed milk without notification to the purchaser. It often contains only minute traces of
fat; whereas it is an offence to sell a cheese containing margarine fat without notification. The varieties of cheese take
their names from the town or district in which they are made;
for example, Cheshire and Cheddar.

There are also on the market so-called margarine cheeses,
which consist of various animal and vegetable fats; filled
cheese is usually manufactured from skimmed milk and hog
or other fat; these are occasionally sold in substitution for
genuine cheese, but as their detection is a comparatively simple
matter, this form of adulteration is not often practised.

Analysis of cheese. Fat. The fat in cheese is best determined by Ratzlaff's method (*Milch. Zeitung*, 1903, vol. v); 6
grams of the cheese are weighed into a small Erlenmeyer flask
about 4 cm. in diameter; 10 c.c. of concentrated hydrochloric
acid are added; a small funnel is placed in the neck of the flask
and the contents are heated on a water bath until they are
dissolved. The flask is now placed on a sand bath; carefully
heated to boiling and kept boiling for three minutes. The flask
is then allowed to cool; 5 c.c. of ether are added and the contents poured into a Stokes tube, the flask is rinsed out once
with 5 c.c. of ether and twice with 5 c.c. of petroleum ether;
the tube is filled to the upper mark with a mixture of equal
parts of ether and petroleum ether and closed with a well-
washed cork. The contents of the tube are thoroughly mixed
and allowed to separate; the volume of the ether layer is then
read off and 20 c.c. are pipetted out into a dried and weighed
fat flask; the ether is evaporated off and the residual fat is
dried in the water oven for 45 minutes and weighed. The

mixture of ether and petroleum ether dissolves the fat only and no other constituent of the cheese.

Example: 5 grams of cheese were taken for the estimation; the volume of the ether layer was 25·5 c.c., the weight of fat obtained from 20 c.c. was 1·976 grams; then the percentage of fat in the cheese was

$$\frac{1·967 \times 25·5 \times 100}{20 \times 5} = 50·39.$$

Water. A portion of the sample is cut into very thin slices and 5 grams are weighed into a platinum dish and dried in an air oven at 105° C. to constant weight; the loss in weight is reckoned as water. The water content should not exceed 35 per cent.

Ash. The dry residue obtained from the water determination is carefully incinerated at a low red heat; the residue is weighed and calculated to a percentage.

Proteids. The proportion of proteids is obtained by multiplying the percentage of nitrogen, as determined by the Kjeldahl process described under milk (p. 106), by 6·38.

Test for starch. A small portion of the sample, from which the fat has been extracted, is boiled with water and filtered; to the filtrate a few drops of a dilute iodine solution are added; when a blue colour is obtained in the presence of starch.

Examination of the fat. It is of course necessary to examine the fat for the presence of other fats than butter fat; and, in order to obtain sufficient fat for this purpose, about 50 grams of the sample are chopped up into small pieces and placed in a muslin bag, which is suspended over a beaker by means of a glass rod; the whole is then placed in a water oven, when the fat will melt out quite clear and should be examined by the Reichert-Wollny process (p. 143).

Estimation of chlorides. Cornish and Golding (*Analyst*, 1915, XL, 197). 1 gram of the sample is placed in a Kjeldahl flask with 20 c.c. of pure sulphuric acid and a few small pieces of pumice; the hydrochloric acid, formed by the action of the sulphuric acid on the chlorides, present in the sample, is driven over into acid silver nitrate solution (50 c.c. of concentrated nitric acid and 50 c.c. of N/10 silver nitrate solution) and precipitated as silver chloride; the silver chloride is filtered off and the precipitate is washed until it is free from nitrates; the filtrate is then titrated with N/10 potassium thiocyanate solution, using 1 c.c. of saturated iron alum solution as an indicator; each c.c. of N/10 silver nitrate solution absorbed by the hydrochloric acid produced represents 0·00585 gram of chlorine as sodium chloride. In order to prevent the silver nitrate solution being sucked back into the Kjeldahl flask, a special apparatus is used and air must be aspirated through it, while the process is being carried on.

Calculation of the composition of the cream (or milk) used in making a cheese. Richmond (*Analyst*, 1910, xxxv, 233). The proteins are divided by 0·3, which will give the equivalent of the solids-not-fat.

The solids-not-fat, thus calculated, are divided by 0·104, which will give the equivalent of water in the original cream.

Water + solids-not-fat + fat represents the original cream, and the fat and solids-not-fat are calculated as percentages.

0·25 per cent. is added to the fat to allow for loss.

Example: A cheese gave 4·1 per cent. of protein.

$$4·1 \div 0·3 \quad = \quad 13·7 \text{ solids-not-fat}$$
$$13·7 \div 0·104 = 132·7 \text{ water}$$
$$\underline{49·5 \text{ fat found}}$$
$$\text{Total} \qquad \underline{195·9}$$

$$\text{Percentage of solids-not-fat} = 13·7 \times \frac{100}{195·9} = 7·0.$$

$$\text{Percentage of fat} = 49·5 \times \frac{100}{195·9} = 25·3 + 0·25 = 25·55.$$

Richmond (*Analyst*, 1919, XLIV, 202) states that the fat and solid-not-fat in the original milk may be calculated from the following formulæ:

$$\text{Fat in original milk} = \frac{100F}{35·4P + F} + 0·25,$$

$$\text{Solids-not-fat in original milk} = \frac{333P}{35·4P + F},$$

where F = percentage of fat in the sample of cheese,
    P = percentage of proteins in the sample of cheese.

CREAM CHEESE

Cream cheese is the product obtained from the souring of milk either with or without rennet, and, according to Moor (*Suggested Standards for Foods and Drugs*, p. 88), should contain at least 40 per cent. of fat. According to Cribb (*Analyst*, 1909, vol. XXXIV, p. 45), in a genuine cream cheese the ratio $\dfrac{\text{fat}}{\text{protein}}$ should exceed 1 (protein = nitrogen number multiplied by 6·38, see p. 107). Numbers of cream cheese are on the market containing only a very small proportion of fat and obviously made from machine-skimmed milk. The sale of these substances as cream cheese without notification can only be regarded as a fraud. According to the standard of the United States of America, cream cheese is a cheese made from milk or cream, or from milk containing not less than 6 per cent. of fat.

The analysis of a cream cheese is carried out precisely as if it were an ordinary cheese.

Typical Analyses of Cheese (in percentages).

	Fat	Water	Casein, etc.	Ash
Camembert	24·52	49·96	20·15	5·37
Cheddar, English	31·57	35·60	28·61	4·32
Cheddar, American	37·09	30·09	29·25	3·57
Cheshire	30·68	37·11	27·79	4·42
Dutch	22·78	41·30	28·82	7·10
Gorgonzola	34·34	31·85	29·23	4·58
Roquefort	34·38	32·26	28·48	4·88
Stilton	39·13	23·57	33·79	3·15
Lard	24·66	31·30	38·87	5·17
Margarine	28·80	30·95	36·27	3·98
Cream	67·15	23·99	8·17	0·69
Cream	47·04	36·61	15·44	0·81
Cream	1·16	70·66	25·37	2·81

The last sample of cream cheese has been made from a machine-skimmed milk.

EDIBLE OILS

General Tests. *Acidity.* 5 grams of the oil are mixed with
50 c.c. of neutral 95 per cent. alcohol; the mixture is just
boiled, a few drops of phenol phthalein solution added, and
the whole is titrated with N/10 potassium hydroxide solution
until a permanent pink colour is obtained; the acidity is returned either (1) as the number of grams of potassium hydroxide required to neutralize the free fatty acids in 1 gram
of the oil, or (2) as the percentage of oleic acid, or (3) as the
percentage of lauric acid; these are calculated from the following formulæ:

(1) $\text{Acidity} = \dfrac{K \times 5 \cdot 61}{5}$,

(2) $\text{Acidity} = K \times 2 \cdot 82 \times 20$ as oleic acid,

(3) $\text{Acidity} = K \times 40$ as lauric acid,

where $K =$ the number of c.c. of N/10 potassium hydroxide
solution used.

Determination of specific gravity. The specific gravity of
oils may be determined in a pycnometer, or by means of a
Westphal balance, or of a hydrometer, but the accuracy of
both these latter types of instrument varies considerably.

Determination of the saponification value. The saponification value is the number of milligrams of potassium hydroxide required to completely saponify 1 gram of oil.

Solutions required:

N/2 alcoholic potassium hydroxide solution; N/2 hydrochloric acid.

The process. 2 grams of the oil are weighed out into a flask
and 25 c.c. of the N/2 alcoholic potassium hydroxide solution
are added from a pipette; a further quantity of 25 c.c. of the
alcoholic potassium hydroxide solution is run out of the same
pipette into another clean and dry flask; the two flasks are
heated on a water bath, under a reflux condenser, for 30
minutes with constant shaking; after 30 minutes' heating, a
few drops of phenol phthalein solution are added and the contents of each flask are titrated with N/2 hydrochloric acid,
until the pink colour just disappears.

The saponification value $= \dfrac{(A - B) \times 0\cdot02805 \times 1000}{2}$, where

> A = the number of c.c. of N/2 hydrochloric acid required for the blank experiment,
> B = the number of c.c. of N/2 hydrochloric acid required for the oil.

Example: 2 grams of an oil required 12·4 c.c. of N/2 hydrochloric acid for neutralization after saponification, the blank experiment required 24·6 c.c., then

the saponification value $= \dfrac{(24\cdot6 - 12\cdot4) \times 0\cdot02805 \times 1000}{2} = 171$.

Determination of iodine absorption. The method for the determination of iodine absorption is given under lard (p. 156).

Determination of unsaponifiable matter. To 10 grams of the oil, 15 c.c. of 50 per cent. sodium hydroxide solution and 50 c.c. of 95 per cent. alcohol are added, and the mixture is saponified under a reflux condenser for 30 minutes; the resultant liquid is transferred to a porcelain dish, the alcohol is evaporated off, about 50 grams of silver-sand, which has been previously extracted with petroleum ether, and 5 grams of sodium bicarbonate, are added and the whole mass is evaporated to dryness; the contents of the dish are thoroughly mixed, and then extracted with petroleum ether in a Soxhlet apparatus; the solvent is evaporated and the residue is dried in the water oven and weighed; the weight of residue obtained multiplied by 10 gives the percentage of unsaponifiable matter.

Determination of bromine absorption.

Solutions required:

A solution of 4 c.c. of dry bromine in 1 litre of dry chloroform or carbon tetrachloride;

A 10 per cent. solution of potassium iodide;

N/10 solution of sodium thiosulphate.

The process. Weigh out 1 gram of oil and dissolve it in chloroform or carbon tetrachloride, and make the solution up to 100 c.c. Into a wide-mouthed stoppered flask, measure out 20 c.c. of the solution, add 20 c.c. of the bromine solution, followed by 25 c.c. of the potassium iodide solution; dilute the mixture with 300 c.c. of water, and titrate with N/10 sodium thiosulphate solution, with vigorous agitation of the flask, until the colour is nearly discharged; a few c.c. of freshly prepared starch solution are then added and the titration is continued until the blue colour is discharged. A blank experiment should always be performed on the materials used. The bromine absorption is obtained from the formula:

$$\frac{T \times 0 \cdot 008 \times 100}{W},$$

where T = the difference in c.c. in the volume of N/10 sodium thiosulphate solution used for the blank experiment and for the oil.

W = the weight of oil taken.

Determination of the Maumené number. The Maumené number is the rise in temperature in degrees Centigrade, which occurs when a definite volume of concentrated (97 per cent.) sulphuric acid is mixed with a definite weight of the oil.

A 150 c.c. beaker is surrounded with cotton wool and placed inside a larger beaker (about 300 c.c. capacity); 50 grams of the oil are then weighed into the smaller beaker and the temperature is noted; 10 c.c. of concentrated (97 per cent.) sulphuric acid (at the same temperature as the oil) are then run into the oil with constant stirring, about one minute being required for the addition of the acid; the stirring is continued until no further rise in temperature takes place; the actual rise in temperature in degrees Centigrade is the Maumené number.

Detection of rancidity. Kerr (*J. Ind. and Eng. Chem.* 1918, X, 471; and *Analyst*, 1918, XLIII, 327). To 10 c.c. of the oil or fat in an 8-inch × 1-inch test-tube add 10 c.c. of concentrated hydrochloric acid and vigorously shake the mixture; 10 c.c. of a 0·1 per cent. ethereal solution of phloroglucinol are then added and the liquid is again vigorously shaken; in the presence of rancidity a red or pink colour appears in the acid layer.

Cloud test (*J. Ind. and Eng. Chem.* 1919, XI, 69; and *Analyst*, 1919, XLIV, 138). The oil is heated at 150° C. and about 45 c.c. is poured into a 4-ounce bottle and then cooled in a suitable bath; the oil is stirred with a thermometer and the temperature at which the first permanent cloud appears is noted. The heating must be done immediately before making the determination, and the cooling must be done as rapidly as possible, but not so rapidly as to freeze the oil on the sides of the bottle.

Determination of acetyl value. Lewkowitsch (*J.S.C.I.* 1897, XVI, 503). The acetyl value is the number of milligrams of potassium hydroxide required to neutralize the acetic acid obtained by saponification of 1 gram of an acetylated oil. 10 grams of the oil are boiled for two hours under a reflux condenser with 20 grams of acetic anhydride; the resulting liquid is poured into a large beaker, and 500 c.c. of boiling water are added, and the boiling is continued for 30 minutes; a slow stream of carbon dioxide is passed in meanwhile, in order to prevent bumping; the water is separated and the residue is again washed three times with boiling water and then filtered through a dry filter paper; 5 grams of the acetylated fat on the filter paper are saponified with N/2 alcoholic potassium hydroxide solution; the alcohol is then distilled off and the residue is dissolved in water, acidified with N/2 sulphuric acid and steam-distilled; about 600 c.c. of distillate are collected and titrated with N/10 potassium hydroxide solution, using phenol phthalein as an indicator.

Acetyl value = No. of c.c. of N/10 potassium hydroxide solution used multiplied by 5·61 and divided by the weight of acetylated fat taken.

Detection of mineral oil in vegetable oil. Pollard (*Analyst*, 1912, XXXVII, 247). 10 grams of solid sodium hydroxide are placed in a nickel crucible and fused over a Bunsen flame; when the sodium hydroxide is just melted, the crucible is removed from the flame and 5 c.c. of the oil are quickly poured in; the contents of the crucible are stirred with an iron rod and allowed to stand in water until quite cold; 50 c.c. of petroleum ether are added and the contents of the crucible are again well stirred with an iron rod; the petroleum ether solution is decanted through a filter paper and then evaporated; the residue is boiled with 3 c.c. of nitric acid, when any residue consists of mineral oil.

Titre test. All tallows and fats, used in the manufacture of soap, margarine, candles, etc., are bought and sold on the titre test; in this test the solidifying point of the fatty acids is determined. About 40 grams of the fat are saponified in a 300 c.c. flask with 30 c.c. of a 25 per cent. solution of sodium hydroxide and 100 c.c. of alcohol, the resulting mass is evaporated on a water bath, with constant shaking, almost to dryness; a further 50 c.c. of alcohol are then added and the mass is again evaporated; the soap is dissolved in 250 c.c. of water and the fatty acids are liberated by the addition of a slight excess of dilute hydrochloric acid; after warming on the water bath until the acids are melted, the water layer is siphoned off and the fatty acids are washed with successive quantities of water, until the washings are free from mineral acid. The liquid fatty acids are then filtered through a dry, double filter paper, in a steam oven, and refiltered until clear. A wide test-tube about 1½ inches in diameter and 6 inches in length is placed, through a cork, in a wide-mouthed bottle; about 20 grams of the fatty acids are placed in the test-tube and the bulb of a short-ranged thermometer is immersed in the centre of the acids. The temperature is raised until the acids are just melted and the mass is then allowed to cool down; and, as soon as crystals begin to appear, the acids are gently stirred with the thermometer; at first, the temperature gradually falls and finally rises sharply and the maximum temperature then obtained is the titre.

The following are general limits for the titre of various fats and oils:

	Degrees Centigrade		Degrees Centigrade
Beef fat	38–46	Palm oil	36–45
Mutton fat	41–48	Palm kernel oil	23–28
Lard	34–42	Olive oil	20–26
Cocoanut oil	21–25	Arachis oil	25–30
Rape oil	15–20	Cottonseed oil	33–37
Linseed oil	14–18	Sesamé oil	23–30

Olive oil. Olive oil is the colourless to yellow oil obtained by extraction or compression from the ripe fruit of *Olea sativa*, which contains about 60 per cent. of oil, and consists chiefly of olein and palmitin. Owing to its high price olive oil is very extensively adulterated, the chief adulterant being Arachis oil, cottonseed oil and mineral oils; the *British Pharmacopœia* requires that the acid value shall not exceed 6 per cent.; it is chiefly used as an edible oil, as a burning oil or lubricant, and in the manufacture of soap.

Test for Arachis oil in olive oil. The sample is saponified with an equal weight of alcoholic potassium hydroxide solution (200 grams of solid potassium hydroxide in 500 grams of 90 per cent. alcohol) on the water bath for 30 to 40 minutes and allowed to cool down to a temperature between 0° and 6° C. In the presence of as little as 5 per cent. of Arachis oil granular masses of potassium arachidate separate on the walls of the test-tube, which are insoluble in alcohol. Large quantities of Arachis oil are indicated by the solidification of the whole mass.

Estimation of Arachis oil. *Solutions required:*

Alcoholic potash solution containing 85 grams of solid potassium hydroxide in 1000 c.c.;

Acetic acid solution, 1·5 c.c. of which exactly neutralize 5 c.c. of the alcoholic potash solution;

Alcoholic hydrochloric acid solution containing 1 per cent. of hydrochloric acid in 70 per cent. alcohol.

The process. Saponify 5 grams of the oil with 25 c.c. of the alcoholic potash solution; exactly neutralize the potash with 7·5 c.c. of the acetic acid solution and rapidly cool the vessel by immersing it in water. At the end of one hour, the precipitate is collected on a filter paper and washed with 70 per cent. alcohol, containing 1 per cent. hydrochloric acid, the temperature being maintained between 15 and 20° C.; the washing is continued until the filtrate does not become turbid on the addition of water. The precipitate, which contains other acids besides arachidic, is dissolved off the filter paper with 25 to 50 c.c. of boiling alcohol (92 to 93 per cent.); from 8 to 16 c.c. of water are added to the solution, in order to reduce the strength of the alcohol to about 20 per cent., and the liquid is cooled for one hour in water at a temperature below 20° C.

The precipitate, which consists of arachidic acid, is collected on a dried and weighed filter paper, washed with 70 per cent. alcohol (free from hydrochloric acid) until the filtrate remains clear on the addition of water, dried at 100° C. and weighed.

Arachis oil contains 4 to 5 per cent. of arachidic acid, consequently the amount of arachidic acid found must be multiplied by 20 to obtain the amount of Arachis oil present.

The various acids obtained in the above process have different melting-points, and it is only by means of the melting-point that exact determinations of the presence of acids higher in the series than stearic and palmitic acids can be obtained. The melting-point of arachidic acid is 77° C., of stearic acid 69·3° C. and palmitic acid 62° C., and the melting-point to be accepted as evidence of the presence of arachidic acid should in every case be over 71° C.

Sesamé oil is expressed from the seeds of *Sesamum Indicum*, which contain about 50 per cent. of oil; it has a pale yellow colour and is practically odourless; the *British Pharmacopœia* requires that the acidity of this oil shall not exceed 8 per cent.; it may be officially used to replace olive oil in pharmacopœial preparations in India, Africa or Australia; it is occasionally adulterated with cottonseed oil or arachis oil; in many countries the addition of sesamé oil to margarine is compulsory, and the detection of the substitution of margarine for butter is thereby greatly facilitated.

Baudouin's test for sesamé oil (*Zeit. Ang. Chem.* 1892, pp. 509–510). *Solution required:* A hydrochloric acid solution of cane sugar, containing 1 gram of cane sugar in 100 c.c. of hydrochloric acid (specific gravity 1·2).

20 c.c. of the oil are mixed with 10 c.c. of the cane sugar solution, the mixture is well shaken and allowed to stand. As little as 2 per cent. of sesamé oil imparts a crimson colour to the aqueous layer.

Villavecchia and Fabri's test (*Zeit. Ang. Chem.* 1893, p. 505). *Solutions required:*

A solution of 2 grams of furfural in 100 c.c. of 95 per cent. alcohol;

Concentrated hydrochloric acid.

The test. 20 c.c. of the oil are mixed with 10 c.c. of hydrochloric acid and a few drops of the furfural reagent in a test-tube; the mixture is well shaken and allowed to stand until it separates into two layers; the lower layer is coloured dark red in the presence of as little as 1 per cent. of sesamé oil. This reaction is a modification of Baudouin's reaction, but is much more sensitive.

Detection of sesamé oil in fats containing colouring matter. Arnold (*Zeit. Unter. Nahr. Genussm.* 1913, XXVI, 655). Occasionally samples of fat are met with which give a red colour with hydrochloric acid alone; this colour is due to the added colouring matter; such samples are treated with hydrochloric acid containing 0·1 gram of stannous chloride per 100 c.c.; the fat is dissolved in petroleum ether and placed in a boiling water bath until the red colour is discharged; the solution of furfural is then added and the test carried out as before.

Cottonseed oil is expressed from the seeds of *Gossypium herbaceum*, which contain about 25 per cent. of oil; it is chiefly used as an edible oil and in the manufacture of soap; it has a strong and characteristic taste; cottonseed oil, on standing at a low temperature, gradually deposits a solid fat known as cottonseed stearine, which has a light yellow colour and is used as an adulterant for butter and lard.

Becchi's reaction for cottonseed oil (*Zeit. Anal. Chem.* 1894, XXXIII, 560). *Solutions required:*

Solution A.

Silver nitrate ..	2 grams	
Alcohol	200	c.c.
Ether	40	,,
Nitric acid (strong)	0·1	,,

Solution B.

Colza oil	15	,,
Amyl alcohol ..	100	,,

6 c.c. of the oil are mixed with 2 c.c. of solution *A* and well shaken; 5 c.c. of solution *B* are then added and the mixture is again well shaken and then immersed in a boiling water bath for 15 minutes; in the presence of cottonseed oil, a red-brown coloration, due to the reduction of the silver, is obtained.

Halphen's test for cottonseed oil has been described under lard (p. 155).

Castor oil is expressed from the seeds of *Ricinus communis*, which contain about 50 per cent. of oil; it is nearly colourless and has a very unpleasant taste; the *British Pharmacopœia* requires that the acid value shall not exceed 4 per cent. and that it shall be soluble in its own volume of absolute alcohol and in 3·5 times its volume of 90 per cent. alcohol; it is chiefly used in medicine and as a lubricant; it has been found adulterated with cottonseed oil.

Almond oil is expressed from the seeds of *Prunus amygdalus*, which contain about 65 per cent. of oil; it is pale yellow in colour and has a slightly nutty flavour; the *British Pharmacopœia* requires that the acidity shall not exceed 6 per cent.; the chief adulterants are arachis, olive, cottonseed or sesamé oils and also the total substitution of peach kernel oil; the analytical constants of the latter are so similar to those of almond oil that it is almost impossible to detect its presence; the *British Pharmacopœia* requires that when 5 c.c. of almond oil are mixed with 1 c.c. of a mixture of equal parts of sulphuric acid, fuming nitric acid and water for 1 minute, the resulting mixture shall be whitish in colour, whereas peach kernel oil under the same conditions gives a bright red colour. Almond oil is chiefly used in medicine and in the manufacture of perfumes.

Arachis oil is expressed from the seeds of *Arachis hypogæa*, which contain about 45 per cent. of oil; it is pale yellow to green in colour with a faint nutty odour; the *British Pharmacopœia* requires that the acidity shall not exceed 6 per cent.; the analytical constants of this oil are very similar to those of olive oil; it is chiefly used as an edible oil and in the manufacture of soap and also as an adulterant of olive oil; it may be officially used as a substitute for olive in pharmacopoeial preparations in India, Africa and Australia.

Cacao butter, or oil of theobroma, is expressed from the seeds of *Theobroma cacao*, which contain about 50 per cent. of oil, and is used chiefly for medicinal purposes; it is yellowish-white in colour and has an agreeable taste and a slight odour of cocoa; the *British Pharmacopœia* requires that the acid value shall not exceed 2 per cent.; it is occasionally adulterated with cocoanut oil, arachis oil, lard and paraffin wax.

Hazel nut oil is obtained from *Corylus avellana*, which contains about 60 per cent. of oil; it is used as an edible oil, as a lubricant and in the manufacture of perfumes.

Maize oil is obtained from *Zea mays*, which contains about 10 per cent. of oil, and is chiefly used as an edible oil and in the manufacture of soap; it has a light yellow colour and a very characteristic taste and odour.

Palm oil is obtained from the fruit of *Elæis guineensis* and from the fruit of *Elæis melanococca*, which contain from 20 to 40 per cent. of oil; it is slightly reddish in colour and is used in the manufacture of candles and soap; this oil gives a characteristic blue colour in the Lieberman-Storch test.

Rape oil is obtained from the seeds of *Brassica campestris*, which contain about 40 per cent. of oil; it has a yellow to dark brown colour and an unpleasant taste; the chief uses of this oil are as a lubricant or burning oil; it is frequently adulterated with cottonseed, linseed or mineral oils.

Detection of hydrogenized fish oils. Tortelli and Jaffé (*Annal. Chim. Applic.* 1914, II, 80; and *Analyst*, 1915, XL, 14). 1 c.c. of the oil is shaken with 6 c.c. of chloroform and 1 c.c. of glacial acetic acid; 40 drops of a 10 per cent. solution of bromine in chloroform are then added; the liquid is vigorously shaken and allowed to stand. In the presence of fish oils, a fugitive rose colour changing to bright green is obtained; vegetable oils remain colourless or give a yellow tint; hemp-seed oil gives a green colour changing to yellow; neat's-foot oil gives a slight rose colour changing to yellow; hydrogenized fish oils give a rose colour changing to pale green and then to emerald green; hydrogenized vegetable oils give no colour or give a slight yellow changing to brown; hydrogenized animal oils give a yellow or light brown colour changing to dark brown; butter gives a yellowish colour, which appears slightly green by reflected light, but is easily distinguishable from fish oils.

Soya bean oil is obtained from *Soja hispida*, which contains about 18 per cent. of oil, and is chiefly used as an edible oil, as a burning oil and in the manufacture of soap; it has a deep brown colour and only a very slight taste and odour.

Detection of soya bean oil. Settimj (*Analyst*, 1913, XXXVIII, 36). 5 c.c. of the oil are shaken with 2 c.c. of chloroform and 3 c.c. of a 2 per cent. solution of uranium nitrate; in the presence of soya bean oil an intense lemon yellow emulsion is produced; arachis, colza, cottonseed, maize and sesamé oils give a white emulsion; olive oil occasionally gives a greenish emulsion, but also occasionally a very slight yellow.

Linseed oil is expressed from *Linum usitatissimum*, which contains about 40 per cent. of oil; the *British Pharmacopœia* requires that the acid value shall not exceed 3 per cent.; it has a yellowish-brown colour and a characteristic odour and is frequently adulterated with cottonseed, rosin or mineral oils; it is chiefly used in the manufacture of soft soap and linoleum and for mixing with paints and varnishes.

Detection of adulteration in linseed oil. Elsdon and Hawley (*Analyst*, 1913, XXXVIII, 3). 2·5 grams of the oil are weighed out into a 25 c.c. graduated flask, sufficient ether is added to dissolve the oil and the contents of the flask are then made up to the mark with ether; 5 c.c. of the ethereal solution are transferred, with a carefully dried pipette, to a fat-free Adams' coil; the solution is carefully and uniformly distributed over the coil, which is then allowed to dry in the air overnight and is finally dried in the water oven for 2 hours; the coil is then extracted with ether (specific gravity 0·720) for three hours; the ether is evaporated, a few c.c. of absolute alcohol are added, and the residue is dried in the water oven for 2 hours, cooled and weighed. A close relationship exists between the percentage extract and the iodine value; the maximum percentage extract permissible for a genuine linseed oil is found from the following equation:

$$\text{Extract} = 81\cdot9 - 0\cdot35I,$$

where I = the iodine value.

Elsdon and Hawley give the following extracts obtained with genuine linseed oils and various mixtures:

Linseed oil	14·0 to 19·2
Colza oil	100·6
Linseed oil and 20 per cent. colza oil ..	21·0
Linseed oil and 20 per cent. whale oil ..	21·2
Linseed oil and 20 per cent. cottonseed oil	19·4
Linseed oil and 20 per cent. seal oil ..	31·6

Lieberman-Storch test for rosin oil (*J.S.C.I.* 1888,

Constants of some oils and fats.

	Specific gravity	Iodine absorption	Saponification value	Unsaponifiable matter	Maumené number	Reichert-Wolny number	Acetyl value	Polenske value
Butter fat ..	0·860–0·870 at 99° C.	26–38	221–233	—	—	24–33	2·0–8·5	1·7–3·5
Lard	0·859–0·864 at 99° C.	50–63	195–197	0·2	24–27	1·1	2·6	—
Beef fat ..	0·943–0·952 at 99° C.	38–46	193–200	—	—	0·5	2·5–8·5	—
Lard oil ..	0·915–0·917 at 15·5° C.	76–81	190–195	—	66–70	—	—	—
Neat's-foot oil ..	0·914–0·916 at 15·5° C.	69–72	195–200	—	47–59	1·0	22	—
Cocoanut oil ..	0·868–0·874 at 15·5° C.	8·0–9·0	250–260	0·15–0·3	—	7·0–8·0	1·0–12·0	15–18
Cacao butter ..	0·850–0·860 at 99° C.	33–37	188–195	0·8–1·0	—	3·5	2·8	—
Cod-liver oil ..	0·922–0·929 at 15·5° C.	125–150	171–210	0·5–1·5	102–115	0·4	4·8	—
Seal oil ..	0·915–0·925 at 15·5° C.	127–152	178–196	0·5–1·5	92–94	0·5	—	—
Whale oil ..	0·930–0·935 at 15·5° C.	110–123	188–193	0·7–3·0	85–90	1·5–7	—	—
Arachis oil ..	0·916–0·921 at 15·5° C.	83–100	190–196	0·4–0·8	47–60	0·5–1·6	9·0	—
Cottonseed oil ..	0·922–0·927 at 15·5° C.	188–200	193–195	0·5–1·8	75–85	0·95	7·0–18·0	—
Linseed oil ..	0·932–0·938 at 15·5° C.	174–200	188–195	1·0–2·0	110–120	0·5–1·5	4·0	—
Maize oil ..	0·922–0·926 at 15·5° C.	114–125	189–194	1·0–3·0	75–85	4·0–9·0	7·5–8·5	0·5
Olive oil ..	0·915–0·918 at 15·5° C.	79–87	187–195	0·5–1·0	39–45	0·6	10·5	—
Palm oil ..	0·859–0·871 at 99° C.	50–57	195–200	—	—	1·0	18	—
Rape oil ..	0·914–0·917 at 15·5° C.	99–105	175–179	0·5–1·0	54–60	0·6	14·5	—
Sesamé oil ..	0·922–0·924 at 15·5° C.	103–110	189–192	0·9–1·2	66–68	1·2	—	—
Castor oil ..	0·960–0·967 at 15·5° C.	83–90	178–185	0·3–0·6	44–48	1·0–2·5	145–151	—

VII, 136). 1 to 2 c.c. of the oil are warmed with acetic anhydride and allowed to cool; the acetic anhydride layer is then removed with a pipette and treated with 1 drop of sulphuric acid (specific gravity 1·53), when, in the presence of rosin oil, a fugitive violet colour is obtained. It must be remembered that this colour is also given by cholesterol.

Burchard's modification (*Zeit. für Anal. Chem.* 1892, 90). A few drops of the oil are dissolved in 2 c.c. of chloroform and 20 drops of acetic anhydride, and 1 drop of sulphuric acid are added, when the violet colour is obtained in the presence of rosin oil.

Bromide of tin test. Bromide of tin is prepared by adding bromine drop by drop to metallic tin in a dry flask, during the operation the flask is kept cold; the product is dissolved in carbon bi-sulphide. 1 drop of the stannic bromide solution is added to 1 c.c. of the oil, when, in the presence of rosin oil, a violet colour is obtained.

CHAPTER IV

TEA—COFFEE—CHICORY—COCOA

TEA

TEA consists of the leaves and leaf buds of species of *Thea*, prepared by fermenting or drying and firing. Tea has been used in China for 6000 years; it was first introduced into Europe by the Portuguese in the middle of the 16th century, and in 1912 it was imported into the United Kingdom to the extent of 361 millions of pounds, 300 millions of which came from India and Ceylon.

There are two chief varieties of tea, green and black; the difference between them is solely in the method of manufacture. Black tea is prepared by allowing the leaves to dry and wither in the sun; they are then rolled, in order to remove the disagreeable juices, fermented and finally dried again either in the sun or artificially; in the preparation of green tea, the leaves are dried artificially immediately after being picked. These varieties are subdivided; green teas into gunpowder, hyson and imperial; black teas into Bohea, Congou, Pekoe and Souchong. Caper tea consists of tea dust made into small hard balls with gum and polished with graphite. Adulteration of tea in this country has practically ceased to exist; 491 samples of tea were examined under the Sale of Food and Drugs Acts in 1911 and all were found to be genuine. This is due to the fact that all tea imported into the United Kingdom is examined by the Customs Authorities acting under the provisions of the Sale of Food and Drugs Acts and the consequent prohibition of the importation of adulterated tea. In the past tea was adulterated by the addition of exhausted leaves, foreign leaves, mineral matter or foreign astringent matter.

Caper tea is said to be manufactured by coating tea leaves with gum and subsequently rolling them into small round granules. This method of manufacture is in itself highly suspicious and lends itself very easily to adulteration. As caper tea has a somewhat extensive use for the purpose of adding flavour to ordinary tea, it should be carefully watched. It is often found adulterated with sandy and earthy matter, and, occasionally, small stones have been found. The total ash should not exceed 8 per cent., and the ash insoluble in hydrochloric acid should not exceed 3 per cent.; an analysis showing higher values than these can only be considered as serious adulteration.

Examination of tea. The complete analysis of tea is very difficult owing to its complex composition, and a partial analysis is generally undertaken.

Detection of foreign leaves. A portion of the sample is soaked for a short time in hot water; the leaves opened out and examined with a hand glass or a low power of a microscope, when the presence of foreign leaves is easily detected, genuine tea leaves being lanceolate in form.

Detection of foreign astringent matter. 1 gram of genuine tea and 1 gram of the suspected sample are extracted with separate portions, of 100 c.c. each, of boiling water; the solutions are strained and a slight excess of lead acetate added; the solutions are then filtered, and to 20 c.c. of each of the filtrates, a few drops of silver nitrate solution are added and the whole carefully warmed; pure tea gives a grey precipitate, but tea containing catechu gives a large brown precipitate of reduced silver. It is claimed that in this way as little as 2 per cent. of catechu may be detected.

Determination of ash. 5 grams of the tea are weighed out into a platinum dish, and carefully incinerated over a Bunsen flame until a white or greyish white residue is obtained; the weight of the residue multiplied by 20 gives the percentage of ash.

Determination of the insoluble ash and silica. The total ash as obtained above is extracted with water and filtered, and the residue well washed with hot water; the filtrate is set aside for the alkalinity determination; the residue on the filter paper is dried in a water oven, incinerated and weighed; from this weight the weight of the ash of the filter paper is subtracted, the difference is the insoluble ash; this insoluble ash is then extracted with dilute hydrochloric acid and filtered; the filter paper is well washed with hot water, dried in a water oven and incinerated; the residue, less the weight of the ash of the filter paper, is silica.

Caper tea is very liable to contain a comparatively large amount of silica, but any percentage above three must be regarded as an adulteration. The soluble ash is obtained by subtracting the insoluble from the total ash; or it may be obtained directly by evaporating the filtrate from the insoluble ash to dryness on the water bath, and heating the residue in the water oven till constant; when the weight of residue obtained multiplied by 20 gives the percentage of soluble ash.

Determination of the alkalinity of the ash. The filtrate from the insoluble ash determination is treated with N/10 sulphuric acid, using methyl orange as an indicator, until the solution has a faint pink colour, when the number of c.c. of N/10 sulphuric acid used multiplied by 0·0047 gives the amount of alkalinity, calculated as K_2O on 5 grams of the tea.

Example: The filtrate from the ash of 5 grams of tea required 14·5 c.c. of N/10 sulphuric acid to produce a permanent pink colour, then $14·5 \times 0·0047 \times 20 = 1·36$ per cent. of alkalinity calculated as K_2O.

Estimation of exhausted leaves. The percentage of exhausted leaves in a sample of tea is calculated either from the soluble ash or from the alkalinity. The soluble ash of a genuine tea should not be less than 3 per cent.; and the alkalinity should not be less than 1·3 per cent. calculated as K_2O.

Examples: A sample of tea gave 2·13 per cent. of soluble ash, then the percentage of exhausted leaves in the sample is $100 - \dfrac{2·13 \times 100}{3} = 29$ per cent. Another sample of tea gave an alkalinity of 0·85 per cent. calculated as K_2O, then the percentage of exhausted leaves in the sample is

$$100 - \frac{0·85 \times 100}{1·3} = 34·6 \text{ per cent.}$$

Analysis of tea. Tatlock and Thomson's method (*Analyst*, 1910, xxxv, 103);

Estimation of moisture. 5 grams of the sample of tea are dried at 100° C. for 1 hour; the residue is weighed and redried and the drying repeated until no further loss occurs.

Estimation of water extract. 1 gram of the powdered sample is boiled with 400 c.c. of water, under a reflux condenser, for 1 hour; the solution is filtered through a weighed filter paper and the residue is washed with 80 c.c. of hot water, dried at 100° C. and weighed; the weight of residue per cent., plus the percentage of water, deducted from 100, gives the percentage of water extract.

Estimation of tannin. The filtrate from the estimation of the water extract is cooled to 15·5° C.; 1 gram of basic quinine sulphate, dissolved in 25 c.c. of water, is added, followed by 2·5 c.c. of N. sulphuric acid; the whole is well mixed and allowed to stand for 10 to 15 minutes; the precipitate is collected on a weighed filter paper, washed with the filtrate, but not with water, allowed to drain, dried at 100° C. and weighed. The weight of quinine tannate obtained multiplied by 0·75 gives the weight of tannin in 1 gram of the sample.

Estimation of caffeine. 2 grams of the sample are exhausted with 800 c.c. of water under a reflux condenser for 1 hour; the extract is filtered and evaporated on the water bath to 40 c.c.; 10 c.c. of N. sodium hydroxide solution are then added and the mixture is extracted three times with chloroform; the chloroform extract is washed with 10 c.c. of N. sodium hydroxide solution to remove traces of tannin, etc., followed by 10 c.c. of water, and is then evaporated to dryness; the residue is heated in the water oven to constant weight; if the caffeine residue is coloured, it should be heated with a little dilute sodium hydroxide solution, and again extracted with chloroform.

Typical Analyses of Tea (in percentages).

	(1)	(2)	(3)	(4)	(5)
Total ash	5·50	4·32	4·92	13·47	6·38
Soluble ash	4·06	0·46	2·12	2·80	3·21
Insoluble ash	1·37	3·58	2·55	4·41	2·49
Silica	0·07	0·28	0·25	6·26	0·68
Alkalinity (as K_2O)	1·67	0·28	0·92	—	1·79

No. (1) is a genuine tea; No. (2) is a sample of exhausted leaves; No. (3) is a sample of tea containing 30 per cent. of exhausted leaves; No. (4) is a sample of adulterated caper tea; while No. (5) is a genuine caper tea.

The following analyses of samples of tea have been kindly supplied by Mr J. West Knights. All these are genuine. The microscopic examination was satisfactory in each sample.

	(1)	(2)	(3)	(4)	(5)	(6)
Soluble ash	3·90	3·20	4·10	3·20	3·75	4·20
Insoluble ash	1·45	2·47	1·75	2·60	2·10	1·90
Total ash	5·35	5·67	5·85	5·80	5·85	6·10

Typical Analysis of the Ash of Tea.

Potash (as K_2O)	30·04
Sand (as SiO_2)	17·78
Phosphate (as P_2O_5)	14·68
Carbonate (as CO_2)	9·58
Lime (as CaO)	8·74
Sulphate (as SO_3)	6·54
Magnesia (as MgO)	4·87
Alumina (as Al_2O_3)	3·42
Oxide of manganese (as Mn_3O_4)	1·37
Soda (as Na_2O)	1·07
Chlorine (as Cl)	1·07
Iron (as Fe_2O_3)	0·84
	100·00

COFFEE

Coffee is the seed of *Coffea arabica* or *Coffea liberica*, roasted and ground or otherwise prepared in a form suitable for a decoction. *Coffea arabica* is indigenous to N.E. Africa and Arabia. Coffee, as a beverage, has been known in Abyssinia from time immemorial, and was introduced into England in the middle of the 17th century. The coffee used in this country consists chiefly of five varieties, Mocha, Jamaican, Indian, Liberian and Brazilian.

As soon as the ripe fruit has been gathered, it is dried and freed from the husk; the raw beans are afterwards roasted in gauze cylinders over a gas or coal fire at a maximum temperature of 200° C.; during this process, the bean loses about 20 per cent. of its weight; the roasted bean is then ground for preparing the infusion.

Coffee has been adulterated by facing with ochre, prussian blue, etc. in order to improve its appearance; but these are easily detected by the increased percentage of ash, which in a genuine coffee should fall between 3·5 and 4 per cent. A number of imitation coffees have been placed on the market; among which may be mentioned black malt, from which pro-

ducts, having the general appearance of coffee beans, are prepared by mixing with gum and moulding. The most common
adulterant is chicory, this is the dried and roasted root of
Chicorium intybus, and its influence on a coffee mixture has
been summed up by Winter Blyth (*Foods: their Composition
and Analysis*, p. 359) as follows: (1) it increases the gum, (2) it
increases the sugar, (3) it decreases the fatty matter, (4) it
decreases the tannin, (5) it modifies the constituents of the ash.

There are on the market a number of semi-liquid substances
known as coffee extracts; they are obtained by extracting
coffee with boiling water and reducing the extract by evaporation to small bulk; they generally contain a sediment of caffeine
tannate, and are also very often either made from chicory or
adulterated with sugar solution.

Detection of chicory. The detection of chicory is a comparatively simple matter. A few grams of the sample are
placed in a beaker and thoroughly extracted with boiling
water; the mixture is kept boiling for about three minutes
with constant stirring, and afterwards allowed to cool and
settle; as soon as the grains have settled to the bottom of the
beaker, the water layer is carefully poured off; if no chicory is
present the grains will remain at the bottom of the beaker,
but, in the presence of chicory, some of the grains will rise up
the sides of the beaker, and these grains should be collected
and examined under the microscope, when the spiral vessels of
the chicory root will be easily recognized. The blunt ends of
the chicory cells are quite distinct from the lanceolate shape
of the coffee cells.

Estimation of chicory. It has been found that the specific
gravity of a 10 per cent. decoction of chicory is much higher
than that of a similar decoction of coffee and from this the
percentage of chicory can be determined. 10 grams of the
sample are weighed out into a 200 c.c. beaker and 100 c.c. of
water are added; the whole is then heated over a Bunsen
flame to boiling and kept at the boil, with constant stirring,
for three minutes; the mixture is allowed to settle and the decoction poured off through a filter paper into a 100 c.c. flask;
the grounds are washed with a very small quantity of hot
water, which is also poured through the filter paper; the filtrate

is now cooled to 60° F. and made up to 100 c.c.; the specific gravity of the decoction is taken either with a Westphal balance or with a specific gravity bottle, and the amount of chicory calculated from this.

Example: The specific gravity of a 10 per cent. decoction of a sample was 1020. The specific gravity of a 10 per cent. decoction of coffee should not exceed 1009·5, that of chicory should not be less than 1024·5, then

$$\frac{(1020 - 1009\cdot5) \times 100}{1024\cdot5 - 1009\cdot5} = 70 \text{ per cent. of chicory.}$$

The above method is not very accurate as the results obtained are influenced by the fineness of the coffee, by the method of working, and also by the variety of the coffee. Since the specific gravity of the 10 per cent. decoction is not constant, this difficulty has been overcome by a method devised by E. W. T. Jones (*Analyst's Laboratory Companion,* p. 133), which gives much more accurate results.

About 10 grams of the sample are placed in the water oven till dry; 5 grams of the dry sample are weighed out into a 300 c.c. beaker; about 200 c.c. of water are added, and the whole boiled for 15 minutes; the mixture is then allowed to settle and the liquid is strained through a wire gauze into a 250 c.c. graduated flask; the grounds are now boiled for five minutes with 50 c.c. of water and the liquid strained off as before; the mixed filtrates are then cooled, made up to the mark and filtered through a dry filter paper; 50 c.c. of the filtrate are measured out into a weighed platinum dish and evaporated to dryness on a water bath and finally dried in the water oven; the residue is calculated as a percentage extract on the dry sample.

Coffee when treated in this way gives a remarkably constant extract of 24 per cent., while the average extract of chicory is 70 per cent. The percentage of chicory in the sample is calculated from the formula

$$X = \frac{E - 24}{0\cdot46},$$

where X = the per cent. of chicory,
E = the per cent. of extract found.

Example: A suspected sample gave a percentage extract of 47, then $\dfrac{47 - 24}{0 \cdot 46} = 50$ per cent. of chicory.

Estimation of caffeine. Fendler and Stüber (*Zeit. Unter. Nahr. Gen.* 1914, XXVIII, 9). 10 grams of the powdered sample are well stirred with 200 c.c. of chloroform and 10 c.c. of 10 per cent. ammonia solution for 30 minutes; the mixture is filtered and 150 c.c. of the filtrate are evaporated to dryness; the residue is boiled with 80 c.c. of water and cooled; 20 c.c. of a 1 per cent. solution of potassium permanganate are added, followed by a slight excess of hydrogen peroxide (containing 1 per cent. of acetic acid); the whole is then digested over a water bath for 15 minutes, and, if a clear solution is not obtained, a further quantity of hydrogen peroxide is added; the solution is allowed to cool and is then filtered; the filter paper is washed with water and the filtrate is extracted with successive quantities of 50, 25 and 25 c.c. of chloroform; the mixed extracts are evaporated to dryness, and the caffeine is dried in the water oven to constant weight.

Of late years a practice has sprung up of selling mixtures of coffee and chicory, which are labelled "coffee" in very large letters and "with chicory" in very small letters; in some cases these mixtures contain very large proportions of chicory, sometimes upwards of 75 per cent.; in one case, in the City of Bristol, a sample was purchased containing at least 95 per cent. of chicory. There is no doubt that mixtures should not be legally sold containing more than 50 per cent. of chicory, as it has been decided by the High Court of Justice (Liddiard *v.* Reece and Horder *v.* Meddings, 44 J.P. 233 and 234) that where, in the opinion of the bench, the excess of chicory is added for the purpose of fraudulently increasing the bulk, an offence is committed. This difficulty is surmounted by the standard in the State of Victoria, where a mixture labelled "coffee and chicory" must contain at least 50 per cent. of coffee, and one labelled "chicory and coffee" must contain at least 50 per cent. of chicory.

The following analyses of various samples of coffee and coffee mixtures have been kindly supplied by Mr West Knights.

	(1)	(2)	(3)	(4)	(5)	(6)
Ash (per cent.) ..	4·40	5·10	4·10	3·90	5·40	5·53
Specific gravity of a 10 per cent. decoction	1009·3	1019·0	1009·0	1009·5	1017·0	1018·0
Chicory (per cent.) ..	none	59·0	none	none	47·0	53·0
Microscopic examination	satisfactory	showed cells of chicory	satisfactory	satisfactory	showed cells of chicory	showed cells of chicory

Analyses of the Ash of Coffee and Chicory.

	Coffee	Chicory
Potash (as K_2O)	53·72	25·80
Lime (as CaO)	6·06	10·61
Magnesia (as MgO) ..	8·34	7·03
Iron (as Fe_2O_3)	0·44	2·71
Sulphate (as SO_3) ..	3·05	10·83
Chlorine (as Cl)	0·72	4·23
Carbonate (as CO_2) ..	16·54	3·21
Phosphate (as P_2O_5) ..	11·13	10·59
Silica (as SiO_2)	—	10·09
Soda (as Na_2O)	—	14·90
	100·00	100·00

The following analyses are given by Ballard (*Compt. Rend.* 1918, CLXVII, 423; and *Analyst*, 1919, XLIV, 30).

	(1)	(2)	(3)	(4)	(5)	(6)
Moisture	3·0	5·6	5·9	8·9	7·2	4·9
Nitrogenous matter ..	14·4	17·4	16·0	12·6	8·9	45·6
Fat	12·5	8·1	8·1	1·3	3·5	21·7
Extractives	51·8	26·5	15·5	71·5	59·7	19·5
Cellulose	13·6	34·5	36·0	—	—	—
Ash	4·7	7·7	18·5	1·8	4·8	5·2
Sugar	—	—	—	3·9	15·9	3·1

No. (1) is a roasted coffee; Nos. (2) and (3) are roasted coffee shell; No. (4) is a mixture of roasted wheat and barley; No. (5) is roasted figs, and No. (6) roasted soya bean.

COCOA

The cocoa of commerce is prepared from the seeds of *Theobroma cacao*; the seeds are contained in a pod and when first picked are white, but gradually darken on exposure to air; after removal from the pod the seeds are sun-dried and roasted;

a process which develops the aroma and flavour; they are then cracked mechanically and the husks removed; the residue being known as cocoa nib. The seeds contain from 7 to 18 per cent. of husk, which is used for adulterating the cheaper forms of cocoa, and also as a useful addition to cattle food.

The following definitions of cocoa are of value: cocoa beans are the seeds of *Theobroma cacao*; cocoa of commerce consists of the powdered beans, more or less deprived of their fat; soluble cocoa or cocoa essence is the product obtained by treating powdered cocoa beans, more or less deprived of their fat, with alkali or an alkaline salt, and should not contain more than 3 per cent. of alkali or alkaline salt, calculated as K_2CO_3. Prepared or compound cocoa is cocoa mixed with other substances such as flour or sugar or both.

The chief adulteration of cocoa is the substitution of prepared cocoa, containing sugar or starch or both for powdered cocoa; the sale of prepared cocoa being perfectly legal provided that the admixture is disclosed on the label.

Analysis of Cocoa

Determination of the cold water extract. Thoroughly mix 5 grams of the cocoa with water in a glass mortar; wash the mixture into a 250 c.c. flask and make up to the mark; the mixture is allowed to stand for 24 hours with intermittent shaking, and it is then filtered; 10 c.c. of the filtrate are evaporated to dryness in a weighed glass dish on the water bath; dried in the water oven and weighed; the weight of the residue obtained multiplied by 500 gives the percentage of the water extract; should this percentage exceed 18 then added sugar is present.

Examples: The dry residue of a sample of cocoa obtained as above was 0·024 gram; then 0·024 × 500 = 12 per cent. of water extract; the sample does not therefore contain added sugar.

Another sample gave a residue of 0·066 gram; then 0·066 × 500 = 33 per cent. of water extract; the sample contains added sugar.

Estimation of fat. Weigh out 4 grams of the sample into a 100 c.c. flask; add 20 c.c. of strong alcohol and boil the whole on a water bath for three minutes; 20 c.c. of dry ether are now added; the flask is warmed on the water bath, well shaken, cooled and made up to 100 c.c. with dry ether; 2 c.c. of the ether are then added to compensate for the volume of the cocoa, and the contents of the flask are well mixed and allowed to settle; as soon as the contents have settled, 50 c.c. of the clear liquid are transferred to a flask with a pipette and evaporated to dryness on the water bath and allowed to cool; the residue in the flask is then taken up with ether and passed through a filter paper into a weighed flask; the filter paper is well washed with ether and the filtrate and washings are then evaporated to dryness on the water bath; the residue is dried in the water oven and weighed; the weight of residue obtained multiplied by 50 gives the percentage of fat.

Example: The weight of fat obtained by the above process was 0·68 gram, then the sample contained 0·68 × 50 = 34·0 per cent. of fat.

A rapid method for the estimation of fat in cocoa and chocolate is suggested by Hughes (*Chem. News*, 1919, CXIX, 104); the cocoa or chocolate is ground so as to pass through a 30-mesh sieve; 2 grams of the powdered sample are placed in a glass cylinder of about 40 c.c. capacity and 30 c.c. of 50 per cent. alcohol are added, and the whole is well mixed, and then subjected to centrifugal action in a Leffman-Beam centrifugal machine; the clear liquid is decanted and rejected, the residue is again washed with 30 c.c. of 50 per cent. alcohol, which is again rejected; to the residue 12·5 c.c. of methylated ether and 12·5 c.c. of petroleum ether are added, and the contents of the tube are well mixed for about 15 minutes and are then subjected to centrifugal action; the clear liquid is poured off into a weighed flask; the residue is treated as before with 12·5 c.c. of methylated ether and 12·5 c.c. of petroleum ether; the ether is distilled off from the mixed extracts and the residue of fat is weighed. This method is stated to give very accurate results, and, as the extracted fat is free from impurities, it is unnecessary to take it up again with ether.

Detection of "green butter" in cocoa butter. Revis and Bolton (*Analyst*, 1913, XXXVIII, 201). As "green butter" is often substituted for cocoa butter in chocolates, Revis and

Bolton have devised the following method of detecting this substitution: 1 gram of the clear fat is dissolved in 2 c.c. of a mixture of equal parts of carbon tetrachloride and petroleum ether (distilling below 40° C.); 2 c.c. of the resulting solution are cooled in water in a test-tube, and a solution of bromine in carbon tetrachloride (made by the addition of bromine to an equal volume of carbon tetrachloride) is added drop by drop, with constant shaking, until the colour of the bromine becomes permanent; very great care must be exercised in the addition of the bromine solution, as only one drop in excess is permissible; the test-tube is corked and allowed to stand for 15 minutes; if the solution is then clear cocoa butter is not present or is less than 10 per cent.; if the solution is turbid, cocoa butter is indicated. Revis and Bolton make this method roughly quantitative, by comparing the turbidity obtained with the sample with that obtained from known mixtures of cocoa butter and solid fat (*e.g.* cocoanut oil); after the turbidity has been compared, 2 c.c. of petroleum ether are added, the contents of the test-tube are mixed by inversion and allowed to stand overnight; the turbidity due to cocoa butter settles out as a very fine canary-coloured precipitate; that from "green butter" as a slight flocculent precipitate.

Estimation of the added cane sugar. 50 c.c. of the filtrate from the cold water extract are placed in a 100 c.c. flask and 5 c.c. of concentrated hydrochloric acid are added; the flask is placed in water, and the temperature is gradually raised until a thermometer in the flask indicates 68° C.; the temperature is maintained between 68 and 70° C. for five minutes; the acid is then neutralized with sodium hydrate solution, and the whole cooled in water and finally made up to 100 c.c.; the copper reducing power is then taken with Fehling's solution, as described under condensed milk (p. 138), and the cane sugar calculated from the weight of cupric oxide obtained by multiplying by 0·4091.

Example: The weight of copper oxide obtained from 25 c.c. of the inverted solution was 0·130 gram, then 0·130 × 0·4091 × 400 = 21·27 per cent. of cane sugar.

Determination of the ash. 5 grams of the sample are placed in a platinum dish and carefully ignited over a Bunsen flame until a white residue is obtained; the weight of this residue multiplied by 20 gives the percentage of ash.

Example: The residue obtained from 5 grams of a sample of cocoa was 0·775 gram, then 0·775 × 20 = 1·55 per cent. of ash.

Estimation of the alkalinity of the ash. The ash obtained above is dissolved in water and washed into a beaker; a few drops of methyl orange are added, and the contents of the beaker are titrated with N/10 sulphuric acid from a burette until a permanent pink colour is obtained. Each c.c. of N/10 sulphuric acid used = 0·0069 gram of alkalinity calculated as K_2CO_3.

Example: The ash of a cocoa required 16·5 c.c. of N/10 H_2SO_4 to produce a permanent pink colour; then

$$16·5 \times 0·0069 \times 20 = 2·28 \text{ per cent.}$$

of alkalinity calculated as K_2CO_3.

Estimation of the soluble ash. The residue from the cold water solids is gently ignited over a Bunsen flame and the ash weighed; the weight is multiplied by 500 to give the percentage; this should not be less than 2 per cent.

Example: The ash of a sample of cocoa obtained as described weighed 0·005 gram, then 0·005 × 500 = 2·5 per cent.

Estimation of added starch. The presence of added starch in cocoa is easily detected by a microscopical examination; but its exact estimation by chemical methods is almost impossible owing to the presence in cocoa of natural starch in varying quantities; the simplest method for the determination is a microscopical one and the results obtained are as near the true amount as those obtained by the most exact chemical methods. Standard mixtures of cocoa and the starch shown under the microscope are made (5, 10, 15, 20 per cent. etc. of starch) and these are compared under the microscope with slides of the sample; with a little practice the standard containing the same percentage of starch as the sample can easily be picked out.

Estimation of starch. Revis and Burnett (*Analyst*, 1915, XL, 429). 5 grams of the fat-free dry sample are thoroughly stirred with 50 c.c. of 10 per cent. (by volume) alcohol, filtered under pressure, washed with two further quantities of 50 c.c.

of 10 per cent. alcohol, and finally with 10 c.c. of 95 per cent. (by volume) alcohol, taking care that at no stage is the cocoa sucked dry. The moist cocoa is then scraped out and washed into a 250 c.c. flask with about 125 c.c. of boiling water; the liquid is well mixed, and the flask is placed in a boiling water bath for 15 minutes, with constant shaking. The contents of the flask are cooled to 38° C. and mixed with 0·05 gram of taka-diastase, 2 c.c. of toluene are added and the flask is shaken, stoppered and placed in an incubator at 38° C. for 24 to 36 hours, with occasional shaking. After incubation, 10 c.c. of N/10 sodium hydroxide solution are added and the flask is cooled to about 15° C., 100 c.c. of water are added, 10 c.c. of acid mercuric nitrate solution are run on to the surface and the volume is made up to 250 c.c. below the toluene, with water; the contents of the flasks are then well mixed and filtered. To 100 c.c. of the filtrate, 0·5 gram of sodium phosphate is added, and, when this has dissolved, 10 c.c. of sodium hydroxide solution are added with constant shaking; the flask is well shaken and the contents are filtered, the copper reducing power is determined on 50 c.c. of the filtrate; polarimetric readings of the filtrate are also taken.

The solution of sodium hydroxide used is so adjusted that 10 c.c. will just neutralize 4 c.c. of the acid mercuric nitrate solution.

Estimation of crude fibre. The residue left after the extraction of fat in the fat determination is washed into a boiling flask of 500 c.c. capacity, with not more than 200 c.c. of water; 50 c.c. of a 5 per cent. solution of sulphuric acid are added and the whole boiled under a reflux condenser for 30 minutes; pass the liquid through a filter paper and wash the residue back into the flask with boiling water, not more than 150 c.c. being used; add 50 c.c. of a 5 per cent. solution of sodium hydroxide and boil under a reflux condenser for 30 minutes; filter through a dried and weighed filter paper and wash the residue with boiling water, then with very dilute hydrochloric acid solution, followed by very dilute ammonia solution; the residue is then washed with boiling water until free from ammonia, dried in the water oven and weighed and multiplied by 25 to bring to the percentage.

Knapp and McLellan's method (*Analyst*, 1919, XLIV, 5).
2 grams of the fat-free cocoa are placed in a 500 c.c. flask and
200 c.c. of 1·25 per cent. sulphuric acid are added; the contents of the flask are boiled under a reflux condenser for exactly 30 minutes, they are then filtered through an ordinary
filter paper and washed with boiling water until free from acid;
the residue is rinsed back into the flask with not more than
200 c.c. of hot water, and 2·5 grams of 98 per cent. sodium
hydroxide are added, and the contents of the flask are again
boiled under a reflux condenser for exactly 30 minutes; they
are then filtered rapidly through a tared filter paper, washed
with boiling water until neutral, dried in a steam oven,
weighed, incinerated and reweighed; the loss in weight is considered as crude fibre.

A rapid method for filtering, during the estimation of crude
fibre is suggested by Pickel (*J. Ind. and Eng. Chem.* 1910, II,
281), in which the filtration is effected by the upward suction
of the fibre against linen, which is tied over the mouth of a
thistle funnel, the stem being connected to a filter pump; the
linen surface is kept in contact with the surface of the liquid
until all the liquid has been removed; the fibre is then washed
off the linen back into a beaker; the wash water is similarly
sucked up; and, finally, the fibre is washed into a tared basin,
the water is evaporated and the fibre is dried, weighed and
ashed.

Crude fibre in a sample of fat-free cocoa should not exceed
6·0 per cent.; any excess over this points to the addition of
cocoa husks, which contain about 18·5 per cent. of crude fibre
in the fat-free sample.

Example: The weight of residue obtained in a crude fibre
determination was 0·094 gram, then 0·094 × 25 = 2·45 per
cent. of crude fibre.

Estimation of cocoa shell. Baker and Hulton (*Analyst*,
1918, XLIII, 199). Use is made of a method, which is a modification by Macara of Filsinger's levigation method (*Zeit.
Offentl. Chem.* 1899, p. 29), but in view of the results obtained
by Knapp and McLellan (*Analyst*, 1919, XLIV, 11) with this
process, the results obtained must be regarded with very
great caution.

The sample is finely ground, and 10 grams are extracted with ether for 24 hours; the final traces of ether are removed by exposure to air and the residue is dried in a water oven, well ground in a mortar, made into a thin paste with water and transferred to a 500 c.c. cylinder; sufficient water is added to make the volume up to 400 c.c., and the whole is well mixed and allowed to settle for 15 minutes; the supernatant liquid is then blown off and the volume is again made up to 400 c.c. with water; the contents of the cylinder are again mixed, allowed to settle for 10 minutes, and the supernatant liquid is again blown off; this procedure is repeated twice, allowing the contents of the cylinder to settle for 5 minutes; if the residue shows much starch, it is finely ground and the process is repeated; the final residue is transferred to a platinum dish, dried, weighed and incinerated, the ash being deducted from the total residue; under these conditions, dry fat-free nib gives a residue of 3 per cent., and dry fat-free shell of 30 per cent. Baker and Hulton calculate the shell from the following formula:

$$S = \left(\frac{100M}{100 - (F + W)} - 3\right) \times \frac{100 - (F + W)}{27},$$

where S = the percentage of shell on the sample,
  M = the percentage of ash-free levigation sediment on the sample,
  F = the percentage of fat on the sample,
  W = the percentage of water on the sample.

Estimation of fibre. Baker and Hulton estimate the fibre on the fat-free sample, using 1·25 per cent. acid and alkali, and calculate the shell from the formula:

$$S = \left(\frac{K \times 100}{100 - (F + W)} - 5\cdot7\right) \times \frac{100 - (F + W)}{11\cdot1},$$

where S = the percentage of shell on the sample,
  K = the percentage of fibre on the sample,
  F = the percentage of fat on the sample,
  W = the percentage of water on the sample;

they assume that the fibre in dry fat-free nib is 5·7 per cent., and in dry fat-free shell is 16·8 per cent.

Estimation of nitrogen. Baker and Hulton estimate the nitrogen by the Kjeldahl method on 1 gram, and calculate the shell from the formula:

$$S = 2\cdot17 \{100 - (F + W)\} - \frac{100N}{2\cdot26},$$

where S = percentage of shell on the sample,
  N = percentage of nitrogen on the sample,
  F = percentage of fat on the sample,
  W = percentage of water on the sample;

they state that the nitrogen in fat-free nib should be 4·9 per cent. and in fat-free shell 2·64 per cent.

Detection of red sandars wood. Reichelman and Leuscher (*Zeit. Offentl. Chem.* 1902, VIII, 203). 2 grams of the sample are well shaken with 10 c.c. of absolute alcohol or acetone; with pure cocoa, the solvent is colourless and the solution gives no colour with ferric chloride solution, but it gives a white precipitate with dilute sodium hydroxide solution; in the presence of red sandars wood, the solvent is coloured, and the solution gives a deep violet colour with ferric chloride solution and with dilute sodium hydroxide solution; if the sandars wood has been previously exhausted, the colour can be obtained by pouring the ferric chloride solution down the side of the tube, when the colour will appear at the junction of the two liquids and disappear on shaking.

Typical Analyses of Cocoa (in percentages).

	(1)	(2)	(3)
Water	5·24	11·40	5·68
Fat	33·50	3·80	21·86
Crude fibre	2·73	15·91	1·41
Ash	4·45	7·40	1·55
Soluble ash	2·31	4·55	0·40
Cold water extract ..	12·00	—	33·00
Theobromine	1·00	—	—
Caffeine	0·32	—	—
Cane sugar	—	—	24·98
Starch	10·47	—	32·03

No. (1) is a genuine cocoa of commerce; No. (2) is an analysis of cocoa nibs; No. (3) is a sample of cocoa adulterated with starch and cane sugar.

The following analysis of the germ of the roasted cacao bean is given by Richards (*Analyst*, 1915, XLIII, 214):

Moisture	7·2	} per cent. on the original germ.
Fat	3·58	
Nitrogen	5·5	
Fibre	3·65	
Total mineral matter	7·3	
Soluble mineral matter	4·0	} on the fat-free dry matter.
Alkalinity (as K_2O)	1·69	
Cold water extract	28·7	
Levigation residue	38·3	

CHAPTER V

WHEAT FLOUR, SELF-RAISING FLOUR, BAKING POWDER—BREAD—RICE—PEARL BARLEY—STARCHES—INFANTS' FOODS

WHEAT FLOUR

WHEAT flour is the clean and sound product of ground wheat from which the husks have been removed; it should not contain more than 15 per cent. of water, nor less than 1·5 per cent. of nitrogen, nor more than 1 per cent. of mineral matter. Owing to the demand on the part of the purchasing public for excessive whiteness poor flours are occasionally bleached with oxides of nitrogen. Flours so treated are to be regarded as adulterated under the Sale of Food and Drugs Acts and are considered to be bleached flours when they contain more than one part per million of nitrite (*Local Government Board Food Reports*, No. 12). There are on the market a number of substances, which are sold under the name of "improvers," and as their sole property is to increase the power of the flour to absorb water, they can only be regarded as adulterations.

Determination of nitrite (Willard, *Bull. Kansas State Board of Health*, 1906, 11, 160). *Solutions required:* A. Weigh out 1 gram of sulphanilic acid and 14·7 grams of glacial acetic acid;

Measure out 286 c.c. of water;

Warm the sulphanilic acid with the acetic acid, diluted with an equal volume of water, until it is dissolved; carefully add the remainder of the water, warming and stirring the mixture to keep the sulphanilic acid in solution.

B. Weigh out 0·2 gram of α-naphthylamine and 14·7 grams of glacial acetic acid;

Measure out 350 c.c. of water;

Warm the naphthylamine with the acetic acid, diluted with twice its volume of water, till it has dissolved, then carefully add the remainder of the water.

The test solution is prepared by mixing equal volumes of A and B.

A cold water extract is made of the sample by digesting the flour with a large quantity of water and filtering; 50 c.c. of the filtrate are placed in a Nessler glass; and in another glass are placed 5 c.c. of a standard potassium nitrite solution (p. 13); the second glass being filled to the mark with water; 2 c.c. of the reagent are then added to each glass and both the standard and sample are allowed to stand for 15 minutes before comparing the pink colour. The depth of tint is then compared by pouring out either the standard solution or the sample, whichever has the deeper tint, until the columns left in the Nessler glasses are of equal tint.

This test is so sensitive that it cannot always be made in the ordinary laboratory owing to the possible presence of nitrites in the atmosphere which sensibly affect the result.

Total nitrogen. The nitrogen is determined by weighing 0·5 gram and proceeding in the usual way by Kjeldahl's method (p. 106).

Total ash. This is estimated by weighing out 5 grams and burning off all the organic constituents in a furnace; cool and weigh and calculate the result on 100 grams.

Estimation of gluten. An approximate estimation of the percentage of gluten in flour is obtained by taking 100 grams of the sample, and making this into a stiff paste with water; the paste is then placed on fine muslin and well kneaded under a stream of running water until no further starch passes through; the muslin bag is then well squeezed to remove as much water as possible, and the contents are transferred to a weighed watch glass and weighed; the weight of wet gluten obtained divided by 2·9 gives the approximate percentage of dry gluten in the sample.

Example: 100 grams of a sample of flour gave:

weight of wet gluten + weight of watch glass = 42·51 grams
weight of watch glass = 10·03 grams
weight of wet gluten = 32·48 grams

therefore the percentage of dry gluten $= \dfrac{32·48}{2·9} = 11·2.$

A good flour should contain from 10 to 12 per cent. of gluten; if the gluten content is less than 10 per cent., the resulting bread will be heavy and of close texture; whereas if the gluten exceeds 50 per cent., the flour is very tenacious and the dough will not rise.

Detection of potassium persulphate improver in flour (Hinks, *Analyst*, 1912, XXXVII, 91). The addition of potassium persulphate improver is detected by means of a 3 per cent. solution of benzidine. A portion of the flour is made into a paste with water and the benzidine solution at once poured over; the particles of potassium persulphate become blue coloured.

Detection of phosphate "improver." Curtel (*Ann. Falsific.* 1910, III, 302). 5 grams of the sample are shaken with 50 c.c. of carbon tetrachloride and centrifuged; the sediment is dissolved in nitric acid and a solution of molybdic acid is added; a yellow precipitate indicates added phosphate "improver" as pure flours do not yield a phosphate reaction when treated by this method.

In connection with the bleaching of flour, the *Reports of the Local Government Board*, 1911 (New Series, No. 49, *Food Reports*, No. 12), by Dr J. M. Hamill "On the bleaching of flour and the addition of so-called improvers to flour," and by Dr G. W. Monier Williams "On the chemical changes produced in flour by bleaching," are of great importance. These reports contain references to the important literature of the subject.

Typical Analyses.

	(1)	(2)	(3)
Carbohydrates ..	72·81	69·05	77·63
Albuminoids ..	11·25	12·83	5·41
Water	12·75	11·60	16·01
Oil	2·14	3·68	0·33
Fibre	0·37	1·48	—
Ash	0·68	1·36	0·62

SELF-RAISING FLOUR

Self-raising flour is wheat flour to which the elements of baking powder have been added. About 8 ozs. of sodium bicarbonate and 18 ozs. of cream of tartar to 1 cwt. of flour is the usual proportion; but occasionally phosphate baking powders are used, and, as these sometimes contain more than the allowable amount of calcium sulphate, it is necessary to determine the amount of calcium sulphate in self-raising flour.

Determination of calcium sulphate. Carefully incinerate 5 grams of the sample; dissolve the ash in dilute nitric acid and warm slightly; filter and determine the phosphate with ammonium molybdate as described under vinegar (p. 240). Well mix a further 5 grams of the sample with 1 gram of lime and carefully ignite the mixture; dissolve the residue in dilute hydrochloric acid and add a little bromine water; filter and precipitate the filtrate with barium chloride solution, filter off the precipitated barium sulphate, wash the precipitate well with hot water; dry in the water oven; incinerate and weigh; from the weight obtained subtract the weight of the ash of the filter paper, deduct the weight of barium sulphate obtained in a blank experiment and multiply the remainder by 0·5837; this gives the calcium sulphate in the sample.

Deduct from the percentage of phosphate found 0·25 per cent. naturally present in flour; multiply the remainder by two which gives pure acid calcium phosphate; add 1/9th, giving an impure phosphate powder containing 10 per cent. calcium sulphate; the calcium sulphate found plus the pure acid calcium phosphate gives the percentage of impure phosphate powder used, and the total calcium sulphate minus the amount constituting the 10 per cent. powder is the excess of calcium sulphate in the self-raising flour.

Example:

Total phosphate found 0·83 per cent.

less 0·25 per cent. natural to flour.

0·58

2

1·16 per cent. pure acid calcium phosphate.

plus 1/9th 0·13

1·29 per cent. of phosphate powder containing 10 per cent. CaSO$_4$.

Pure acid calcium phosphate .. .. 1·16 per cent.
CaSO$_4$ found .. .. 2·32 per cent.
Impure phosphate powder used in flour 3·48 per cent.
Total CaSO$_4$ .. .. 2·32 per cent.
Due to 10 per cent. phosphate powder 0·13 per cent.
Excess CaSO$_4$ .. .. 2·19 per cent.

Now 3·48 grams of impure phosphate powder contained 2·32 grams of calcium sulphate, then the original phosphate powder contained 66 per cent. of calcium sulphate.

Estimation of sulphates. Thomson's method (*Analyst*, 1914, XXXIX, 519). 20 grams of the sample of flour are heated in boiling water with 250 c.c. of water and 15 c.c. of hydrochloric acid (specific gravity 1·16) until the gelatinous starch is liquid; the mixture is then boiled for a few minutes, cooled and filtered; the precipitate is washed with dilute hydrochloric acid and the filtrate is evaporated to small bulk; the sulphate in the filtrate is precipitated with barium chloride solution as described above.

Cripps and Wright's method (*Analyst*, 1914, XXXIX, 429). 100 grams of the sample of flour are shaken with 1000 c.c. of 1 per cent. acetic acid solution for 1 hour, and then allowed to stand overnight; 50 c.c. are decanted and boiled with a little hydrochloric acid, nearly neutralized with ammonia solution, the proteins are then precipitated by the addition of tannin solution; the precipitate is filtered off and well washed, the filtrate is evaporated to small bulk, and the sulphate is precipitated with barium chloride solution.

Elsdon's method (*Analyst*, 1915, XL, 142). 10 grams of the sample are added to 25 c.c. of concentrated hydrochloric acid in a 250 c.c. beaker; the beaker is gently warmed on a water bath for a few minutes, with frequent shaking, until the liquid is a deep purple colour, and it is then heated on the water bath for about one hour, being placed on the metal cover so as not to come in contact with the steam; 100 c.c. of water are then added, and, after standing for a few minutes, the liquid is filtered and the filter paper is washed once with cold water. The filtrate is boiled, barium chloride solution is added and the precipitate of barium sulphate is collected and weighed.

Howard (*J. Ind. and Eng. Chem.* 1915, VII, 807) modifies the above method by using 200 c.c. of 5 per cent. hydrochloric acid, instead of 25 c.c. of concentrated acid.

Detection of maize starch. Occasionally the self-raising ingredients are added mixed with maize starch. White (*Analyst*, 1900, XXV, 317) gives the following qualitative test for maize starch; the sample is thoroughly mixed in a mortar and 1 gram is weighed out into a test-tube with 10 c.c. of water and well shaken; 15 c.c. of a 1 per cent. solution of sodium hydroxide are then added and the mixture allowed to stand for four hours; the whole of the wheat starch becomes gelatinized and a drop of the emulsion examined under the microscope shows the granules of maize starch very distinctly.

Estimation of maize starch (Embrey, *Analyst*, 1900, XXV, 310).

Solutions required:

(1) Potassium hydroxide solution containing 18 grams of potassium hydroxide in 1000 c.c.;

(2) Iodine solution containing iodine, 0·25 gram; potassium iodide, 1·00 gram; water to 250 c.c.;

(3) Hydrochloric acid solution containing hydrochloric acid (specific gravity, 1·16), 50 c.c.; distilled water, 150 c.c.

Weigh out:

(1) 0·2 gram of the sample.

(2) 0·18 gram of pure wheat starch and 0·02 gram of pure maize starch = 10 per cent. maize starch.

(3) 0·17 gram of pure wheat starch and 0·03 gram of pure maize starch = 15 per cent. maize starch.

(4) 0·16 gram of pure wheat starch and 0·04 gram of pure maize starch = 20 per cent. maize starch.

(5) 0·15 gram of pure wheat starch and 0·05 gram of pure maize starch = 25 per cent. maize starch.

(6) 0·14 gram of pure wheat starch and 0·06 gram of pure maize starch = 30 per cent. maize starch.

Place each of the above mixtures in a test-tube, fitted with a cork, add to each mixture 20 c.c. of the potassium hydroxide solution and shake for three minutes; then add to each 12 drops of the hydrochloric acid solution and centrifuge the mixture; remove 1 c.c. of the liquid, avoiding the deposit; make up to 50 c.c. with water in a Nessler glass and add two drops of the hydrochloric acid solution followed by 1 c.c. of the iodine solution; thoroughly mix the liquids and compare the tints; in this way the amount of maize starch can be estimated to within 5 per cent.

BAKING POWDER

Baking powder is a substance which gives off carbon dioxide on moistening and heating. A number of compounds are used for the purpose, all of which are to a greater or less extent mixed with starch. The following are typical compounds used: sodium bicarbonate or ammonium carbonate mixed with cream of tartar, tartaric acid, acid potassium sulphate, acid sodium phosphate, and acid calcium phosphate. The use of acid calcium phosphate and acid potassium sulphate is very objectionable, since the former often contains large quantities of calcium sulphate, and the latter, since with the sodium bicarbonate it forms potassium sulphate and sodium sulphate, both of which have a purgative action. The most satisfactory baking powder is a mixture of sodium bicarbonate or ammonium carbonate with cream of tartar and starch. Until the Sale of Food and Drugs Act of 1899, baking powder was not subject to analysis as a food, but the definition of food was altered in that Act expressly to include this substance. Adulterations of baking powder are the presence of alum and sulphates (especially calcium sulphate) and excess of starch; calcium sulphate is generally found in baking powders containing acid calcium phosphate, and the presence of this substance in amounts larger than 10 per cent. is to be looked upon as an adulteration (*Local Government Board Food Reports*, No. 13). J. White (*Analyst*, 1902, XXVII, 119) reports the substitution for cream of tartar of a substance having the following composition in percentages:

Moisture	..	4·10	Tartaric acid	..	47·07
Silica	..	0·30	Phosphate	..	6·97
Potash	..	15·50	Sulphate	..	12·70
Lime	..	9·10	Rice starch	..	5·00

and from which he deduces that the composition was:

Cream of tartar	..	..	64
Superphosphate	..	..	31
Rice starch..	..	..	5

The *British Pharmacopœia* requires that 1 gram of dry cream of tartar should require at least 10·5 c.c. of N/2 sodium hydroxide solution for neutralization, which corresponds to the presence of 98·77 per cent. of cream of tartar; the above sample required 4·8 c.c. of N/1 sodium hydroxide solution, corresponding to 90·24 per cent. of cream of tartar. Occasionally a substance known as "baking soda" is sold, it consists of sodium bicarbonate, and is very seldom, if ever, adulterated.

Estimation of available carbon dioxide. A Shrotter's carbon dioxide apparatus is carefully cleaned and dried; concentrated sulphuric acid is poured into the exit tube, in order to dry the carbon dioxide as it escapes; water is poured into the inlet tube and the whole apparatus is then weighed; about 1 gram of baking powder is inserted into the bulb and the apparatus is again weighed, the increase in weight is the amount of baking powder taken. The water is now allowed to run into the bulb, when a gentle stream of carbon dioxide is evolved; after the action has ceased air is sucked through the apparatus, which is then cooled and weighed; the loss in weight is due to the available carbon dioxide, which has escaped. Dilute hydrochloric acid is now placed in the inlet tube and the apparatus again weighed; the hydrochloric acid is then run into the bulb and the apparatus warmed on a water bath; when the reaction has ceased air is again sucked through the apparatus, which is allowed to cool and is then weighed; the loss in weight is due to unavailable carbon dioxide which, with the available carbon dioxide, constitutes the total carbon dioxide present.

Example: In an experiment 0·801 gram of baking powder was used, after the addition of water there was a loss in weight of 0·1065 gram, then the available carbon dioxide

$$= \frac{0 \cdot 1065 \times 100}{0 \cdot 801} = 13 \cdot 29 \text{ per cent.}$$

After the addition of hydrochloric acid there was a further loss of 0·016 gram, then the unavailable carbon dioxide

$$= \frac{0 \cdot 016 \times 100}{0 \cdot 801} = 1 \cdot 99 \text{ per cent.}$$

and the total carbon dioxide = 1·99 + 13·29 = 15·28 per cent. Baking powder should contain at least 8 per cent. of available carbon dioxide.

Estimation of carbon dioxide. Macara (*Analyst*, 1915, XL, 272) suggests that the "apparent" available carbon dioxide should be determined; he defines this as "the amount of carbonic acid liberated on boiling with water only for 30 minutes"; the method is as follows:

5 grams of baking powder (or 10 grams of self-raising flour) are placed in a dry litre distillation flask with a few pieces of pumice; this is connected with an absorption flask, containing 50 c.c. of a saturated solution of barium hydroxide, and 100 c.c. of well boiled and cooled water; 100 c.c. of alcohol are run into the distillation flask, and the mixture is well shaken to break down any lumps; 100 c.c. of water are added and the mixture is again shaken; 100 c.c. of liquid paraffin are then added and the contents of the flask are heated, with constant shaking, until the liquid boils briskly; the boiling is continued for 15 minutes; 400 to 500 c.c. of boiling water are then carefully added, and the boiling is continued for a further 15 minutes; the absorption flask should be well shaken, during the earlier part of the process, and a shallow basin of water placed under it, as soon as it begins to get hot. The absorption flask is then disconnected, closed, and cooled under running water. The excess of barium hydroxide is neutralized with 20 per cent. hydrochloric acid until the liquid is slightly acid to phenol phthalein; N/2 sodium hydroxide solution is then run in until the liquid is just alkaline; the flask is well shaken and the liquid is carefully neutralized with N/2 or N/10 hydrochloric acid; methyl orange is added and the titration is completed; with a little care, the barium carbonate can thus be titrated direct; but occasionally a little scale forms, in which case excess of acid must be added and the liquid heated for a few minutes, the excess of acid being determined by titration with N/10 sodium hydroxide solution.

The total carbon dioxide may be similarly determined by the addition of 20 to 25 c.c. of hydrochloric acid; the alcohol and paraffin are not necessary in this case.

Each c.c. of N/2 hydrochloric acid represents 0·011 gram

of carbon dioxide or each c.c. of N/10 hydrochloric acid represents 0·0022 gram of carbon dioxide.

Estimation of sulphates. 5 grams of the sample are dissolved in dilute hydrochloric acid by continuous boiling; a slight excess of barium chloride solution is added and the precipitate of barium sulphate allowed to settle; the solution is then carefully filtered, the precipitate is well washed, dried in a water oven, incinerated and weighed; the weight of ash, less the weight of the ash of the filter paper, multiplied by 0·3434 gives the weight of sulphates (as SO_3) in 5 grams of the sample.

Estimation of calcium. 5 grams of the sample are dissolved, with boiling, in dilute hydrochloric acid; a slight excess of ammonia is added, followed by a slight excess of acetic acid; any precipitate is filtered off, and to the filtrate is added an excess of ammonium oxalate; the precipitate of calcium oxalate is collected on a filter paper, washed, dried in a water oven, incinerated, ignited over a blowpipe, cooled, and weighed; the weight of the ash is the weight of calcium (as CaO) in 5 grams of the sample.

Estimation of tartaric acid. White's modification (*Analyst*, 1902, XXVII, 119) of Goldenberg's method (*Analyst*, 1896, XXI, 333). 2 grams of the sample are dissolved in 20 c.c. of hot water and 5 c.c. of dilute hydrochloric acid and made up to 100 c.c.; of this, 50 c.c. are made faintly alkaline with solid potassium carbonate, boiled for two minutes, cooled and made up to 100 c.c. Place 50 c.c. (= 0·5 gram of the powder) in a 500 c.c. flask with 10 c.c. of glacial acetic acid and 250 c.c. of a mixture of equal parts of alcohol (90 per cent.) and ether (sp. gr. ·730); close the flask with a well fitting cork; shake the contents well and allow them to stand for three hours; filter, wash the precipitate with the alcohol and ether mixture until the washings are neutral to litmus; dissolve the precipitate off the filter paper with boiling water and finally titrate with N/10 sodium hydroxide solution; each c.c. of N/10 sodium hydroxide solution used represents 0·0075 gram of tartaric acid or 0·0188 gram of cream of tartar.

Estimation of lead in tartaric acid and cream of tartar, and citric acid (Tatlock and Thomson, *Analyst*, 1908, XXXIII, 173). 10 grams of cream of tartar are treated with 50 c.c. of water and 40 c.c. of 2N ammonia (in the case of tartaric acid 81 c.c. of 2N ammonia and 9 c.c. of water, and in the case of citric acid 85 c.c. of 2N ammonia and 5 c.c. of water are used); agitate the mixture well until solution is complete; filter through a dry filter paper; to 50 c.c. of the filtrate add 0·1 gram of potassium cyanide and 1 c.c. of a strong colourless solution of ammonium sulphide, and compare with the colours obtained from a standard lead solution (see p. 19).

The *Report of the Local Government Board*, 1911 (New Series, No. 46, *Food Reports*, No. 13), by Dr J. M. Hamill "On the presence of calcium sulphate in baking powder and self-raising flour" should be consulted.

BREAD

Bread is the substance obtained by moistening, kneading and baking wheat flour, and to which porosity has been imparted by means of carbonic acid gas, obtained from baking powder, or by means of fermentation produced in the dough by the addition of yeast. Bread should not contain more than 45 per cent. of moisture, nor more than 1·5 per cent. of ash, nor more than 0·2 per cent. of ash insoluble in hydrochloric acid. In estimating the moisture in bread care must be taken to obtain a representative sample, as bread contains less moisture on the outside than in the middle of the loaf. The addition of foreign starches, in the form of boiled potatoes, is sometimes practised, but this adulteration is difficult if not impossible to detect owing to the alteration in the starch granules produced by the baking process. Occasionally alum is added to bread to produce that whiteness which the purchasing public considers to be synonymous with purity.

Detection of alum. *Solutions required:*

(1) Logwood solution; a freshly prepared alcoholic extract of logwood chips;

(2) A saturated solution of ammonium carbonate.

Dilute 5 c.c. of the logwood extract and 5 c.c. of the ammonium carbonate solution to 100 c.c., and pour the mixture over about 10 grams of bread crumbs in a small porcelain dish;

allow the mixture to stand for about five minutes; pour off the excess of liquid and dry the residue in the water oven; in the presence of alum, a lavender blue colour is produced, and in its absence, a reddish brown colour is obtained. Care must be taken that the bread has not become sour before the test is performed, as sour bread will occasionally give the alum colour. Care must also be taken that the logwood extract is always freshly made.

Estimation of alum. Carefully incinerate 100 grams of bread crumbs over a Bunsen flame, completing the process by the addition of a small quantity of sodium carbonate and potassium nitrate; dissolve the residue in water and acidify with dilute hydrochloric acid and evaporate to dryness in a platinum dish; moisten the residue with hydrochloric acid and dissolve in water; filter and wash the precipitate well with hot water; dry in the water oven, ignite, weigh and record the weight as silica (SiO_2).

The filtrate from the silica determination is poured into an excess of concentrated sodium hydroxide solution, boiled and filtered; acidify the filtrate with hydrochloric acid; add a few drops of sodium phosphate solution, followed by excess of ammonia, filter, well wash the precipitate, dry in a water oven, ignite and weigh; the weight obtained multiplied by 1·0397 gives the grains of ammonium alum per four pound loaf; allowance must be made for the aluminium phosphate naturally present in the bread, amounting to about 15 to 18 grains per four pound loaf.

Detection of potato starch. Schutz and Wein (*Chem. Zeit.* 1915, xxxix, 143; and *Analyst*, 1915, xl, 235). A few crumbs of the sample are steeped in water and well kneaded; a portion is placed between two cover slips, which are then forced apart; the cover slips are dried in the air, passed three times quickly through a flame and then treated with a drop of concentrated thionine solution, diluted with twice its volume of water, for 3 minutes and the excess of stain is removed by washing. Cereal starches remain unstained, while potato starch is coloured a deep reddish violet. Quantitative estimation may be made by comparison with mixtures of known composition.

Estimation of sugar in bread and biscuits (*Analyst*, 1917, XLII, 294). *Preparation of the sample:*

Biscuits. These are rapidly ground in a mortar or mincing machine and thoroughly mixed.

Bread. A slice of not less than ½ an inch in thickness is dried until the moisture is about 10 per cent.; it is then weighed again, ground and thoroughly mixed.

Buns and cakes. Several buns or cakes are coarsely broken, dried until the moisture is about 10 per cent., weighed again, ground and thoroughly mixed.

Articles containing fruit, etc., in which sugar is naturally present. A large portion is weighed and broken, and the fruit is removed and weighed; the cake is then treated as above, and the fruit is reserved for a determination of the sugar.

The process:

Estimation of moisture. 5 grams of the sample are dried to constant weight at 100° C.; the loss is corrected for previous drying, and also for removal of fruit, if necessary.

Estimation of sugar. 10 grams of the sample are ground up with about 200 c.c. of cold water, and transferred to a 250 c.c. flask; the flask is well shaken at intervals during 30 minutes; if necessary basic lead acetate solution, followed by sodium sulphate solution, or alumina cream, or copper sulphate solution, is added as a clearing agent; the liquid is then made up to 250 c.c. and filtered. 50 c.c. of the filtrate in a 100 c.c. flask are inverted as follows: 5 c.c. of 38 per cent. hydrochloric acid are added, and the solution is placed in a water bath at 70° C. until it reaches 69° C.; it is then maintained at 69° C. for 7 to 7½ minutes; the total time of heating being 10 minutes; the liquid is then cooled and neutralized, the volume is made up to 100 c.c. and the solution is filtered. The copper reducing power of the filtrate is determined with Fehling's solution and calculated as cane sugar. The amount of cane sugar estimated is corrected to the original moisture, and to the cake plus fruit, and from the quantity thus found, that due to added fruit is deducted. The amount due to fruit is estimated by determining the sugar in the fruit removed and the loss sustained, on the basis of the following average amount in water-free natural dried fruits: raisins 80, currants 80, figs 70, dates

(without stones) 70; 3 per cent. is deducted from the total
for sugars due to the flour, and an allowance of 2 per cent. is
made for variations in sampling, methods of analysis and
amount of sugar in materials employed.

The *Report of the Local Government Board* (New Series, No.
55) by Dr Hamill "On the nutritive value of bread made from
different wheat flours" is of considerable value as regards the
subject of nutrition. Dr Plimmer's *Analyses and energy values
of foods* (1921), should also be consulted.

RICE

Rice is the hulled grain of *Oriza sativa*; the lower grades are
sometimes polished to give them an appearance of higher
quality, and this is produced by the application of talc to the
grains; the talc is generally mixed with glucose, glycerine and
starch paste, and occasionally with mineral oil. Talc is a sili-
cate of magnesium with small quantities of the silicates of iron,
aluminium and potassium, and its general use for this purpose
is not advisable; should the ash of a sample of rice exceed 0·3
per cent. it is advisable to look for a coating of talc. The limit
of steatite or talc suggested by the Local Government Board
is 0·5 per cent.

Estimation of talc. A number of methods have been devised for the estimation of talc, but the simplest is that recommended by E. W. T. Jones (*Chem. News*, 1913, CVIII, 176)
in which 5 grams of rice are placed in a squat 150 c.c. beaker,
20 c.c. of ether are added and the whole agitated for a few
minutes; the ether is poured into a 100 c.c. beaker, containing
about 2 c.c. of water, and then evaporated off on a water bath;
the remaining ether is also evaporated from the rice grains
and about 15 c.c. of cold distilled water added; the whole is
agitated and the water added to the ether residue and repeated
four or five times until the water comes away clear; the mixed
washings are allowed to stand overnight; the clear supernatant
liquid is poured off, leaving the talc and a little fine rice behind,
which is transferred to a weighed platinum dish with methylated spirit, evaporated to dryness on a water bath, ignited

and weighed; the weight obtained is the weight of talc in 5 grams of the sample.

The following analyses of various samples of rice have been supplied by Mr J. West Knights. The numbers represent percentages.

	(1)	(2)	(3)	(4)	(5)	(6)
Ash	0·44	0·54	0·42	0·54	0·90	1·20
Steatite washed from the surface of the rice	0·14	0·16	0·09	0·23	0·47	0·75

All the samples except (6) are within the limit; No. (6) is of questionable genuineness.

PEARL BARLEY

Pearl barley is occasionally faced with talc; the ash of genuine pearl barley should not exceed 1·0 per cent.; the talc, if present, may be determined by the methods given under rice; rice powder is also frequently used as a facing and can be estimated by shaking a weighed quantity of the sample in a sieve, the rice powder passes through the sieve and can be collected and weighed; the powder should then be examined under a microscope and compared with slides containing known proportions of barley starch and rice starch in order to determine the proportion of rice powder in the dust.

STARCHES

The general appearance of the various starches under the microscope is an essential part of the examination of foods. A small portion of the starch should be placed in a small glass mortar and well mixed with water; a drop of the mixture is then placed on a glass slide, covered with a slip and examined under a 2/3 and 1/6 lens of a microscope. After a little practice the characteristic appearance of the various commoner starches becomes familiar and mixtures of starches can readily be distinguished.

Microscopical Appearance of the Commoner Starches.

1. *Potato.* This starch consists of oval granules, having an annular hilum at the smaller end and very distinct and complete rings; some of the granules are very large and some are very small; gives a good play of colours with polarized light and selenites; normal dimensions 0·06 to 0·1 mm.

2. *Arrowroot.* Not unlike potato, but the hilum is usually at the larger end, and the granules are chiefly of medium size only; and, in consequence, have a more uniform appearance; gives a play of colours with polarized light and selenites; average dimensions 0·036 mm.

3. *Wheat.* The granules are circular and flat; they seldom exhibit a hilum and are very variable in size; some are very large and some very small with a few intermediate in size.

4. *Maize.* The granules are various in shape from round to polyhedral; the hilum is prominent and often appears as an irregular cross. Average dimensions 0·018 mm. Concentric rings are practically invisible; with polarized light a fairly definite cross is exhibited, but not much colour with selenites.

5. *Barley.* This starch has circular granules, very similar to those of wheat, but slightly smaller; they exhibit no hilum, but some have rings.

6. *Rye.* The granules are not unlike barley, and some of them show a broken hilum.

7. *Rice.* Very similar to maize, in that the granules are angular, a starred hilum is sometimes visible, the granules are much smaller than maize and are very regular in size. Normal dimensions 0·005 to 0·0075 mm. There is practically no colour with selenites and polarized light, and only a very faint cross.

8. *Oat.* This starch also consists of polygonal granules, slightly larger than those of rice; there are usually a number of compound granules and under a very high power they exhibit a hilum.

9. *Sago.* The granules of this starch are oval and they exhibit a circular hilum and have faint rings; gives a good play of colours with polarized light and selenites.

10. *Tapioca.* All the granules are truncated at one end, so when resting on the flat end, they appear circular. The hilum,

which sometimes appears as though split into an irregular star, is generally not in the centre but nearer to the curved than to the flat surface. Normal dimensions 0·01879 mm. to 0·014 mm. Tapioca displays a fairly marked cross with polarized light and a slight iridescence with selenites.

11. *Pea* or *Bean*. The large pea granules have a broken longitudinal hilum in the centre and the bean granules are similar, except that perhaps they are a little larger and more uniform.

INFANTS' FOODS

The following methods of analysis of infants' foods are given by J. L. Baker (*Local Government Board Food Reports*, No. 20).

Estimation of starch. 5 grams of the sample are ground in a mortar with 10 to 15 c.c. of water, and 15 to 20 c.c. of hydrochloric acid (specific gravity 1·15) are added, 5 c.c. at a time; the mixture is allowed to stand for 30 minutes, and is then transferred to a 200 c.c. flask, containing 10 c.c. of a 4 per cent. solution of phosphotungstic acid and 20 c.c. of hydrochloric acid (specific gravity 1·15); the mortar is washed out, and the volume is made up to 200 c.c. with hydrochloric acid (specific gravity 1·1); the mixture is well shaken, allowed to stand for 30 minutes and then filtered; the rotation is taken in a 200 mm. tube at 20° C. and the percentage of starch is calculated from the formula:

$$P = \frac{R \times 40}{11 \cdot 6},$$

where P = the percentage of starch,
  R = the reading.

If sugars are present, the following corrections must be made before using the formula:

the percentage of cane sugar × 0·028 is added to the reading,
the percentage of dextrose × 0·07 is deducted from the reading,
the percentage of lactose × 0·07 is deducted from the reading.

Estimation of cold water extract. 10 grams of the sample are extracted, with frequent shaking, for 3 hours at 15·5° C. with 200 c.c. of water (if the fat exceeds 5 per cent., fat-free material should be used); the solution is filtered, and the specific gravity, rotatory power and soluble carbohydrates are determined on the filtrate.

Estimation of reducing sugar, other than lactose. The copper reducing power of the cold water extract is determined with Fehling's solution (see p. 138), and calculated as dextrose, a correction being made in the presence of lactose.

Estimation of cane sugar. A portion of the cold water extract is boiled with a 2 per cent. solution of citric acid, in order to invert the cane sugar; the copper reducing power is then taken, the reducing sugar, already determined, is deducted and the remainder, less 1/20th, gives the cane sugar.

Estimation of lactose. The aqueous extract is boiled with a 2 per cent. solution of citric acid, exactly neutralized, and a little diastatic malt extract added. In the presence of 2 or 3 per cent. of sugars, 0·5 gram per 100 c.c. of brewers' yeast is then added; the vessel is closed with a cotton wool plug, and the contents are incubated at 27° C. for 3 days; the resulting solution is cleared with alumina, filtered, boiled, made up to volume and titrated with Fehling's solution. 1 c.c. of Fehling's solution corresponds to 0·0075 gram of pure lactose.

Estimation of fat. The fat cannot be always estimated by extraction with ether in a Soxhlet apparatus, and is therefore determined by the Werner-Schmidt or the Rose-Gottlieb method (see pp. 104, 105).

Estimation of proteins. The nitrogen is determined on 0·5 gram of the sample by the Kjeldahl method (see p. 106), and the amount multiplied by 6·25 gives proteins.

Estimation of moisture. 5 grams of the sample are dried in the water oven for 5 hours, the loss in weight being taken as moisture.

Estimation of mineral matter. 5 grams of the sample are incinerated at a low red heat. In some cases the incineration is very difficult, and the sample should then be treated with sulphuric acid, and 1/10th of the ash should be deducted as a correction.

Estimation of cellulose. 5 grams of the sample (fat-free, if more than 1 per cent. of fat is present) are made into a thin paste with cold water, diluted to about 200 c.c. and boiled for 30 minutes; the solution is then cooled to 80° C. and 5 c.c. of diastatic malt extract are added; the mixture is allowed to stand for 5 minutes, and is then brought to the boil and cooled to 60° C., and a further quantity of 25 c.c. of diastatic malt extract is added, and the whole is maintained at 60° C. for 4 hours; the mixture is filtered, the residue is well washed with water at 60° C., and, when quite free from reducing sugars, with alcohol and ether; the residue is dried and weighed, and the proteins are determined. A duplicate experiment is at the same time carried out, except that the ash is determined instead of the proteins; the weight of the residue, less the weight of ash and proteins, is calculated as cellulose.

CHAPTER VI

PEPPER, CAYENNE, MUSTARD—NUTMEG, CINNAMON, GINGER

PEPPER

PEPPER is the dried berry of *Piper nigrum*; black pepper is the immature whole berry, sun-dried or roasted and ground; white pepper is the mature berry from which the outer coating has been removed.

The chief adulterants of pepper are: excess of mineral matter (sand, etc.), starch (chiefly rice), long pepper, added husk, and ground olive stones or pepperette or poivrette. It must be stated that the public themselves are primarily responsible for the adulteration of pepper, since of late years a craze has grown for excessive whiteness in pepper.

The following standard for pepper is in force in the Commonwealth of Australia (*Analyst*, 1917, XLII, 255):

Black pepper.

Not more than 5 per cent. of white berries.

Not more than 15 per cent. of waste material.

Not more than 7 per cent. of total ash.

Not less than 6 per cent. of extract soluble in ether.

Not less than 8 per cent. of extract soluble in ethyl alcohol.

White pepper.

Not more than 5 per cent. of black berries.

Not more than 7 per cent. of immature berries.

Not more than 3·5 per cent. of ash.

Not less than 6 per cent. of extract soluble in ether.

Not less than 7 per cent. of extract soluble in ethyl alcohol.

Detection of adulteration. The addition of starch is detected under the microscope and the amount of foreign starch determined by comparison with standard slides as described under cocoa (p. 188); ground olive stones and long pepper may also be detected by a microscopical examination, olive stones showing bright with a red tint under polarized light, and long pepper a bluish tint. In a routine analysis the determinations usually made are the total ash, the ash insoluble in hydro-chloric acid and the crude fibre; the total ash of a black pepper should not exceed 5·5 per cent. and of a white pepper 3 per cent.; the crude fibre should not exceed 5 per cent. Campbell Brown (*Analyst*, 1887, XII, 24) has shown that the crude fibre of poivrette is 48·48 per cent., of ground almond shells 51·68 per cent. and of olive stones 45·38 per cent.

Detection of poivrette (Martelli, *Staz. Sper. Ag. Ital.* XXVIII, 53). Digest for two or three days 1 gram of phloro-glucinol in 50 to 60 c.c. of hydrochloric acid (specific gravity 1·1) and decant the clear solution. To about 0·5 gram of the sample of pepper add sufficient of the reagent to cover it and heat cautiously until fumes of hydrochloric acid begin to come off; poivrette and similar substances (*e.g.* almond shells, wal-nuts, etc.) give a very intense cherry red colour easily dis-tinguished by the naked eye from the yellow colour of pepper. On adding to the mass a little water and decanting the liquid a violet red powder is left, which consists almost entirely of poivrette stained by the reagent.

Detection of turmeric (Parry, *Chem. and Drugg.* 1914, LXXXIV, 34). *Solution required:*

Weigh 1 gram diphenylamine;

Measure 20 c.c. of 90 per cent. alcohol,
         25 c.c. of sulphuric acid.

Dissolve the diphenylamine in the alcohol, add the sul-phuric acid and cool. One drop of the reagent is placed on a microscopical slide, and a small quantity of the sample on a cover glass; the cover glass is then mounted over the slide so that the sample falls on the reagent; the particles of turmeric will be found to be coloured a fine purple. The proportion of turmeric present in the pepper is estimated by comparison with slides containing a known amount.

Typical Analyses of Pepper (in percentages).

				A	B	C
Water ..			..	9·83	10·60	9·71
Ash ..			..	3·70	1·34	1·35
Volatile oil		..		1·60	1·26	1·47
Starch ..			..	37·30	43·10	31·45
Crude fibre		..		10·02	4·20	3·92

A is a sample of Singapore black pepper, B of Singapore white pepper, C of commercial white pepper.

CAYENNE

Cayenne is the dried and powdered or ground fruit of *Capsicum fastigiatum, Capsicum frutescens*, or of *Capsicum annum*; it is very rarely adulterated in England, but occasionally foreign starch, mineral matter and ground olive stones have been found. The presence of foreign starch is detected by a microscopical examination; excessive mineral matter by the ash, and the ash insoluble in hydrochloric acid; the ash of a genuine sample of cayenne should not exceed 7 per cent. and the ash insoluble in hydrochloric acid 0·5 per cent.; a determination of the crude fibre will show the presence of ground olive stones, genuine cayenne having a crude fibre of not more than 28 per cent.

A typical Analysis (in percentages) of a genuine Cayenne by Richardson (U.S. Dept. of Agric. Bull. XII, p. 211).

Water	..	..	5·74
Ash	..	..	5·24
Volatile oil		..	17·90
Fixed oil		..	1·58
Crude fibre		..	18·10
Albuminoids	..	..	11·20

MUSTARD

Mustard is the ground seed of *Sinapis alba, Brassica juncea* or *Brassica nigra*; after grinding the mass is sifted and a large part of the oil removed; the pungent properties of mustard are due to the presence of allyl isothiocyanate, which is produced by the action of the enzyme myrosin and water on the potassium myronate present in the seed. The most common adulterants of mustard are starch and turmeric; in the natural state mustard should contain no starch, but a practice has arisen of mixing mustard with comparatively large quantities of starch, the manufacturer stating that the presence of starch is necessary to prevent decomposition and caking and that the customers prefer it so mixed; but this contention has no foundation in fact and the mixture is usually sold as "Mustard Condiment."

In the routine examination of mustard, the presence of

starch is detected by the microscope and the percentage by comparison with standard slides.

Detection of turmeric. A small portion of the sample is treated with ammonia and examined under a magnifying glass, in the presence of turmeric some of the grains will be coloured red; or a strip of filter paper may be soaked in an alcoholic extract of the sample, then in a solution of borax, finally acidified with hydrochloric acid and allowed to dry; in the presence of turmeric a rose red colour is produced, which becomes a deep blue when treated with ammonia, or a green when treated with dilute potassium hydroxide solution.

Estimation of oil. 5 grams of the mustard are placed in a Soxhlet thimble in a Soxhlet extractor and treated with ether on a water bath until the ether passes over colourless, when the flask is removed and the ether evaporated off, and the residue dried in a water oven to constant weight.

In a sample from which the oil has not been removed, the percentage of mustard may be calculated roughly from the formula

$$\frac{\text{per cent. of oil} \times 100}{30}.$$

Typical Analyses of Mustard (in percentages).

			A	B	C
Moisture	..	..	5·55	6·83	6·43
Total ash ..	..	..	5·58	5·03	4·37
Ether extract	..	..	17·46	13·81	27·45
Alcohol extract	..	..	25·31	14·21	16·31
Volatile oil ..	..	..	3·98	2·26	0·00
Crude fibre ..	..	..	3·28	10·90	4·95

A was a sample of commercial English brown mustard flour, freed from husk, and with a portion of the fixed oil removed; B was a sample of English brown mustard husk; C was a sample of whole ground mustard seed.

NUTMEG

Nutmeg is the fruit of *Myristica fragrans*, artificially dried or sun-dried and deprived of its testa; when the fruit contains its testa it is known as mace; owing to the fact that nutmeg is generally sold as a whole fruit, adulteration is practically impossible and only becomes possible when the sample is ground. In the routine examination of nutmeg the usual determinations are the ash, which should not exceed 5 per cent.; the ash insoluble in hydrochloric acid, which should not exceed 0·5 per cent.; and the crude fibre, which should not exceed 10 per cent.

Caraway Seeds. These are the seeds of *Carum carui* and should contain at least 5 per cent. of oil, and not more than 7 per cent. of mineral matter; they are sometimes adulterated by the removal of the oil by distillation, the seeds being subsequently dried.

Cloves. Cloves are the dried calxy and buds of *Eugenia caryophyllata* and are chiefly obtained from Zanzibar and the East Indies; they contain about 15 per cent. of volatile oil and about 5 per cent. of non-volatile oil; the *British Pharmacopœia* requires that the ash of cloves shall not exceed 7 per cent.; cloves are occasionally adulterated by removal of a portion of the oil, which can be detected by the determination of the ether extract; they are also adulterated occasionally by the partial or total substitution of pimento, which is easily detected by the microscope, and by the determination of the ether extract, as pimento rarely contains more than 5 per cent. of volatile oil.

CINNAMON

Cinnamon is the bark of *Cinnamomum zeylanicum,* from which the outer layers have been removed, for which cassia or the dried bark of *Cinnamomum cassia* is occasionally substituted; this substitution is easily detected by the naked eye, cinnamon being thin and containing no outer bark, whereas cassia is thick and contains the outer bark. The larger portion of cinnamon is obtained from Ceylon, cassia being grown in China or India; cinnamon is chiefly required for the volatile oil which it contains. Dyer and Gilbard (*Analyst,* 1895, xx, 129) have found cinnamon adulterated with ground walnut shells. In the routine examination of cinnamon, the ash, which should not exceed 6 per cent., is determined and the sample is examined microscopically.

Typical Analyses (in percentages).

				A	B
Moisture	..	..	..	12·41	9·97
Total ash	..	..	..	4·22	0·87
Ash soluble in water		..		0·46	0·37
Ash insoluble in water		..		2·76	0·50
Fibre	..	..	..	34·25	47·67

These analyses are by Dyer and Gilbard (*Analyst*, 1895, xx, 129); A is of cinnamon and B of ground walnut shells.

GINGER

Ginger is the dried rhizome of *Zingiber officinale*, from India, China or Jamaica, washed and sun-dried, and sometimes scraped and immersed in a solution of lime which prevents the destruction of the rhizome from the attacks of insects. The most common adulterants of ginger are exhausted ginger, excessive mineral matter, foreign starches, turmeric and capsicum. The usual determinations are crude fibre (not more than 8 per cent.), total ash (not more than 8 per cent.), lime (not more than 1 per cent.), ash insoluble in hydrochloric acid (not more than 3 per cent.) and the aqueous extract.

Detection of capsicum (Garnett and Crier, *Pharm. Jour.* 1909, vol. LXXXVII, 441). A small portion of the sample is heated with a dilute solution of potassium hydroxide which destroys the pungent odour of ginger but not of capsicum.

Determination of the ash. 5 grams of the sample are incinerated in a platinum dish over a Bunsen flame and weighed; the weight of ash multiplied by 20 gives the percentage of total ash; the ash is then extracted with hot water, the solution is filtered, the residue on the filter paper is well washed with hot water, dried in a water oven and incinerated; the weight of the ash, less the weight of the ash of the filter paper, multiplied by 20 gives the percentage of insoluble ash, and this deducted from the total ash gives the percentage of soluble ash.

Determination of the cold water extract (Winton, Ogden and Mitchell, *U.S. Dept. of Agric. Bull.* LXV, 59). Four grams of the sample are placed in a 200 c.c. graduated flask and water is added to the mark; the mixture is shaken at intervals for 8 hours and then allowed to stand for 16 hours. The contents of the flask are then filtered and 50 c.c. of the filtrate are evaporated to dryness, dried in the water oven and weighed; the weight of the residue multiplied by 100 gives the cold water extract.

Detection of exhausted ginger. Commercially there are two varieties of exhausted ginger, one the product left after the alcoholic extraction for the preparation of ginger extract, and the other the product of the water extraction in the preparation of ginger beer, etc. Dyer and Gilbard (*Analyst*, 1893, XVIII, 197) have shown that the ash soluble in water is a reliable method of detecting exhausted ginger, since the water soluble ash of a genuine ginger varies from 1·9 to 3 per cent., whereas an exhausted ginger gives a water soluble ash of from 0·2 to 0·5 per cent.

Detection of foreign starches, etc. The microscopic appearance of ginger is so characteristic that adulteration with foreign starches has fallen into disuse; but a microscopical examination should always be made for foreign substances.

Typical Analyses (in percentages).

			(1)	(2)
Moisture ..	..	..	13·6	12·1
Volatile oil	..	..	0·7	0·8
Fixed oil	..	..	3·0	5·2
Alcoholic extract		..	3·1	1·2
Total ash	..	..	3·1	2·1
Soluble ash	..	..	2·4	0·4
Insoluble ash	..	..	0·7	1·7

No. (1) is a genuine ginger and No. (2) is an exhausted ginger.

CHAPTER VII

CANE SUGAR—GOLDEN SYRUP AND TREACLE—
HONEY—JAM

CANE SUGAR

CANE sugar is found in the sap and fruits of a very large number of plants. Its chief manufacturing sources are the beet (*Beta vulgaris*), the sugar cane (*Saccharum officinarum*) and the sugar maple (*Acer saccharinum*). When heated to 160° C. cane sugar forms a light amber coloured mixture of dextrose and lævulose, known as "barley sugar," and when heated above this temperature it forms caramel. Adulteration of cane sugar is very rare; occasionally ultramarine blue is added to correct the yellow colour, and coloured crystals are sold in substitution for Demerara sugar, which is or should be manufactured in Demerara. The sale of yellow crystallized cane sugar, regardless of the place of origin, as Demerara sugar is now legal (Anderson *v.* Britcher 78 J. P. 65). The colour is imparted to Demerara sugar by the addition of tin chloride, which fixes the natural colour on the sugar crystals and is itself almost completely removed in the molasses. In the manufacture of sugar, the beet or sugar cane is first cleansed from mud and stones and then sliced; and the juice extracted by pressure or diffusion. The juice is then clarified by the addition of lime to the warm solution; the excess of lime is precipitated by means of CO_2; the juice, which has now an amber colour, is concentrated with exhaust steam and finally crystallized in "vacuum pans"; the crystals are separated from the molasses by centrifugal force and the molasses then treated with strontium hydroxide, which forms with the saccharose a precipitate of insoluble strontium saccharate; this is decomposed with CO_2 giving a further crop of cane sugar crystals.

Detection of ultramarine blue. 50 grams of the sample of sugar are dissolved in water and allowed to stand overnight, when the colouring matter will sink to the bottom and should be washed by decantation; the residue is then treated with hydrochloric acid, when the blue colour will be discharged with evolution of sulphuretted hydrogen.

Detection of dyed crystals. The sample is extracted with alcohol (90 per cent.); the solution is filtered and evaporated to dryness and the residue taken up with alcohol; a skein of wool is then placed in the solution and the whole placed on a water bath for 30 minutes; the wool is then removed and dried; in the presence of artificial dye the wool will be coloured yellow.

GOLDEN SYRUP AND TREACLE

Golden syrup and treacle are bye products in the manufacture of cane sugar and consist principally of cane sugar, dextrose and lævulose. They contain from 30 to 35 per cent. of cane sugar, which cannot be separated by direct crystallization and they should not contain more than 20 per cent. of water. They are frequently adulterated by the addition of starch-glucose, which is the product obtained by the hydrolyzing of starch until the greater part has been converted into dextrose.

Analysis of golden syrup and treacle. The most convenient method of analysis for these products is that devised by E. W. T. Jones (*Analyst*, 1900, XXV, 67).

Estimation of total solid matter. 25 grams of the sample are dissolved in water and made up to 250 c.c.; the specific gravity of this solution (which should not be less than 1032, indicating 20 per cent. of water) is taken with the specific gravity bottle, and the excess gravity over 1000 is divided by four, giving the total solid matter. Jones finds that this gives a more accurate practical figure than that obtained by dividing by 3·86 which is theoretically correct. The percentage of total solid matter subtracted from 100 gives the water.

Example: The specific gravity of a 10 per cent. solution of a sample of golden syrup was 1032·7, then the sample contained $\frac{32\cdot7}{4} = 8\cdot175 \times 10 = 81\cdot75$ per cent. of solid matter, and $100 - 81\cdot75 = 18\cdot25$ per cent. of water.

The amount of water in the sample cannot be determined

in the usual way by drying a weighed quantity of the sample in the water oven, owing to the impossibility of removing all the water.

Estimation of cane sugar and starch glucose. The temperature of the 10 per cent. solution is raised to 17·5° C.; the solution is examined in the polarimeter tube (100 mm.) and the angle of rotation noted; 50 c.c. of the 10 per cent. solution are then heated with 5 c.c. of N/1 hydrochloric acid in a 100 c.c. flask in a boiling water bath for 20 minutes; the solution is then cooled; 5 c.c. of N/1 sodium hydroxide solution are added and the whole is made up to 100 c.c. at 15·5° C.; the resulting solution is then raised to 17·5° C. and the reading taken in the polarimeter and multiplied by two to correspond to the 10 per cent. solution. If the sample after inversion has a dextro-rotation, starch glucose is present and its amount is calculated from the formula

$$\frac{([\alpha]_D \text{ after inversion} + 11) \times 100}{120}.$$

The amount of cane sugar is calculated from the alteration in the specific rotatory power after inversion. The specific rotatory power of cane sugar is $[\alpha]_D + 66\cdot5°$, and that of invert sugar is $[\alpha]_D - 19\cdot6°$; then the amount of cane sugar in a sample is calculated from the formula

$$\frac{100 \times ([\alpha]_D \text{ after inversion} - [\alpha]_D \text{ before inversion})}{[\alpha]_D \text{ of cane sugar} - [\alpha]_D \text{ invert sugar}}.$$

Example: A sample of syrup gave a specific rotatory power after inversion of $[\alpha]_D = + 11\cdot07$,

then $\dfrac{(11\cdot07 + 11) \times 100}{120} = 18\cdot4$ per cent.

of starch glucose in the sample. The sample was said by the manufacturers to contain 18 per cent. of glucose syrup.

A sample of syrup gave $[\alpha]_D$ before inversion $+ 19\cdot0$, and after inversion $[\alpha]_D - 12\cdot5$; then the cane sugar in the sample was

$$\frac{100 (19\cdot0 - 12\cdot5)}{66\cdot5 - 19\cdot6} = 36\cdot62 \text{ per cent.}$$

Determination of the copper reducing power. 10 c.c. of the 10 per cent. solution are made up to 100 c.c., and 20 c.c. of this solution are added to 50 c.c. of Fehling solution, diluted with 30 c.c. of water, in a boiling water bath; the mixed solutions are allowed to remain in the water bath for 12 minutes and then filtered; the precipitate is well washed, dried in a water oven, ignited in a porcelain crucible and weighed as CuO; the weight of CuO obtained multiplied by 0·4307 gives the invert sugar.

Example: The weight of CuO obtained in an experiment was 0·210, then 0·210 × 0·4307 = 0·090447 × 500 = 45·22 per cent. of invert sugar.

10 c.c. of the 10 per cent. solution are now inverted as described above and made up to 100 c.c.; 20 c.c. of this solution are added to 50 c.c. of Fehling solution as before. The weight of CuO obtained in the first experiment is deducted from that obtained in the second experiment, and the difference multiplied by 0·4091 gives the cane sugar.

Example: After inversion the sample of syrup gave 0·366 gram of CuO, then 0·366 − 0·210 = 0·156 × 0·4091 = 0·0638196 × 500 = 31·91 per cent. of cane sugar.

Estimation of water. Testoni (*Staz. Sper. Agraire. Italiana,* 1904, XXXVII, 366). 50 grams of the sample are placed in a 400 c.c. distillation flask with 200 c.c. of oil of turpentine and distilled; the distillate, passing over below 150° C., is collected in a graduated cylinder; the volume of the water layer multiplied by 2 gives the percentage of water in the sample.

HONEY

Honey is the saccharine exudation of plants which has been collected, modified and stored in the honeycomb by the honey bee (*Apis mellifica*). It consists principally of dextrose and lævulose in roughly equal proportions and a small quantity of cane sugar. It should not contain more than 25 per cent. of water. Honey is extensively adulterated chiefly with cane sugar or starch glucose. A 10 per cent. solution of honey examined in the polarimeter should always show a lævo-rotation. In the event of a sample showing a dextro-rotation, either it contains added cane sugar, or it is artificial honey, or it contains starch glucose. The analysis of honey is carried out exactly as if it were a sample of golden syrup. A solution of the sample should be tested for calcium with ammonia and ammonium oxalate, and for sulphates with hydrochloric acid and barium chloride, as the presence of calcium sulphate is an indication of the presence of starch glucose.

Some typical analyses of various sugars (in percentages).

	(1)	(2)	(3)	(4)	(5)	(6)
Cane sugar	32·71	22·39	1·78	36·49	85·92	2·29
Invert sugar	44·91	20·45	77·12	32·14	6·84	71·43
Starch glucose	—	35·35	—	—	—	—
Water	18·29	20·06	20·75	20·32	5·37	21·64
Ash	3·00	1·40	0·22	8·45	1·37	4·15
Total solid matter	81·71	79·94	79·27	79·56	94·63	78·36

No. (1) is a sample of golden syrup; No. (2) is a sample of golden syrup containing 35 per cent. of starch glucose; No. (3) is a sample of honey; No. (4) is a sample of treacle; No. (5) is a commercial cane sugar; and No. (6) is an artificial invert sugar.

JAM

Jam is a mixture prepared by boiling fruit pulp. Jams of the highest quality contain nothing but the pulp and juice of the fruit, after which they are named, and pure cane sugar. The pulp mixed with the necessary proportion of water is boiled, and varying amounts of sugar are added, from one-third to one-half of the whole; the final product is solid, caused by the gelatinization which has taken place owing to the presence of pectin in the juice.

Adulterations. In the case of some fruits, notably raspberry and strawberry, there is present only a small quantity of pectin, and it is therefore necessary, in order to obtain the correct consistency in the finished product, either to boil the mixture for a considerable time, which spoils the appearance, or to add some fruit juice rich in pectin, as for example apple or gooseberry juice. Provided that this addition is notified on the label, it cannot be regarded as an adulteration, since it is not added for the purpose of increasing the bulk. At the same time it must be noticed that some manufacturers take advantage of this fact to add comparatively large quantities of apple pulp, and this must be regarded as an adulteration. Occasionally, for the sake of cheapness, commercial glucose is used instead of cane sugar.

Estimation of water. The determination of water in jam is exceedingly difficult, owing to the practical impossibility of driving off the last traces of water. The sugars, estimated by Fehling's process, plus 6 per cent. allowed for fibre and other constituents, deducted from 100, give a fair approximation of the amount present. A jam should not contain more than 35 per cent. of water.

Estimation of insoluble matter. 25 grams of the sample are heated in a 200 c.c. flask on a water bath for 30 minutes, and filtered through a weighed filter paper; the residue is returned to the flask and twice extracted with water and filtered; the residue on the filter paper is well washed with hot water, dried at 105° C. and weighed; the weight obtained, less the weight of the filter paper, multiplied by 4 gives the percentage of insoluble matter.

Estimation of glucose. 10 grams of the jam are dissolved in about 70 c.c. of water in a 200 c.c. flask; 7 c.c. of concentrated hydrochloric acid are added; the mixture is heated to 68° C. and kept at that temperature for five minutes; the solution is then cooled and neutralized with sodium hydroxide solution; 10 c.c. of lead subacetate solution are added to clarify the mixture which is then made up to 200 c.c., well shaken and filtered; the filtrate is placed in a polarimeter tube and the angle of rotation observed at 87° C., at which temperature the reading of invert sugar is 0, all rotation therefore is due to glucose. The average specific rotatory power $[a]_D$ of glucose is 150, and from this the percentage of glucose is calculated.

Example: A sample of jam had a specific rotatory power $[a]_D$ of 30° at 87° C., then the glucose in the sample

$$= \frac{30 \times 100}{150} = 20 \text{ per cent.}$$

Detection of apple pulp. About 5 grams of the jam are

boiled with 25 c.c. of water and then cooled; a few drops of
iodine solution are added, when, in the presence of apple pulp,
some of the cells appear blue, owing to the presence of starch
in the cells of apple pulp. The microscopic appearance of apple
pulp should be carefully studied, and the percentage estimated
by comparison, under the microscope, with jams containing a
known amount of the pulp.

Detection of agar-agar. Hartel and Solling (*Zeit. Unt.
Nahr. Gen.* 1911, XXI, 168). 30 grams of the sample are boiled
with 270 c.c. of water for 15 minutes, filtered and cooled; in
the presence of agar-agar, a precipitate forms within 24 hours;
the precipitate is collected, dissolved in a little hot water and
cooled; if agar-agar is present, the solution sets to a jelly.

Estimation of salicylic acid. Harry and Mummery
(*Analyst*, 1905, XXX, 124) have devised a convenient method
of estimating salicylic acid in jam. 50 grams of the sample
are placed in a 300 c.c. flask; a small quantity of water is
added, followed by 15 to 20 c.c. of a saturated solution of basic
acetate of lead, and the whole is then made alkaline with 15
to 20 c.c. of N/1 sodium hydroxide solution; the alkali throws
down excess of lead, and afterwards dissolves the hydroxide
and some albuminous material; and, in order to reprecipitate
these, 15 to 20 c.c. of N/1 hydrochloric acid are added; the
contents of the flask are now made up to 300 c.c., well shaken
and filtered; 200 c.c. of the filtrate are acidified with hydrochloric acid, filtered, if necessary, and extracted three times
with ether; the mixed ether extracts are evaporated and the
salicylic acid is dissolved in a small quantity of dilute alcohol
and made up to 100 c.c.; 50 c.c. of this solution are placed in
a Nessler glass, 2 c.c. of neutral ferric chloride solution are
added, and the amount of salicylic acid present estimated by
comparison with the colour obtained from known quantities
of a standard solution of salicylic acid.

In view of the volatility of salicylic acid in water vapour,
and as ether usually contains a considerable quantity of water
in proportion to the amount of acid, it is better to extract the
salicylic from the ethereal solution by caustic soda solution,
run off the ethereal layer, add dilute sulphuric acid to the
watery solution to neutralize the soda, and distil the acidified

aqueous solution. The salicylic acid comes over with the water vapour and can be estimated as above.

Example: 50 c.c. of the alcoholic solution gave a colour exactly matched by 1·5 c.c. of standard salicylic acid solution (containing 0·1 per cent. of salicylic acid); then the amount of salicylic acid in the sample is

$$\frac{1 \cdot 5 \times 0 \cdot 001 \times 2 \times 3 \times 2}{2} = 0 \cdot 009 \text{ per cent.}$$

or 0·63 grain per pound.

Table containing the specific rotatory powers of various sugars.

	$[a]_D$
Cane sugar ($C_{12}H_{22}O_{11}$)	+66·6
Maltose ($C_{12}H_{22}O_{11}$)	+138
Lactose Anhydrous ($C_{12}H_{22}O_{11}$) ..	+55·4
Lactose (cryst. $C_{12}H_{22}O_{11}H_2O$) ..	+52·6
Dextrose ($C_6H_{12}O_6$)..	+51·3
Lævulose ($C_6H_{12}O_6$)	−95·4
Invert sugar ($C_6H_{12}O_6$)$_2$ (at 17·5° C.)	−19·6

Table containing the weights of various sugars equivalent to 50 c.c. of Fehling's solution, and to 1 gram of CuO.

50 c.c. of Fehling's solution = 0·2375 gram of dextrose.

50	,,	,,	,,	= 0·2572	,,	lævulose.
50	,,	,,	,,	= 0·2470	,,	invert sugar.
50	,,	,,	,,	= 0·3380	,,	lactose.
50	,,	,,	,,	= 0·3890	,,	maltose.

1 gram of CuO = 0·7435 gram maltose.

1	,,	,,	= 0·4535	,,	dextrose.
1	,,	,,	= 0·4715	,,	invert sugar.
1	,,	,,	= 0·4897	,,	lactose.
1	,,	,,	= 0·4911	,,	lævulose.

CHAPTER VIII

ALCOHOLIC BEVERAGES—WHISKEY, RUM, GIN, BRANDY—BEER—CIDER

SPIRITS

Whiskey. Whiskey is principally manufactured in Scotland from malted and unmalted barley, and from malted and unmalted barley and other grains in Ireland. The flavour and bouquet of the spirit are due to the presence of "impurities," higher alcohols, esters, etc. The spirit is produced by the distillation of a fermented extract of the grain. In Ireland the spirit as distilled has an alcoholic strength of about 30 degrees over proof, and in Scotland about 25 degrees over proof. The distillation is carried out either in a "pot" or a "patent" still, and the character of the distillate is dependent on the still used. "Patent" still spirit is comparatively free from the higher alcohols, esters, etc., and it was considered by analysts to be adulterated until the Royal Commission on Whiskey and other Potable Spirits, 1908–9, reported to the contrary. The crude distillate is allowed to mature in wooden casks for a number of years. The Sale of Food and Drugs Act, 1879, as amended by the Licensing Act, 1921, requires that whiskey shall not be sold at a greater dilution than 35 degrees under proof, and, practically, the only adulteration now is an excessive dilution, since the Royal Commission on Whiskey and other Potable Spirits, 1908–9, reported that "Whiskey is applicable to a spirit manufactured from malt or from malted and unmalted barley or other cereals" and that "Whiskey is a spirit obtained by distillation from a mash of cereal grains saccharified by the diastase of malt." The amount of alcohol in whiskey may vary between 50 and 55 per cent.

Proof spirit is that spirit which when mixed with gunpowder will just allow the gunpowder to be ignited; if the gunpowder burns with a flash the spirit is over proof, and if the gunpowder cannot be ignited the spirit is under proof.

Rum. Rum is produced in the West Indies, principally

Jamaica, from molasses by fermentation and distillation. The "impurities" in rum are usually comparatively high; the colouring matter consists of caramel, and the average alcoholic strength of imported rum is 25 degrees over proof. The Sale of Food and Drugs Act, 1879, as amended by the Licensing Act, 1921, requires that rum shall not be sold at a greater dilution than 35 degrees under proof; and, practically, the only adulteration is excessive dilution. The amount of alcohol in rum varies between 50 and 60 per cent.

Gin. Gin is manufactured by the distillation of spirit, obtained by the fermentation of grain extract, with Juniper berries. The chief grains used are maize, malt and rye. Sweetened gin is obtained by adding syrup to plain gin. The Sale of Food and Drugs Act, 1879, requires that gin shall not be sold at a greater dilution than 35 degrees under proof, and adulteration other than excessive dilution is very uncommon. The amount of alcohol in gin is usually between 45 and 55 per cent.

Brandy. Brandy is, or should be, made from the juice of the grape. It contains higher alcohols, esters, volatile oil, tannin and colouring matter. The colour is obtained by storing the colourless fresh spirit in oak casks. When it is first distilled brandy has an alcoholic strength of about 25 degrees over proof; the standard alcoholic strength for brandy in the United States of America is 19 degrees over proof. The Sale of Food and Drugs Act, 1879, as amended by the Licensing Act, 1921, requires that brandy shall not be sold at a greater dilution than 35 degrees under proof. The most common adulterations are excessive dilution and blending with "silent" spirit. British brandy is a spirit obtained from grains with flavouring ingredients added. The amount of alcohol in brandy is between 45 and 55 per cent.

Estimation of the alcoholic strength of spirits. The specific gravity of the sample at 60° F. is taken with a specific gravity bottle; 100 c.c. of the sample are placed in a distilling flask of not more than 250 c.c. capacity; 25 c.c. of water are added and the contents of the flask distilled until about 95 c.c. have passed over; the distillate is collected in a 100 c.c. flask, cooled to 60° F. and made up to the mark; the specific gravity of the distillate is then taken with a specific gravity bottle.

The contents of the distilling flask are now washed into a 100 c.c. flask, cooled to 60° F. and made up to the mark; the specific gravity is then taken as before; to the specific gravity of the original spirit, add 1000 and deduct the specific gravity of the residue; the difference should be the specific gravity of the distillate, and the percentage of alcohol is obtained by reference to the alcohol tables (see Addenda, p. 317).

Example: The specific gravity of a sample of rum was 953·5; the specific gravity of the distillate was 948·5, and the specific gravity of the residue was 1005·0; then

$$953·5 + 1000 = 1953·5 - 1005·0 = 948·5;$$

and, by reference to the alcohol tables, the rum was 26·20 degrees under proof and contained 35·25 per cent. of alcohol by weight and 42·12 per cent. of alcohol by volume.

Estimation of the total solid matter. 20 c.c. of the sample are placed in a platinum dish and evaporated to dryness on a water bath; the residue is dried in a water oven and cooled and weighed; the weight of the residue multiplied by five gives the total solid matter in percentages.

Example: The weight of the residue obtained from 20 c.c. of a sample of rum was 0·058 gram; then the total solid matter in the sample was 0·058 × 5 = 0·29 per cent.

Calculation of the alcoholic strength from the total solid matter and the specific gravity. One per cent. of total solid matter raises the specific gravity by 3·86; therefore, the specific gravity of the sample, less the total solid matter, multiplied by 3·86, will give the specific gravity from which to obtain the alcoholic strength.

Example: The specific gravity of a sample of rum, containing 0·29 per cent. of total solid matter, was 946·81; then 946·81 − (0·29 × 3·86) = 945·7; and, by a reference to the alcohol tables, the sample was 23·12 degrees under proof, and contained 36·82 per cent. of alcohol by weight, and 43·87 per cent. of alcohol by volume.

Estimation of the percentage of the excess of water. In order to obtain the percentage of the excess of water by volume in a sample of whiskey, rum, brandy, or gin, multiply the number of degrees under proof over 35 by 1·54.

Example: A sample of gin was 66 degrees under proof, then the percentage of the excess of water by volume in the sample was (66 − 35) × 1·54 = 47·74 per cent.

The amount by weight of alcohol in percentages is obtained by the use of the formula

$$\frac{\text{percentage by volume} \times 0\cdot7938}{\text{specific gravity}},$$

and therefore the percentage volume can be obtained by the formula

$$\frac{\text{percentage by weight} \times \text{specific gravity}}{0\cdot7938}.$$

The percentage of proof spirit may be obtained from the percentage of alcohol by volume × 1·75.

Detection of methyl alcohol. Vivario (*J. Pharm. Chim.* 1914, X, 145). 100 c.c. of the sample of whiskey, brandy, rum or gin are distilled over anhydrous sodium carbonate until 30 c.c. of the distillate have been collected; 15 grams of potassium hydroxide and 1 gram of hydroxylamine hydrochloride are then added to the distillate, and the whole is boiled under a reflux condenser for seven hours; after being allowed to cool, the mixture is made slightly acid with dilute sulphuric acid and distilled in steam; in the presence of methyl alcohol, the resulting distillate will contain hydrocyanic acid. The method is capable of detecting less than 10 per cent. of methyl alcohol. Furfural, if present, must first be removed by treatment with metaphenylene diamine hydrochloride.

Hasses' method (*Analyst*, 1920, XLV, 234). A small quantity of the sample is distilled, and 0·5 c.c. of the distillate, which must not contain more than 0·025 c.c. of alcohol, is treated with 1 c.c. of potassium permanganate solution (5 per cent.), and 2·5 c.c. of dilute sulphuric acid (8·7 per cent.); the mixture is allowed to stand for two minutes and is then decolorized with 1 c.c. of oxalic acid solution (10 per cent.); to 0·5 c.c. of the resulting solution are added 1 drop of peptone solution, containing 0·0025 gram of peptone, and 1 c.c. of sulphuric acid, containing iron; a deep blue colour is obtained in the presence of 1 per cent. of methyl alcohol, a red blue in the

presence of as little as 0·3 per cent. Pure ethyl alcohol gives a
yellowish-red colour.

Estimation of methyl alcohol in ethyl alcohol. Schryver
and Wood (*Analyst*, 1920, XLV, 164). 10 c.c. of the ethyl
alcohol containing methyl alcohol are diluted with 50 c.c.
of water; 5 c.c. of the resulting solution are mixed with 5 c.c.
of a 1 per cent. solution of ammonium persulphate in a test-
tube; this is then provided with a short air condenser and
heated in a boiling water bath for 10 minutes. At the end of
this period, 1 c.c. of the mixture is added to 1 c.c. of a 1 per
cent. solution of phenyl hydrazine hydrochloride, with which
it is heated in a boiling water bath for 5 minutes. After cooling
1 c.c. of a 2·5 per cent. solution of potassium ferricyanide is
added, followed by 3 c.c. of concentrated hydrochloric acid;
in the presence of methyl alcohol, a pink colour is produced,
and this colour is compared with those produced in a similar
way from ethyl alcohol containing known amounts of methyl
alcohol; it is possible by this method to estimate the percentage of methyl alcohol within 1 per cent.

Beer. This is a fermented extract of malt and hops. About
35,000,000 barrels of beer are now produced in the United
Kingdom annually. Since the middle of the last century beer
has been made on scientific principles; the malt is produced
by steeping barley in hard water for from three to five days;
the water is then drained off and the barley allowed to ger-
minate; it is then transferred to a kiln and dried; during the
process the diastase is developed. In the production of beer
the malt is crushed between rollers, and then mixed with water
at a suitable temperature for about two hours, during which
time the diastase acts on the starch forming maltose and other
carbohydrates; the extract is then drawn off and the residue
"sparged" with water at a suitable temperature to wash out
the last traces of extract; the extract or "wort" is then
passed to the copper where it is boiled and the hops are added;
in the copper the diastase is destroyed, and the wort concentrated, sterilized and aerated; the wort now passes to the "hop
back," where the hops are allowed to settle and act as a filter;
after about 20 minutes the extract is drained off and passes to
the coolers, where albuminous matter is deposited; from here

it passes to the fermenting tuns, where the yeast is added, which acts on the maltose and other carbohydrates to form alcohol and carbon dioxide; when the fermentation is complete the yeast is removed, and the fermented extract is run into barrels, where the "fining" materials of isinglass, etc. are added, which remove all suspended matter and give a clear, bright, finished product.

The principal adulterations of beer are the use of hop substitutes, the addition of excessive quantities of salt, and, where invert sugar has been used to prime the beer, the presence of excessive quantities of arsenious oxide, which may be dissolved in the impure sulphuric acid used for the inversion. The salt in beer should not exceed 50 grains per gallon, and the arsenic 1/100th of a grain per gallon.

Determination of acidity. *Solution required:* N/10 solution of ammonia.

The process. 50 c.c. of the sample are diluted with water in a porcelain dish, the N/10 solution of ammonia is gradually added, until a drop of the mixture shows a faint blue colour when placed on a piece of red litmus paper. The number of c.c. of ammonia solution used multiplied by 0·012 gives the amount of acidity (calculated as acetic acid) per 100 c.c. of the sample.

Determination of the original gravity. 150 c.c. of the beer are gently poured from one beaker into another, until as much as possible of the gas has been driven off; 100 c.c. of the resulting liquid are placed in a 250 c.c. flask and distilled, the distillate is collected in a 100 c.c. flask, and, after cooling, is made up to 100 c.c.; the residue in the distillation flask is washed out into a 100 c.c. flask, cooled and made up to the original volume; the specific gravity of the two solutions is then taken; the specific gravity of the distillate subtracted from 1000 gives the "spirit indication," this shows, from the table, the degrees of gravity of the original wort, lost during fermentation; to the "spirit indication," when the acidity exceeds 0·1 gram per 100 c.c., must be added a correction for the acidity, which is found from the table; the specific gravity of the residue plus the degrees of gravity lost gives the original gravity of the sample.

Example: The following results were obtained from a sample of beer:

Present gravity = 1009·5,
Specific gravity of the distillate = 993·7,
Specific gravity of the residue = 1016·4,
Acidity = 0·85 gram per 100 c.c. (as acetic acid),
therefore the spirit indication = 1000·0 − 993·7   = 6·30
add for excess acidity over 0·1gr. per 100c.c.(from table) = 0·97
                                       true spirit indication = 7·27

Degrees of gravity lost (from the table) = 32·27,
therefore the original gravity of the sample was

$$1016·4 + 32·25 = 1048·65$$

and the present gravity should be 1016·4 − 7·27 = 1009·13.

Specific gravity of wort lost during fermentation.

Spirit indication	0	1	2	3	4	5	6	7	8	9
0	0·00	0·42	0·85	1·27	1·70	2·12	2·55	2·97	3·40	3·82
1	4·25	4·67	5·10	5·52	5·95	6·37	6·80	7·22	7·65	8·07
2	8·50	8·94	9·38	9·82	10·26	10·70	11·14	11·58	12·02	12·46
3	12·90	13·34	13·78	14·22	14·66	15·10	15·54	15·98	16·42	16·86
4	17·30	17·75	18·21	18·66	19·12	19·57	20·03	20·48	20·94	21·39
5	21·85	22·30	22·76	23·21	23·67	24·12	24·58	25·03	25·49	25·94
6	26·40	26·86	27·32	27·78	28·24	28·70	29·16	29·62	30·08	30·54
7	31·00	31·46	31·93	32·39	32·86	33·32	33·79	34·25	34·72	35·18
8	35·65	36·11	36·58	37·04	37·51	37·97	38·44	38·90	39·37	39·83
9	40·30	40·77	41·24	41·71	42·18	42·65	43·12	43·59	44·06	44·53
10	45·00	45·48	45·97	46·45	46·94	47·42	47·91	48·39	48·88	49·36
11	49·85	50·35	50·85	51·35	51·85	52·35	52·85	53·35	53·85	54·35
12	54·85	55·36	55·87	56·38	56·89	57·40	57·91	58·42	58·93	59·44
13	59·95	60·46	60·97	61·48	61·99	62·51	63·01	63·52	64·03	64·54
14	65·10	65·62	66·14	66·66	67·18	67·70	68·22	68·74	69·26	69·78
15	70·30	70·83	71·36	71·89	72·42	72·95	73·48	74·01	74·54	75·07

Correction of spirit indication for acidity.

Acetic acid over 0·1 gram per 100 c.c.	0·00	0·01	0·02	0·03	0·04	0·05	0·06	0·07	0·08	0·09
0·0	0·00	0·02	0·04	0·06	0·07	0·08	0·09	0·11	0·12	0·13
0·1	0·14	0·15	0·17	0·18	0·19	0·21	0·22	0·23	0·24	0·26
0·2	0·27	0·28	0·29	0·31	0·32	0·33	0·34	0·35	0·37	0·38
0·3	0·39	0·40	0·42	0·43	0·44	0·46	0·47	0·48	0·49	0·51
0·4	0·52	0·53	0·55	0·56	0·57	0·59	0·60	0·61	0·62	0·64
0·5	0·65	0·66	0·67	0·69	0·70	0·71	0·72	0·73	0·75	0·76
0·6	0·77	0·78	0·80	0·81	0·82	0·84	0·85	0·86	0·87	0·89
0·7	0·90	0·91	0·93	0·94	0·95	0·97	0·98	0·99	1·00	1·02
0·8	1·03	1·04	1·05	1·07	1·08	1·09	1·10	1·11	1·13	1·14
0·9	1·15	1·16	1·18	1·19	1·21	1·22	1·23	1·25	1·26	1·28
1·0	1·29	1·31	1·33	1·35	1·36	1·37	1·38	1·40	1·41	1·42

Estimation of salt. 25 c.c. of the beer are evaporated to dryness in a platinum dish, and carefully incinerated at a low temperature; the residue is extracted with hot water, filtered, and well washed on the filter paper with hot water; the filtrate is cooled, and a few drops of potassium chromate solution are added, followed by N/10 silver nitrate from a burette until a permanent reddish colour is obtained. Each c.c. of N/10 silver nitrate solution used = 0·00585 gram of sodium chloride.

Example: 25 c.c. of beer treated as described required 4·6 c.c. of N/10 silver nitrate to produce a permanent red colour, then 0·00585 × 4·6 × 4 = 0·10764 × 700 = 75·35 grains of salt per gallon.

Estimation of arsenic. About 5 grams of arsenic-free zinc are placed in Marsh's arsenic apparatus; a little distilled water and a few drops of arsenic-free hydrochloric acid added and the whole allowed to stand for a few minutes; a small quantity of solid cadmium sulphate is then added; after 15 minutes, during which time the cadmium becomes deposited on the zinc, the water is poured off and the zinc covered with arsenic-free hydrochloric acid; the top of the apparatus is fitted on and the reaction allowed to proceed for 15 minutes; the hydrogen gas, escaping from the end of the arsenic tube, and a small gas flame, so situated that it plays on the neck of the arsenic tube, are lighted; 10 c.c. of the beer are now added, together with a little amyl alcohol, and after two or three minutes a small quantity of stannous chloride; the reaction is allowed to proceed for 15 minutes and the deposit is compared with standard deposits from known quantities of arsenic. Care must be taken that the reagents used themselves give no deposit of arsenic.

Detection of hop substitutes. The most convenient method for the detection of hop substitutes is that proposed by Chapman (*Analyst*, 1900, xxv, 36). The method is to take 500 c.c. of the sample and evaporate on a water bath in a porcelain dish; recently ignited sand is added towards the end of the evaporation with constant stirring; the residue is dried in the air oven and finally powdered, and extracted with ether in a stoppered bottle; the ether extract is filtered into a flask and evaporated; the residue is carefully oxidized with an alkaline solution of potassium permanganate (containing 40 grams of potassium permanganate and 10 grams of potassium hydroxide per 1000 c.c.) with vigorous shaking; the excess of potassium permanganate is reduced with a few drops of a hot solution of oxalic acid; the colourless solution is filtered and evaporated to dryness in a glass dish; the dry residue is acidified with dilute sulphuric acid, when, in the case of genuine hops, the odour of valeric acid is obtained, and in the presence of quassia, acetic acid is liberated; camomile gives the odour of valeric acid, but chiretta does not.

Estimation of sulphites. 25 c.c. of the sample are diluted with 100 c.c. of water; 2 grams of phosphoric acid are added and the mixture distilled; about 80 c.c. of the distillate are collected in bromine water, and heated on a sand bath until all the bromine has been expelled; the solution is then acidified with hydrochloric acid, and barium chloride solution is added; the precipitate of barium sulphate is allowed to settle and is then filtered, well washed, dried in the water oven, incinerated and weighed. The weight of barium sulphate obtained multiplied by 0·2747 gives the weight of sulphite (calculated as SO_2) in 25 c.c. of the beer.

Example: The weight of barium sulphate obtained from 25 c.c. of beer was 0·041 gram; then

$$0\cdot041 \times 0\cdot2747 = 0\cdot0112627 \times 4 = 0\cdot045 \text{ per cent.}$$

of sulphite (calculated as SO_2).

Estimation of alcohol in beer. Take 300 c.c. of the beer; place in a distilling flask; add a spoonful of tannic acid to stop the frothing when it is boiled; distil about 200 c.c. and make up the volume to the original 300 c.c.; mix well and take the specific gravity of this distillate in a specific gravity bottle at 15° C. From the specific gravity read off the amount of alcohol from the alcohol tables (p. 317). In the lighter beers the alcohol is about 3 to 4 per cent. and in the heavier beers and porters about 5 to 8 per cent.

Cider. This is an alcoholic beverage produced by the fermentation of apple juice. Perry is a similar beverage produced by the fermentation of pear juice. Cider contains from 2 to 8 per cent. of alcohol. In this country there is no standard for either cider or perry, but both should certainly be alcoholic

liquors, and the sale of spurious cider, consisting of a coloured
and ærated solution of cane sugar, should be considered an
offence under the Sale of Food and Drugs Act. The sale of
spurious ciders was very common in some seaside resorts, but
it has now almost ceased owing to the action of the local authorities. Numerous attempts have been made to suggest
chemical standards for cider, but, so far, none of them is
satisfactory.

Detection of spurious cider (Russell and Barker, *Analyst*,
1909, XXXIV, 125). 100 c.c. of the sample are evaporated to
about 10 c.c. on a water bath; the residue is shaken in a test-
tube with an equal volume of ethyl acetate for five minutes
and the two liquids are allowed to separate; the ethyl acetate
is then drawn off and carefully run down the side of a test-tube
on to the surface of a small quantity of lime water; in the
presence of a genuine cider, a yellow band is produced at the
junction of the two liquids by the action of the lime water on
the tannins of the apple juice.

Some Typical Analyses.

	(1)	(2)	(3)
Specific gravity	1025·0	1007·0	1010·0
Acid per cent.	0·45	·034	0·466
Tannin per cent.	0·19	0·18	—
Alcohol per cent.	4·20	5·07	3·64
Total solid matter per cent.	7·85	3·88	4·50
Ash per cent.	0·368	0·322	0·30
Alkalinity of the ash	0·10.	0·108	—
Phosphate per cent.	0·20	0·0191	—

Nos. (1) and (2) are analyses of genuine ciders by Russell
and Barker (*Analyst, loc. cit.*) and No. (3) is an analysis of a
sample of perry by Embrey (*Analyst*, 1891, XVI, 41).

CHAPTER IX

VINEGAR—LIME AND LEMON JUICE

VINEGAR

VINEGAR has been defined (*Local Government Board's Annual Report for* 1911–12) as "a liquid derived wholly from alcoholic and acetous fermentations; it shall contain not less than 4 grams of acetic acid (CH_3COOH) in 100 cubic centimetres of vinegar; it shall not contain arsenic in amounts exceeding 0·0143 milligram per 100 c.c. of vinegar; nor any sulphuric acid or other mineral acid, lead or copper; nor shall it contain any foreign substance or colouring matter except caramel. Malt vinegar is derived wholly from malted barley or wholly from cereals, the starch of which has been saccharified by the diastase of malt. Artificial vinegar is any vinegar or substitute for vinegar containing, or derived from any preparation containing, any added acetic acid which is not wholly the product of alcoholic and subsequent acetous fermentation; it shall contain not less than 4 grams of acetic acid (CH_3COOH) in 100 c.c. of artificial vinegar; it shall not contain arsenic in amounts exceeding 0·0143 milligram per 100 c.c. of artificial vinegar, nor any sulphuric acid or other mineral acid, lead or copper, nor shall it contain any foreign substance or colouring matter except caramel."

There are two chief varieties of vinegar sold in this country, malt vinegar and "wood" vinegar. "Wood" vinegar is obtained by diluting concentrated acetic acid with water and adding a little caramel as colouring matter. Malt vinegar should be obtained from malted barley or from a mixture of malted and unmalted barley; the malt or the mixture is ground and mashed with successive quantities of hot water, which is then run off and treated with yeast; this causes fermentation with the production of alcohol. This is subsequently oxidized to acetic acid by passing the wort over birch twigs, which have been impregnated with *Mycoderma aceti*. Malt vinegar contains traces of alcohol, gum, sugar, extractive, acetates, ethers, aldehyde, phosphates, etc. and is usually sold at 18, 20, 22 or 24; the last contains 6 per cent. of acetic acid and has a specific gravity of 1019; the figures denote that one fluid ounce will neutralize 18, 20, 22 or 24 grains respectively of pure dry sodium carbonate.

Malt vinegar is usually adulterated by the partial or total substitution of "wood" vinegar or by the addition of mineral acid. The detection of "wood" vinegar in malt vinegar was formerly possible by the determination of the nitrogen figure; but of late years manufacturers of malt vinegar, in order to minimize fermentation, have removed a portion of the nitrogen by precipitation, and this figure has in consequence become of no practical importance. The presence of artificial vinegar is now detected by the amount of phosphate present; the percentage of phosphate in genuine malt vinegar should not be less than 0·05 per cent. calculated as P_2O_5 (Russell and Hodgson, *Analyst*, 1910, XXXV, 346).

Determination of the total solid matter. Evaporate 25 c.c. of the vinegar in a platinum dish and dry the residue in a water oven until constant; the weight of the residue multiplied by four gives the percentage of the total solid matter per 100 c.c.

Example: The residue from 25 c.c. of a sample of vinegar weighed 0·586 gram; then 0·586 × 4 = 2·344 grams of total solid matter per 100 c.c.

Ash. The residue obtained above is carefully incinerated over a Bunsen flame until a white ash is obtained; the weight of this ash multiplied by four gives the weight of ash per 100 c.c.

Example: The weight of ash obtained from 25 c.c. of vinegar was 0·078, then 0·078 × 4 = 0·312 gram of ash per 100 c.c.

Estimation of acetic acid. Dilute 10 c.c. of the vinegar to about 200 c.c., add a few drops of phenol phthalein solution, and titrate with N/1 sodium hydroxide solution until a permanent pink colour is obtained; each c.c. of the N/1 sodium hydroxide solution used = 0·06 gram of acetic acid.

Example: 10 c.c. of a sample of vinegar required 10·3 c.c. of N/1 sodium hydroxide solution to produce a permanent pink colour; then $10\cdot3 \times 0\cdot06 \times 10 = 6\cdot18$ grams of acetic acid per 100 c.c.

Calculation of original solids. Theoretically 60 grams of acetic acid are produced from 90 grams of glucose; therefore the acetic acid found multiplied by $1\cdot5$ gives the amount of sugar from which the acetic acid was derived; to this is added the amount of total solid matter contained in the vinegar, giving the original solid matter.

Example: A sample of vinegar contained $4\cdot8$ grams of acetic acid and $2\cdot34$ grams of total solid matter per 100 c.c., then the original solids were $(4\cdot8 \times 1\cdot5) + 2\cdot34 = 7\cdot20$ grams per 100 c.c.

Estimation of phosphate. Evaporate 50 c.c. of the vinegar to dryness; incinerate the residue and dissolve the ash in dilute nitric acid; a few c.c. of a solution of ammonium molybdate are added and the mixture is kept at 60° C. for two hours; in the presence of phosphate the characteristic canary yellow precipitate is obtained; this is filtered off and washed with water containing ammonium molybdate; the washed precipitate is then dissolved off the filter paper with dilute ammonia, and a few c.c. of a cold magnesia mixture added; the mixture is allowed to stand for 12 hours; the precipitate is then filtered off, washed with dilute ammonia water, dried in the water oven, incinerated, ignited over a blowpipe and weighed as magnesium pyrophosphate ($Mg_2P_2O_7$); the weight of magnesium pyrophosphate obtained multiplied by $0\cdot6396$, and then multiplied by two, gives the weight of phosphate (as P_2O_5) in 100 c.c. of the vinegar.

Example: 50 c.c. of vinegar gave $0\cdot0295$ gram of magnesium pyrophosphate, then $0\cdot0295 \times 0\cdot6396 \times 2 = 0\cdot038$ gram P_2O_5 per 100 c.c.

Detection of free mineral acid. When acetates and other salts of organic acids are incinerated, alkaline carbonates are formed; but when the salts of mineral acids are ignited the residue has a neutral reaction; therefore, if the ash of a vinegar is alkaline, mineral acids are not present; but if the ash is neutral, mineral acids have probably been added.

Estimation of free mineral acid. Qualitative tests for chlorides and sulphates are first performed, and 25 c.c. of vinegar are placed in a platinum dish with 20 c.c. of N/10 sodium hydroxide solution; the whole is evaporated to dryness and incinerated; the ash is dissolved in water and a few drops of methyl orange are added; N/10 sulphuric acid is then added until a permanent pink colour is obtained; in the absence of mineral acids 20 c.c. of N/10 sulphuric acid would be used; the amount of mineral acid present is calculated from the difference between the acid used and 20 c.c.

Example: A sample of vinegar treated as described above required 15 c.c. of N/10 sulphuric acid to produce a permanent pink colour; qualitative tests showed sulphates to be present; then $20 - 15 = 5$; each c.c. represents 0·0049 gram of sulphuric acid or 0·00365 gram of hydrochloric acid, therefore the sample contained $5 \times 0·0049 = 0·0245 \times 4 = 0·098$ gram of H_2SO_4 per 100 c.c.

Schidrowitz's method (*Analyst*, 1903, XXVIII, 233). *Solutions required:*

N. sodium hydroxide solution;

N. alcoholic solution of sulphuric acid;

The process. To 40 c.c. of the sample of vinegar 5 c.c. of the N. solution of sodium hydroxide are added, and the mixture is evaporated to dryness; the residue is dissolved in 5 c.c. of 50 per cent. alcohol, a few drops of methyl orange are added, and the alcoholic solution of sulphuric acid is added drop by drop until a faint permanent pink colour is obtained; the number of c.c. of sodium hydroxide solution added, less the number of c.c. of sulphuric acid used, gives the number of c.c. of sodium hydroxide solution neutralized by the free mineral acid present in the sample.

Example: Qualitative tests showed hydrochloric acid to be present in the sample. 5 c.c. of N. sodium hydroxide solution were added to 40 c.c. of the sample, and 3·2 c.c. of sulphuric acid were required for neutralization. Then the amount of hydrochloric acid present in the sample

$$\frac{(5·0 - 3·2) \times 0·0364 \times 1000}{40} = 0·1638 \text{ gram per 100 c.c.}$$

Typical Analyses of Vinegar (in percentages).

	(1)	(2)	(3)	(4)	(5)
Total solid matter (grs. per 100 c.c.)	2·70	1·47	2·36	0·472	1·54
Ash (grs. per 100 c.c.)	0·60	0·42	0·23	0·041	0·20
Alkalinity of ash (as K_2O) (grs. per 100 c.c.)	0·032	0·037	0·035	0·014	0·07
Phosphates (as P_2O_5) (grs. per 100 c.c.)	0·051	0·078	0·020	nil	0·005
Acetic acid (grs. per 100 c.c.)	4·80	6·15	4·80	2·20	3·50
Specific gravity	1019·3	1018·0	1017·0	1012·1	1010·0

Nos. (1) and (2) are genuine malt vinegars; No. (3) is a malt vinegar admittedly "made without the use of malt"; No. (4) is a "wood" vinegar; and No. (5) is a sugar vinegar.

The following analyses in percentages are given by Jamieson (*Analyst*, 1915, XL, 106).

	(1)	(2)	(3)
Specific gravity	1·019	1·020	1·013
Total solids	3·66	3·28	1·64
Ash	0·36	0·34	0·36
Nitrogen	0·009	0·014	0·06
Phosphoric acid	0·02	0·02	0·05
Acetic acid	4·20	0·50	4·59
Original solids	9·96	10·03	8·52

No. (1) was prepared from germinated maize and pasteurized; No. (2) is the same vinegar, before pasteurization; No. (3) is an ordinary malt vinegar.

LIME AND LEMON JUICE

Lime juice is the expressed juice of *Citrus medica acida,* and lemon juice of *Citrus medica limonum.* According to the official description of lime juice in the *British Pharmacopœia* it should contain from 7 to 9 per cent. of citric acid and should have a specific gravity at 60° F. of 1030 to 1040; it should contain about 14 per cent. of total solids and the ash should not exceed 3 per cent. of the total solids. Commercially these syrups are sold as lime juice cordial and lemon squash in order that they may not be subject to the provisions of the Sale of Food and Drugs Acts, and they usually contain from 2 to 4 per cent. of citric acid, and from 30 to 40 per cent. of total solid matter, the latter consisting chiefly of added sugar, but it is doubtful whether or not the sale of such substances is an offence under the Act.

Estimation of free citric acid. Dilute 10 c.c. of the lime juice to about 100 c.c. and titrate with N/10 sodium hydroxide solution, using phenol phthalein as an indicator; each c.c. of N/10 sodium hydroxide solution used represents 0·007 gram of citric acid.

Example: 10 c.c. of a sample of lime juice required 44·3 c.c. of N/10 sodium hydroxide solution to produce a permanent pink colour; then 44·3 × 0·007 × 10 = 3·10 per cent. of citric acid.

Estimation of combined citric acid. Exactly neutralize 10 c.c. of the lime juice with N/10 sodium hydroxide solution, and evaporate the neutral solution to dryness on a water bath; incinerate the residue over a Bunsen flame and extract the ash with hot water; to the water extract add 20 c.c. of N/1 sulphuric acid and titrate with N/1 sodium hydroxide solution, using methyl orange as an indicator, until an orange colour is obtained; from the number of c.c. of N/1 sulphuric acid used deduct the number of c.c. of N/1 sodium hydroxide solution required, and multiply the difference by 0·07; this gives the total citric acid in 10 c.c. of the lime juice.

Example: 10 c.c. of a sample of lime juice treated as above required 13·7 c.c. of N/1 sodium hydroxide solution to produce an orange colour; then 20·0 − 13·7 = 6·3 c.c. of N/1 sulphuric acid used; 6·3 × 0·07 × 10 = 4·41 per cent. of total citric acid; the sample contained 3·08 per cent. of free citric acid; therefore the sample contained 4·41 − 3·08 = 1·33 per cent. of combined citric acid.

Mineral acid. The addition of mineral acid to lime juice has become common, the manufacturers' view being that it is necessary to prevent decomposition. The presence of mineral acid is detected and the amount estimated as described under vinegar (pp. 240, 241).

Preservatives. Most samples of lime juice cordial and lemon squash which do not contain mineral acid, contain instead some other preservative; the most common being salicylic acid and sulphite; the methods for the estimation of these substances will be given later (p. 260).

Typical Analyses of Lime Juice (in percentages).

	(1)	(2)
Total solid matter	12·56	6·65
Free citric acid ..	7·33	3·08
Combined citric acid	1·41	1·33
Ash	0·16	0·20
Sulphite	—	0·06

No. (1) is a genuine lime juice; No. (2) is deficient in solids and citric acid and contains sulphite preservative.

CHAPTER X

MEAT AND MEAT PRODUCTS

EXTRACT OF MEAT

MEAT extract was first popularized by Liebig about 1850, and consists essentially of evaporated beef tea. A genuine "Liebig" extract should be practically free from fat and contain no gelatine. Vast areas in South America are now devoted to the feeding of cattle used in the preparation of meat extract; about 1000 pounds of beef being required in the preparation of about 30 pounds of extract. In the preparation of the extract, the meat is hung for twelve hours, the fat and "grisle" are then removed and the residue is chopped and minced; the finely minced meat is extracted with warm water, the fat being continually skimmed off during the extraction, and the resulting liquid is concentrated *in vacuo* with constant stirring; the final extract should not contain more than 20 per cent. of water, nor more than 21 per cent. of ash; the nitrogen content should be about 9·5 per cent.; the creatin 1·85 per cent., and the creatinin 4·85 per cent.; the fat should not exceed 0·2 per cent.

Yeast extracts, somewhat similar in appearance to meat extract, have been put on the market, and are occasionally sold in partial or total substitution for meat extracts. As the nutritive value of these extracts is very much lower than that of meat extract, such substitution can only be regarded as a serious adulteration.

Determination of water. 10 grams of the sample are dried in a platinum dish in the water oven, and finally in the air oven at 105° C. to constant weight.

Determination of ash. The dry residue, obtained from the water determination, is thoroughly charred, extracted with water and filtered; the residue on the filter paper is returned to the platinum dish and incinerated to a white ash; the filtrate is then added and the whole is evaporated to dryness on a water bath, the residue is gently ignited and weighed.

The phosphate (as P_2O_5), chlorine, lime and alkalinity should be determined on the ash; if the lime exceeds 0·2 per cent., added casein should be looked for, and if the ash requires more than 10 c.c. of normal acid for neutralization, added albumin should be looked for.

Detection of starch. A portion of the sample is treated with iodine, when, in the presence of starch, a blue colour will be obtained; a portion of the sample should also be examined microscopically for starch grains.

Determination of fat. 10 grams of the dry sample are extracted with petroleum ether in a Soxhlet apparatus for 6 hours, the fat is then dried in a water oven to constant weight.

Determination of albuminoids. 1 gram of the dry and fat-free sample is weighed out and the nitrogen is determined by Kjeldahl's method (p. 106); the percentage of nitrogen obtained multiplied by 6·25 gives the percentage of albuminoids.

Determination of creatinin. Folin (*Zeit. Phys. Chem.* 1904, XLI, 223). *Solutions required:*

A saturated solution of picric acid;

A 10 per cent. solution of sodium hydroxide;

A normal solution of hydrochloric acid;

A solution of potassium bichromate, containing 24·565 grams per 1000 c.c.

The process. 5 grams of the sample are dissolved in 500 c.c. of water; to 20 c.c. of the solution, 20 c.c. of the saturated picric acid solution and 5 c.c. of the 10 per cent. sodium hydroxide solution are added; the mixture is well shaken, allowed to stand for 5 minutes and then made up to 500 c.c.; the resulting solution is compared with a column of the potassium bichromate solution 8 mm. in depth; the colour of this depth of the potassium bichromate solution is the same as that obtained with 0·01 gram of creatinin.

Determination of creatin. To 15 c.c. of the solution obtained above, are added 10 c.c. of the normal solution of hydrochloric acid; the liquid is then evaporated to dryness on a water bath, the residue is dissolved in 15 c.c. of water, treated with 20 c.c. of saturated picric acid solution and 5 c.c. of the sodium hydroxide solution; the liquid is well stirred, allowed to stand for 5 minutes, diluted with water to 500 c.c.

and compared with the potassium bichromate solution as before; the percentage of creatinin, already found, is deducted and the remainder multiplied by 1·16 gives the percentage of creatin.

In view of the results obtained by Chapman (*Analyst*, 1909, XXXIV, 475), the above method must be used with caution.

Determination of gelatine. Stutzer (*U.S. Department of Agriculture Bull.* 13). 10 grams of the sample are dissolved in the smallest possible quantity of hot water in a porcelain basin; freshly ignited sand is then added in sufficient quantity to absorb the whole of the liquid, and the basin is dried to constant weight in a water oven; the contents of the basin are then ground in a mortar, transferred to a beaker and extracted four times with 50 c.c. of absolute alcohol, the liquid being each time filtered through asbestos; the funnel should be kept cold during the filtration; the residue in the beaker is stirred for a few minutes with successive portions of 100 c.c. each of a mixture of 100 grams of absolute alcohol, 300 grams of ice and 600 grams of cold water, the liquid being each time passed through the asbestos filter; the washing is continued until the filtrate comes through colourless. The asbestos bed of the filter is then transferred to a Kjeldahl flask, and the nitrogen is determined in the usual way. The percentage of nitrogen obtained multiplied by 5·55 gives the percentage of gelatine.

SAUSAGES

Sausages are generally made from meat and water with the addition of bread, rice or potatoes as a "filler," salt, seasoning materials and preservatives. In 1918, the Food Controller ordered that first quality sausages uncooked should contain at least 67 per cent. of meat, and second quality, at least 50 per cent. of meat.

Methods of analysis. Stubbs and More (*Analyst*, 1919, XLIV, 125).

Preparation of the sample. Remove the meat from the skin, and closely examine the skin for evidence of dirt; make a general examination of a few pieces of the meat and thoroughly mix and mince the remainder; the minced meat is immediately placed in a stoppered bottle.

Determination of the water. 5 grams of the minced meat are thoroughly mixed with 20 grams of ignited sand in a porcelain dish, and dried at 100° C. to constant weight.

Determination of the fat. 5 grams of the minced meat are dried in the water oven for 30 minutes, being stirred with a glass rod at intervals; the dry residue is then macerated with ether in the dish, the ether solution is filtered through a dried and weighed filter paper, which is finally washed free from fat with ether; the fat-free residue in the dish and on the filter paper is dried to constant weight, giving the non-fatty solids; the ethereal solution is evaporated, dried and weighed, giving the fat. The percentage of fat plus the percentage of non-fatty solids is deducted from 100, giving the percentage of water, which should agree with the direct determination.

Determination of nitrogen. The percentage of nitrogen is determined by Kjeldahl's process (p. 106).

Determination of ash. The dry residue from the water determination is incinerated, the residue represents mineral matter.

Microscopical examination. A portion of the sample should be examined under the microscope in order to determine the nature of the "filler."

Calculation. The percentage of proteins plus the percentage of ash is deducted from the percentage of non-fatty solids, the result gives the amount of carbohydrates and crude cellulose, and this, multiplied by 2, gives the approximate percentage of bread or other "filler," containing 40 per cent. of water.

From the total percentage of nitrogen deduct 1 per cent. of the "filler" (which may be taken as nitrogen due to "filler"), the balance gives the nitrogen due to meat; the percentage of nitrogen due to meat multiplied by 100/3·75 (in the case of beef or mutton) or by 100/4 (in the case of pork) or by 100/3·87 (in the case of mixed meats) gives the percentage of defatted meat, and this, added to the percentage of fat obtained, gives the percentage of meat in the sample.

The percentage of "filler" plus the percentage of meat is deducted from 100 giving the percentage of added water.

The analysis should be checked as follows: 40 per cent. of the "filler" found, plus 75 per cent. of the defatted meat found, plus the added water (if any), should be equal to the percentage of water found within an error of not more than 2 per cent.

This method is based on the considerations that meat is free from carbohydrates and crude cellulose; that the percentage of nitrogen in fat-free meat is 3·75 for beef and mutton and 4 per cent. for pork; that "fillers" contain about 40 per cent. of water, about 50 per cent. of carbohydrates and crude cellulose, and 1 per cent. of nitrogen.

Stokes' method (*Analyst*, 1919, XLIV, 127). The total solids, water, and ash are determined as usual. 10 grams of the sample are boiled for one hour under a reflux condenser with a 5 per cent. alcoholic solution of sodium hydroxide; in this way the fat and meat are dissolved and the starch is unaltered. The liquid is filtered through a plug of slag-wool, and the residue is washed with hot alcohol; the filtrate is cooled and made up to 250 c.c., 25 c.c. of the solution are evaporated, in order to remove the alcohol, and the fat is determined in the residue by the Werner-Schmidt method (p. 104); the filter plug and the residue are returned to the original flask and shaken with 100 c.c. of cold, aqueous, 5 per cent. sodium hydroxide solution for one hour, the volume is then made up to 500 c.c. and the liquid is again filtered through a plug of slag-wool. To 50 c.c. of the filtrate, 100 c.c. of alcohol (90 per cent.) are added and the liquid is well stirred and allowed to stand for 30 minutes; the precipitated starch is filtered through a weighed filter paper, dried and weighed.

Calculation. The fatty acids obtained represent 95 per cent. of the fat present; the percentage of fat plus the percentage of starch is deducted from the percentage of total solids, the balance represents "dry" meat; to the "dry" meat is added 2·33 times its weight (representing natural water) giving fat-free flesh; to the percentage of starch obtained is added 0·66 times its weight (representing natural water) giving the percentage of bread.

MEAT PASTES

Meat pastes are usually sold in tins or pots under the names of ham, tongue, chicken, ham and tongue, chicken and ham, etc. Stokes (*Analyst*, 1919, XLIV, 129) employs the same methods of analysis as described for sausages.

TINNED FOODS

A large quantity of foods are on the market in sealed tins and are used especially as rations and emergency rations for army purposes; the methods of analysis described above are used for their examination by Stokes (*Analyst*, 1919, XLIV, 130). The army rations are required to contain not more than 12 per cent. of fat, nor more than 70 per cent. of water, nor more than 2 grains of tin per pound, nor to have an acidity greater than 72 c.c. of N/10 sodium hydroxide solution per 100 parts; Stokes picks out the meat and shreds it finely; the vegetables are then mashed and mixed and the shredded meat is added, the whole being well mixed; 5 grams of the sample are then shaken with 100 c.c. of cold water for one hour and filtered, a portion of the filtrate being titrated with N/10 sodium hydroxide solution.

PRESERVATIVES

Determination of salt. 1 gram of the finely divided sample is boiled with 100 c.c. of water under a reflux condenser and filtered; the filtrate is cooled and made up to 100 c.c. and the chlorine, as chlorides, is determined in 25 c.c. of the solution by titration with N/10 silver nitrate solution.

Detection of potassium nitrate. 20 grams of the dry fat-free sample are boiled with 50 c.c. of water and filtered; to a portion of the filtrate, an equal volume of concentrated sulphuric acid is added; a solution of ferrous sulphate is then carefully poured down the side of the test-tube, when, in the presence of nitrates, a brown or black ring will appear at the junction of the two liquids.

Determination of boric acid. The boric acid may be determined either by the method of Thompson (p. 118) or by the method of Fresenius and Popp (p. 261).

Determination of formaldehyde. 50 grams of the sample are distilled with phosphoric acid; the distillate is added to milk (free from formaldehyde), and the proportion of formaldehyde is determined by Shrewsbury and Knapp's process (p. 121), or the method described on p. 263 may be used.

Determination of sulphur dioxide. 50 grams of the sample are distilled with phosphoric acid and the sulphur dioxide is determined as described on p. 260.

Typical Analyses.

The following typical analyses are given by Stokes (*Analyst*, 1919, XLIV, 128).

	(1)	(2)	(3)	(4)	(5)	(6)
Fat	0·9	20·2	9·5	6·9	20·9	11·2
Bread	9·5	16·7	5·3	32·2	29·4	20·3
Flesh	89·1	72·2	71·0	51·1	26·0	60·2
Water	66·8	48·1	66·0	58·4	53·6	58·6

	(7)	(8)	(9)	(10)	(11)	(12)
Fat	3·6	16·6	15·4	13·4	11·1	13·2
Bread	11·0	3·0	6·7	13·8	13·6	8·7
Flesh	61·0	85·3	63·2	45·1	41·1	63·6
Water	71·6	55·9	61·6	65·0	69·0	62·6

	(13)	(14)	(15)	(16)	(17)
Fat	11·7	4·9	8·2	8·2	8·1
Water	67·5	73·0	67·4	68·0	68·4
Acidity	16·0	32·0	48·0	32·0	30·0
Ash	1·2	1·3	1·4	1·3	1·6

Nos. (1), (2), (3), (4) and (5) are analyses of single samples of sausages; No. (6) is the average analysis of 60 samples; Nos. (7), (8), (9) (10) and (11) are analyses of individual samples of meat pastes; No. (12) is the average analysis of 14 samples; Nos. (13), (14), (15), (16) and (17) are the analyses of samples of army rations.

CHAPTER XI

POISONOUS METALS IN FOODS

THE most common poisonous metals found in foods are tin, copper and arsenic. Tin appears in canned foods owing to the action of the acid juices, or owing to the action of putrefactive gases on the container. The proportion of tin should not exceed 2 grains per pound (*Local Government Board Food Reports*, No. 7). Copper is used in the so-called "greening" of preserved vegetables with the object of bringing out the deep green colour, especially of preserved peas. The Departmental Committee on Preservatives and Colouring Matters in Food, 1901, suggested that "the use of copper salts in the so-called greening of preserved foods be prohibited." Arsenic appears in beer from the use of impure sugar, and also in a number of other foods. The Royal Commission on Arsenical Poisoning, 1903, reported that "In our view it would be entirely proper that penalties should be imposed under the Sale of Food and Drugs Acts upon any vendor of beer or any other liquid food, or of any liquid entering into the composition of food, if that liquid is shown by an adequate test to contain 1/100th of a grain or more of arsenic in the gallon, and with regard to solid food—no matter whether it is habitually consumed in large or in small quantities or whether it is taken by itself (like golden syrup) or mixed with water or other substances (like chicory or 'carnos')—if the substance is shown by an adequate test to contain 1/100th grain of arsenic or more in the pound."

Determination of tin in canned foods (Buchanan and Schryver, *Local Government Board Food Reports*, No. 7). *Solutions required:* Stannous chloride solution containing 1·428 grams of stannous chloride per 500 c.c.;

Solution of dinitrodiphenylaminesulphoxide containing 0·2 gram in 100 c.c. of N/10 sodium hydroxide solution.

Preparation of dinitrodiphenylaminesulphoxide. Ten parts of nitric acid (specific gravity 1·48) are mixed with 10 parts of nitric acid (specific gravity 1·40) and the mixture cooled with ice and salt; 1 part of thiodiphenylamine is then added in small quantities at a time, with continual stirring; the temperature should not be allowed to rise above 5° C., and such small quantities should be added at a time that the hissing sound is hardly perceptible when the solid matter comes into contact with the liquid mixture. The thiodiphenylamine dissolves at first in the nitric acid to form a clear red solution, which gradually thickens owing to the separation of the nitro body. The solution is allowed to stand for some hours (not more than half a day); the nitro body is then sucked off on an asbestos filter and washed, first with concentrated nitric acid and then with nitric acid of gradually diminishing strength, and finally with pure water; it is then extracted with hot alcohol, in which it is not appreciably soluble.

The process. 50 grams of the meat or fruit are introduced into two 700 c.c. round-bottomed Jena flasks (25 grams in each); 10 grams of powdered potassium sulphate and 30 c.c. of concentrated sulphuric acid are added; the contents of the flasks are then heated till colourless as described in Kjeldahl's method for the estimation of nitrogen (p. 106). When the flasks are cold, the contents are diluted with water to about 100 c.c. and mixed; sulphuretted hydrogen is then passed through the solution, the mixture is allowed to stand overnight in a well-corked flask; the contents of the flask are slightly warmed on a water bath and filtered through a filter paper (4 cm. in diameter); the precipitate is washed with water, and the precipitate and filter paper are transferred to a test-tube and boiled with 5 c.c. of concentrated hydrochloric acid to dissolve the sulphide; the solution is filtered through a small conical Buchner funnel into a wide-mouthed test-tube with a side tube near the top, by means of which the test-tube is connected with a filter pump; the filter paper is sucked as dry as possible, and washed with 25 c.c. of concentrated hydrochloric acid; the test-tube is then connected with a carbonic acid gas apparatus, and gas is passed through the solution by means of a tube passing through the cork placed in the mouth of the test-tube and reaching down to the surface of the liquid; the side tube serves as an exit for the gas. Whilst the solution is still hot 0·75 gram of zinc foil is thrown into the strongly acid liquid, and, as soon as the last traces of zinc are dissolved, 2 c.c. of the reagent are added, by means of a pipette, to the hot liquid; the cork of the tube is momentarily lifted for the insertion and carbonic acid gas is passed the whole time. On the addition of the reagent, the nitro body is at first precipitated but afterwards redissolves; the solution is then boiled for two minutes and diluted to 100 c.c. with cold water; this diluted solution is filtered with the aid of the filter pump from the unchanged nitro body and usually turns violet during the filtration; a drop of dilute ferric chloride solution is added to bring out the maximum colour, which is then matched with known quantities of the standard tin solution.

Gravimetric estimation. The organic matter is destroyed as described above; and, when the incineration is complete, the contents of the flask are diluted, mixed and further diluted to about 600 c.c.; excess of sulphuretted hydrogen gas is now passed through the solution and the mixture is allowed to stand overnight in a well-corked flask; the contents of the flask are then slightly warmed, and the mixture of sulphide and sulphur filtered through a filter paper (7 cm. in diameter); the precipitate is washed with warm water and dissolved off the filter paper with a small quantity (10 to 20 c.c.) of a hot 10 per cent. solution of sodium hydroxide; from the yellow solution thus obtained, the sulphide is reprecipitated by means of glacial acetic acid and filtered; the precipitate is washed with hot water, dried in a water oven, incinerated and weighed as oxide.

Determination of copper in preserved peas. 10 grams of the sample are incinerated in a porcelain dish; the residue is dissolved in 3 c.c. of concentrated nitric acid; filtered, and the filtrate diluted to 100 c.c.; an electric current is then passed through this diluted solution contained in a platinum dish so that the dish is the kathode and the copper is deposited on the platinum dish; as soon as all the copper is deposited the anode is removed, and the solution in the platinum dish is at once poured off the copper, which is well washed with distilled water, dried in a water oven and weighed.

Example: 10 grams of a sample of peas were incinerated and the residue made up to 100 c.c. and from 50 c.c. of this solution 0·024 gram of copper was deposited; then

$$0·024 \times 20 = 0·48 \text{ per cent.}$$

of copper in the sample.

Detection of lead. Warren (*Analyst*, 1919, XLIV, 199). 10 grams of the sample are incinerated in a small dish; the ash is dissolved in 1 c.c. of nitric acid, and a small quantity of water, and then filtered; any residue on the filter paper is well washed with water; to the colourless filtrate, a slight excess of ammonia is added and the precipitate is filtered off and well washed; practically the whole of the lead will be found in the precipitate, which is washed into a Nessler cylinder with water, 5 c.c. of dilute acetic acid are added, followed by 5 c.c. of hydrogen sulphide solution, and the colour produced is matched against that of a standard lead solution.

Detection of arsenic. (1) *Reinsch's test.* When a clear, bright piece of copper foil is boiled in a hydrochloric acid solution of an arsenic compound, a grey film appears on the copper; the foil is gently washed and dried; placed in a tube of hard glass and gently heated; crystals of arsenious oxide will appear on the cold parts of the tube; a blank test should always be carried out with the acid used. This test is used in toxicological examinations and is capable of detecting one part of arsenic in 250,000 parts of solution.

(2) *The electrolytic test.* The apparatus for this test consists of a platinum cathode in a glass cylinder, which is open at one end and fits into a porous cell; this is surrounded by an anode and stands in a glass vessel; the upper portion of the cylinder is fitted with a ground-glass neck for insertion of the drying tube and funnel; a hard glass capillary tube fits into the end of the drying tube, and is surrounded at the shoulder by a piece of platinum gauze, which can be heated by a small Bunsen flame.

The process. Carefully wash the apparatus with distilled water; fill the outer cell with a 30 per cent. solution of sulphuric acid and partially fill the inner cell; a current of electricity (not exceeding 5 amperes) is then passed through the apparatus, and, as soon as all the air has been expelled, the escaping hydrogen is lighted, and also the small Bunsen flame; the current is run for 15 minutes; if no deposit appears in the capillary tube in that time, the materials are free from arsenic. A solution of the food to be tested is made in 30 per cent. sulphuric acid, and passed through the funnel into the inner cell; the current is again turned on, and, after passing for 15 minutes, the capillary tube is fused off at the shoulder and the deposit obtained is compared with standard deposits.

Preparation of the standard deposits. Weigh out 0·1 gram of pure dry finely ground oxide of arsenic (As_2O_3); wash it into a 1000 c.c. flask and make up to the mark. Each c.c. of this solution represents 0·0001 gram of oxide of arsenic. Measure out 100 c.c. of this solution and dilute it to 1000 c.c. Each c.c. of this dilute solution contains 0·00001 gram of oxide of arsenic. Standard deposits of 0·00001 gram, 0·000008 gram, 0·000006 gram, and 0·000004 gram of oxide of arsenic are obtained by placing 1 c.c., 0·8 c.c., 0·6 c.c., and 0·4 c.c. respectively of the dilute arsenic solution in the apparatus, and, after the deposit is obtained, the capillary tube is sealed at both ends; the deposit will keep for some time, but should be renewed occasionally.

(3) *The Gutzeit test.* Goode and Perkin's modification (*Jour. Soc. Chem. Ind.* 1906, xxv, 507). The apparatus consists of a conical flask of 250 c.c. capacity fitted with a dropping funnel and attached to a U-tube, containing a 10 per cent. solution of acid cuprous chloride; the exit from the U-tube is restricted by inserting a rubber bung, through which passes a glass tube of 5 cm. diameter. About 5 grams of ammonium chloride are first placed in the flask; then 1 to 2 grams of magnesium turnings, and 5 to 10 grams of the food are added, and 10 c.c. of water are run on to the mixture; the apparatus is gently shaken and placed in a basin of cold water. A piece of filter paper, soaked in a strong alcoholic solution of mercuric bromide, is placed over the outlet, and kept there for one hour or, in the presence of arsenates, for one and a quarter hours; the paper is then placed on a watch glass, moistened with a few drops of concentrated hydrochloric acid, warmed and the acid poured off; the paper is then washed with a little water and allowed to dry; in the presence of arsenic a red stain will be produced on the filter paper; it is claimed that by this method 0·000001 gram of arsenic is easily detected.

B.P. test for arsenic. From the *British Pharmacopœia*, 1914, p. 501.

Apparatus required: A wide-mouthed bottle, about 120 c.c.

capacity and fitted with a rubber cork, through which passes a glass tube; the latter has a total length of 200 mm., and an internal diameter of 5 mm. and is open at both ends; the upper end is slightly widened to a diameter of 8 mm., and the lower end is drawn out to a diameter of 1 mm.; a hole, of diameter 2 mm., is blown in the side at the constriction.

Lead papers are pieces of thin white paper 100 mm. by 40 mm., soaked in solution of lead acetate and dried.

Mercuric chloride papers are circles of smooth white filter paper 5·5 cm. in diameter, soaked in a saturated aqueous solution of mercuric chloride and dried.

Solutions and reagents required:

Brominated hydrochloric acid. 1 c.c. of bromine is mixed with 100 c.c. of hydrochloric acid;

Calcium hydroxide. 10 grams give no visible stain, when tested.

Citric acid. 10 grams give no visible stain, when tested.

Hydrochloric acid containing not more than 0·1 part per million of arsenic and free from iron.

Nitric acid. 10 c.c. give no visible stain, when tested.

Potassium chlorate. 5 grams give no visible stain, when tested.

Arsenic solution containing 0·00001 gram of arsenic.

Solution of bromine containing 30 grams of bromine and 30 grams of potassium bromide in 100 c.c.; it should not contain more than 1 part per million of arsenic.

Solution of stannous chloride containing not more than 1 part per million of arsenic.

Zinc. Granulated zinc, which conforms to the arsenic requirements of the control test and is free from iron.

General test. A strip of lead paper is rolled up and placed in the glass tube so that the upper end is not less than 2 cm. below the top of the tube. A piece of mercuric chloride paper is placed over the top and secured by a rubber ring. The tube is inserted in the rubber cork. The solution to be examined is placed in the wide-mouthed bottle, and 10 grams of zinc are added. The cork is placed in position, the lower end must be clear of the liquid and the hole in the tube clear of the cork. The action is allowed to proceed for 30 minutes in the dark.

In the presence of arsenic a yellow stain is obtained on the mercuric chloride paper, which is compared with stains obtained by using known quantities of arsenic. The standard stains must be freshly prepared, as they fade on keeping.

Standard stains. 1 c.c. of the arsenic solution is added to 50 c.c. of hot water, and 10 c.c. of stannated hydrochloric acid and then treated as described under "general test," the stain produced on the mercuric chloride paper is the standard stain.

Control test for reagents:

Hydrochloric acid. 0·2 c.c. of bromine solution is added to 50 c.c. of the hydrochloric acid; the solution is evaporated on the water bath to 16 c.c.; 50 c.c. of hot water and 5 drops of stannous chloride solution are added and the "general test" is carried out; the stain so obtained should not exceed 0·1 part per million of arsenic.

Solution of bromine. 10 c.c. are evaporated nearly to dryness; 50 c.c. of hot water and 10 c.c. of hydrochloric acid are added and sufficient stannous chloride to remove the remainder of the bromine; the "general test" is then carried out. The stain should not exceed 1 part per million of arsenic.

Solution of stannous chloride. 6 c.c. of water and 10 c.c. of hydrochloric acid are added to 10 c.c. of the stannous chloride solution; the whole is distilled and 16 c.c. are collected; 50 c.c. of water are added to the distillate and the "general test" is carried out; the stain should not show more than 1 part per million of arsenic.

Zinc. The "general test" is carried out with 10 c.c. of stannated hydrochloric acid, 50 c.c. of hot water and 10 grams of zinc; no visible stain should be produced on the mercuric chloride paper.

The method of preparing the solution of the substance for the "general test" varies with different substances, but the majority of the substances are dissolved in hot water and hydrochloric acid.

B.P. test for lead. From the *British Pharmacopœia*, 1914, p. 497.

Solutions required:

Solution of lead. Dissolve 0·16 gram of lead nitrate in distilled water, add 50 c.c. of nitric acid, and dilute with water to 100 c.c. This solution contains 0·001 gram of lead per c.c.

Dilute solution of lead. Dilute 1 c.c. of the above solution, measured from a burette, to 100 c.c. with distilled water.

Solution of potassium cyanide. Dissolve 10 grams of potassium cyanide in distilled water, add 2 c.c. of hydrogen peroxide solution and dilute to 100 c.c. with distilled water. This solution, after being allowed to stand, when tested by the quantitative-limit-test for lead gives no colour with the dilute solution of lead.

Solution of sodium sulphide. Dissolve 10 grams of sodium sulphide in distilled water and make up to 100 c.c. with distilled water.

The process. Two solutions of the substance under examination are made in hot distilled water:

(1) The primary solution, containing 12 grams of the substance.

(2) The auxiliary solution, containing 2 grams of the substance.

Each solution is filtered, if necessary, and made alkaline with solution of ammonia and treated with 1 c.c. of the solution of potassium cyanide. If the colours of the solutions differ much, the difference may be rectified by the cautious addition of a highly diluted solution of burnt sugar. The quantity of the dilute solution of lead, which must be added to the auxiliary solution, in order that the colour produced in both solutions on the addition to each of the solutions of two drops of sodium sulphide solution, is then determined. In these circumstances, each c.c. of the dilute solution of lead required corresponds to 1 part per million of lead in the substance examined.

We are indebted to the Pharmacopœia Committee of the General Medical Council for permission to publish the B.P. tests for arsenic and lead.

The detection of poisonous metals in water is described in Chap. I, pp. 19–20.

The reports of the Royal Commission on Arsenical Poisoning, 1903 (Cd. 1869, Cd. 1845, and Cd. 1848), are of importance in connection with arsenic in foods; the final Report, part I (Cd. 1848), sums up and discusses the evidence.

CHAPTER XII

PRESERVATIVES—DISINFECTANTS

PRESERVATIVES IN FOODS

Sulphite preservative is generally present in the form of calcium or sodium bisulphite; it is often found in preserved meat, in beer and wines from the "sulphuring" of the casks. The Departmental Committee's Report on Preservatives and Colouring Matters in Food (1901) made no recommendation as to the use of this preservative in foods or drinks. In the United States of America the Federal rules limit it to 350 milligrams per litre, provided that not more than 70 milligrams are in a free state. In France the amount permitted in wines and ciders is limited to 100 milligrams of the acid per litre whether "free" or "combined." In Austria-Hungary it is limited to 80 milligrams per litre. Durham (*Jour. of Hygiene*, 1909, vol. XVII, 17) suggests that in cider and perry more than a trace of sulphite should be labelled with a declaration to that effect; and that the word "trace" should be defined as "less than 10 (or possibly) 20 milligrams of SO_2 per litre."

Estimation of sulphite. 50 grams of the sample, or, in the case of a liquid, 50 c.c., are made into a paste with water and transferred to a distilling flask; the mixture is acidified with phosphoric acid and the distillate collected in a large excess of N/10 iodine solution; the excess of N/10 iodine solution is then titrated with N/10 sodium thiosulphate solution; using starch solution as an indicator. Each c.c. of N/10 iodine solution used = 0·0032 gram of sulphite, calculated as sulphur dioxide. The presence of more than 0·03 per cent. of sulphite must be regarded as an adulteration.

Example: In an experiment carried out as described above, 50 grams of meat gave sufficient sulphur dioxide to neutralize 32 c.c. of N/10 iodine solution; then 32 × 0·0032 × 2 = 0·205 per cent. of sulphite (calculated as sulphur dioxide).

Salicylic acid is sometimes added to beer and very often to British wines, lime and lemon juice. The most convenient method for the estimation is that proposed by Harry and Mummery (*Analyst*, 1905, XXX, 124).

The process. 100 c.c. of the sample are placed in a 300 c.c. flask, and made alkaline with N/1 sodium hydroxide solution; the mixture is evaporated until all the alcohol has been driven off; the residue is then cooled and neutralized with N/1 sulphuric acid; at least 20 c.c. of a saturated solution of lead subacetate are then added; the whole is made alkaline with 20 c.c. N/1 sodium hydroxide solution; made up to the mark with water and filtered; 100 c.c. of the filtrate are made acid with hydrochloric acid; the precipitate of lead chloride is filtered off and the filtrate is extracted three times with ether; the mixed ethereal residues are evaporated, and the residue dissolved in dilute alcohol, washed into a Nessler cylinder and made up to the mark; the salicylic acid is then estimated colorimetrically as described under Jam (p. 226).

Estimation of boric acid in meat. Fresenius and Popp (*Chem. Centr.* 1897, II, 69). The meat is finely chopped and 10 grams are well mixed with 40 to 80 grams of anhydrous sodium sulphate; dried in a water oven; and, when perfectly dry, finely powdered and washed into a 300 c.c. conical flask with 100 c.c. of methyl alcohol; the mixture is allowed to stand for 12 hours; the alcohol is then distilled off, and the residue is washed with a further quantity of 50 c.c. of methyl alcohol, which is also distilled off; the mixed distillates are made up to 150 c.c. with methyl alcohol, and to 50 c.c. are added 50 c.c. of water and 50 c.c. of a 50 per cent. solution of glycerine and a few drops of phenol phthalein solution; the solution is then titrated with N/10 sodium hydroxide solution until a permanent pink colour is obtained. Each c.c. of N/10 sodium hydroxide solution used corresponds to 0·0062 gram of boric acid.

Detection of benzoic acid. *In milk, cream, and butter.* Hinks (*Analyst*, 1913, XXXVIII, 555). For a qualitative text 25 c.c. of milk or 10 to 20 grams of cream or butter are heated with an equal volume of concentrated hydrochloric acid (as in the Werner-Schmidt method of estimating fat in milk, p. 104) and cooled; the solution is extracted with 20 c.c. of a mixture of ether (1 vol.) and petroleum ether (2 vols.); the ethereal solution is separated, and one drop of ammonia solution and 5 c.c. of water are added to it; the mixture is shaken and the aqueous layer separated; the ammonia is expelled by heating on a water bath, and a few drops of a neutral solution of ferric chloride are added; in the presence of benzoic acid a buff coloured precipitate is obtained.

For a quantitative test the same volume of milk or weight of cream as above is heated with hydrochloric acid under a reflux condenser, cooled and extracted three times with 20 c.c. of the ether mixture; the mixed ethereal extracts are made alkaline with ammonia, and 10 c.c. of water are added; the mixture is well shaken, the aqueous layer is separated and acidified with hydrochloric acid and extracted with the mixed ether as before; the ethereal extract is allowed to evaporate spontaneously and the residue is dried to a constant weight in a desiccator; the weighed residue is placed in an air oven at 100° C. for two hours, cooled and reweighed; the loss in weight represents benzoic acid. Boric acid does not interfere with the reaction.

In meats. Fischer and Gruenert (*Zeit. Untersuch. Nahr. Genussm.* 1910, XX, 580). 50 grams of the finely divided meat are shaken with 150 c.c. of a 1 per cent. solution of sodium bicarbonate at the melting point of the fat; the hot aqueous solution is separated and neutralized with dilute sulphuric acid; 10 c.c. of Fehling's copper solution, and 10 c.c. of a 3·1 per cent. solution of potassium hydroxide are added and the mixture is filtered; the filtrate is acidified with dilute sulphuric acid and extracted with ether; the ether extract is evaporated at a low temperature; the residue is dissolved in water containing ammonia and evaporated to 1 c.c.; and one drop of a dilute neutral solution of ferric chloride is added; in the presence of benzoic acid a buff coloured precipitate is obtained.

Detection of fluorides in butter and margarine. Monier-Williams (*Local Government Board Food Reports*, No. 17). Advantage is taken of the bleaching action of fluorides on peroxidized titanium solution. 10 grams of the butter or margarine are melted and shaken in a separating funnel with ether and a small quantity of water; the water layer is run off into a test-tube; a few drops of hydrogen peroxide are added and 1 c.c. of a 2 per cent. solution of titanium sulphate in a 10 per cent. solution of sulphuric acid; in the presence of fluorides the yellow colour of the titanium solution is partially discharged, a fact which is easily seen when the solution is compared with that obtained at the same time from genuine butter.

Estimation of formaldehyde in meats, etc. Romijn (*Zeit. Anal. Chem.* 1897, XXXVI, 18). To 100 grams of the finely chopped meat 100 c.c. of water and 1 c.c. of sulphuric acid (1 in 3) are added in a distillation flask; the mixture is carefully distilled over a low flame until 20 c.c. of distillate have been collected; this distillate contains one-third of the total formaldehyde present; to the distillate (which should not contain more than 0·3 per cent. of formaldehyde) are added 25 c.c. of N/10 iodine solution in a stoppered flask; a dilute solution of potassium hydroxide is then added drop by drop until the solution is yellow; the mixture is allowed to stand for 15 minutes; concentrated hydrochloric acid is then added until the red colour is restored, and the excess of iodine is titrated with N/10 sodium thiosulphate solution. The weight of iodine absorbed multiplied by 0·118 gives the weight of formaldehyde in the distillate, and this multiplied by three gives the weight (per cent.) of formaldehyde.

Detection of fluorides in sausages. 25 grams of the sample are mixed in a platinum dish with 25 c.c. of lime water, and the mixture is evaporated to dryness and incinerated; the dish is covered with a clock glass coated with vaseline, from parts of which the vaseline coat has been removed; about 1 c.c. of water and 1 c.c. of concentrated sulphuric acid are added to the contents of the dish, which are then strongly heated; in the presence of fluorides, the glass will be etched on the exposed parts.

The detection of various preservatives in milk and cream is described in Chap. II, pp. 118 and 129.

The Report of the Departmental Committee on the use of Preservatives and Colouring Matters in the preservation and colouring of food, 1901 (Cd. 833), contains the minutes of the evidence taken before the Committee as well as a full discussion.

DISINFECTANTS

A disinfectant is a solid or a liquid which is used for the purpose of destroying injurious organisms, and is, generally, though not necessarily, an antiseptic and deodorant. The actual germ-killing power of a disinfectant cannot be determined by chemical means, but the proportion of the active substance can be determined. A large number of commercial disinfectants are of little or no practical value for the purpose for which they are intended, and local authorities are largely to blame for the rubbish which is supplied to them as disinfectants, as it is a common practice to advertise for tenders for the supply of disinfectants "containing 10 per cent. or more of liquid carbolic acid." The local authority expects to be supplied with a disinfectant containing 10 per cent. or more of absolute phenol, the price of which would of course be positively prohibitive. The methods of analysis of only a few of the more important disinfectants are described here.

Estimation of hydrogen peroxide. The amount of hydrogen peroxide can be stated as the amount of "available" oxygen either by volume or by weight. A solution of the substance containing 3 per cent. by weight of H_2O_2 corresponds to a solution which liberates 10 times its volume of available oxygen. And 100 c.c. of such a solution which gives off 1000 c.c. of oxygen at $0°$ C. and 760 mm. is called a ten-volume solution.

The method of estimation is to add 5 c.c. of dilute sulphuric acid to about 500 c.c. of water in a dish; $N/10$ potassium permanganate is run in until the faint pink colour is permanent; now add 5 c.c. of the hydrogen peroxide solution and run in the permanganate solution till the faint pink colour again becomes permanent. If the first drop of permanganate causes a permanent coloration add a little more sulphuric acid; and if the colour still persists for a few minutes it means that no hydrogen peroxide is in solution. The equation representing the change is of course

$$5H_2O_2 + 2KMnO_4 + 4H_2SO_4 = 2MnSO_4 + 2KHSO_4 + 8H_2O + 5O_2.$$

Hydrogen peroxide is usually of three different strengths, and contains 5, 10 or 20 times its own volume of "available"

XII]   DISINFECTANTS   265

oxygen. The "ten-volume" solution gives off ten times its volume of oxygen, and this is equivalent to 3·04 per cent. of H_2O_2, and to 1·43 per cent. by weight of "available" oxygen. It is used in medicine, and for killing pathogenic and other organisms in milk and other foods. It is generally used in the form of a 1 per cent. solution.

Sulphur dioxide destroys vermin but not spores; the dry gas has little or no effect and it must be used in a moist condition. It is generally obtained by burning sulphur candles and is used to disinfect verminous houses, for sterilizing beer barrels, and, in the form of bisulphite, as a food preservative.

Estimation of available sulphur dioxide. Muter (*Analyst*, 1890, xv, 63). 2 grams of the powder are placed on a filter and washed with anhydrous ether to remove tarry matters; the residual ether is evaporated from the powder, which is then added to 50 c.c. of N/10 iodine solution and allowed to stand for 30 minutes with frequent shaking; the contents of the bottle are then titrated with N/10 sodium thiosulphate solution, using starch solution as an indicator. Each c.c. of iodine used represents 0·0032 gram of available sulphur dioxide.

Sulphite disinfectants oxidize rapidly, and if kept badly may depreciate very rapidly; it is necessary therefore to estimate this "reversion."

Estimation of the "reverted" sulphur dioxide. Muter (*Analyst*, 1890, xv, 63). 20 grams of the sample are placed in a bottle and 200 c.c. of water are added; the mixture is shaken occasionally, allowed to settle and filtered; 20 c.c. of the filtrate (= 2 grams of the sample) are mixed with an excess of bromine and filtered; the filtrate is treated with an excess of barium chloride solution and the precipitate is collected on a filter paper, dried in a water oven, incinerated and weighed; the weight of barium sulphate obtained multiplied by 0·2747 gives the amount of total sulphur dioxide in 2 grams of the sample; the available sulphur dioxide deducted from this gives the "reverted" sulphur dioxide.

Lime and chloride of lime are excellent disinfectants for large quantities of material; they kill bacteria but not spores, and are used for the disinfection of enteric fever and cholera discharges. Chloride of lime depends for its activity on the liberation of chlorine, and it is therefore necessary to know the proportion of available chlorine in a sample.

Estimation of available chlorine in chloride of lime. Penot's method (*J. Prakt. Chem.* 1896, LIV, 59). *Solutions required: N/10 sodium arsenite solution.* Weigh out 4·95 grams of pure powdered arsenious oxide and dissolve in 250 c.c. of water; 20 grams of sodium carbonate are added and the whole warmed and shaken until solution is complete, and finally diluted to 1000 c.c.

N/10 iodine solution. Weigh out 12·7 grams of pure resublimed iodine, and 18 grams of pure potassium iodide, and dissolve them together in 250 c.c. of water; dilute the solution to 1000 c.c.

The process. Weigh out 7·09 grams of the chloride of lime, mix it with water in a mortar until a smooth cream is formed; wash the cream into a 1000 c.c. flask and dilute it to 1000 c.c.; to 50 c.c. of this solution (= 0·3545 gram of the powder) add excess of the sodium arsenite solution; the excess of sodium arsenite is then determined by titration with the N/10 iodine solution, using starch solution as an indicator, until a permanent blue colour is obtained. Each c.c. of the sodium arsenite solution used represents 1 per cent. of available chlorine.

Pontius' method (*Chem. Zeit.* 1904, XXVIII, 54). *Solution required: N/10 potassium iodide solution.* Weigh out 16·6 grams of pure potassium iodide, dissolve it in water, and dilute the solution to 1000 c.c.

The process. Dissolve 7·09 grams of the chloride of lime in 1000 c.c. of water as above; to 50 c.c. of this solution (= 0·3545 gram of the powder) add 3 grams of solid sodium carbonate, and 2 to 3 c.c. of starch solution; this solution is immediately titrated with the N/10 potassium iodide solution until the blue colour is permanent. Each c.c. of N/10 potassium iodide solution used represents 0·0213 gram of available chlorine.

This method is very convenient and rapid and is applicable to the determination of available chlorine in powders of unknown strength, but the results are only approximate.

Permanganates of potassium and sodium must always be used in excess; the presence of excess of the permanganate is shown by the permanent pink colour; they are excellent

deodorizers but are very costly and occasionally imperfect.
"Condy's fluid" is a solution of sodium permanganate.

The estimation of the strength of a solution of potassium
permanganate depends upon the following chemical changes:

$$2KMnO_4 + 5C_2H_2O_4.2H_2O + 3H_2SO_4 = 10CO_2$$
$$+ K_2SO_4 + 2MnSO_4 + 18H_2O.$$

A $N/10$ solution of the oxalic acid is made by dissolving
6·301 grams of the pure crystals in one litre of pure water.

50 c.c. of the oxalic acid solution are placed in a beaker and
a few c.c. of sulphuric acid added together with about 300 c.c.
of water; warm to about 60° C. and the solution of potassium
permanganate run in till the faint pink tint remains permanent.
The strength of the solution can then be calculated from the
above equation.

Mercuric chloride. "Corrosive sublimate" is one of the
most powerful disinfectants; it should not be used for the disinfection of sputum or excreta or with hard water or sulphides.

Formaldehyde or "formalin" is used in the form of a
spray and has the advantage that it is easily applied and it is
very effective.

Estimation of formaldehyde. The commercial "formalin"
should contain about 40 per cent. of formaldehyde. It is estimated by oxidizing it to formic acid by iodine in an alkaline
solution according to the following equation:

$$H.COH + H_2O + I_2 = 2HI + H.COOH.$$

Dilute 10 c.c. of the solution to 400 c.c. with pure water;
then place 10 c.c. of this 1 per cent. solution in a beaker and
mix with 100 c.c. $N/10$ iodine; add sodium hydroxide drop by
drop till the colour becomes bright yellow; allow to stand for
about 10 minutes, acidify with dilute hydrochloric acid, and
titrate the liberated iodine with $N/10$ sodium thiosulphate. Each
c.c. of the $N/10$ iodine which disappears when the formaldehyde
is oxidized to formic acid = 0·00015 gram of formaldehyde.

Coal tar disinfectants rely for their effectiveness chiefly
on the proportion of phenol or cresols which they contain.
They are in the form of liquids and powders, and occasionally
contain little or no phenol, but comparatively large quantities
of tar oils.

Estimation of tar oils. Muter (*Analyst*, 1890, xv, 63). 50 grams of the powder, or 50 c.c. of a liquid, are shaken with 200 c.c. of a 10 per cent. solution of sodium hydroxide and the bottom layer run off; the upper layer is washed with a 5 per cent. solution of sodium hydroxide and the whole is rapidly filtered; the precipitate on the filter paper is washed into a beaker with water and filtered again through a weighed filter paper; the filter paper is cautiously dried between blotting paper, placed in a desiccator for 12 hours and weighed; the increase in weight represents tar oils.

Estimation of phenol. *In a powder containing no lime.* 50 grams of the sample are placed in a Soxhlet apparatus and completely extracted with ether; the ethereal solution is shaken twice with 20 c.c. of a 20 per cent. solution of sodium hydroxide; the alkaline solution is then evaporated to about 10 c.c., poured into a burette, acidified with dilute sulphuric acid and allowed to stand till perfectly cold; a layer of phenol separates and its volume is read off in c.c. The number of c.c. of phenol obtained multiplied by 1·05 gives the number of grams of phenol in the 50 grams of powder taken.

In a powder containing lime. 50 grams of the sample and 5 c.c. of water are placed in a large mortar; dilute sulphuric acid (50 per cent. by volume) is then added a few drops at a time until the solution is acid to litmus; this addition should take several hours and the temperature should not be allowed to rise, otherwise some of the phenol will be lost by evaporation; the residue is then placed in a Soxhlet apparatus and treated as described above.

In liquid preparations. 100 c.c., or less, according to the supposed strength of the sample, are placed in a litre distilling flask with 150 c.c. of distilled water, acidified with dilute sulphuric acid, and distilled; 100 c.c. of hot water are then added and the mixture is again distilled; the mixed distillates are made up to 500 c.c. and the phenol determined by Wilkie's method (*Jour. Soc. Chem. Ind.* 1911, xxx, 398). To 100 c.c. of the distillate are added equal volumes of N/10 sodium carbonate solution and N/10 iodine solution; after standing for 5 minutes, the sodium carbonate is neutralized with N/10 sulphuric acid, and the excess of iodine is titrated with N/10

sodium thiosulphate solution, using starch solution as an indicator. Each c.c. of N/10 iodine solution absorbed = 0·0127
× 0·1235 gram of phenol.

**Koppeschaar's method of estimating the amount of
phenol.** Shake up bromine with water until the latter is saturated; 0·25 gram of pure dry crystalline carbolic acid is
weighed; place in a well-stoppered flask; dissolve in 100 c.c.
of distilled water; run in the bromine water from a burette,
with constant shaking, till the bromine colour remains; allow
to stand for half an hour; if the colour disappears run in more
bromine water from the burette; shake again and allow to
stand; note the total amount added; then add excess of a
solution of potassium iodide; and determine the liberated
iodine with a standard solution of thiosulphate in the usual
way, as described on p. 7. The free iodine is equivalent to the
excess of bromine and must be subtracted from the total
bromine which was added. The amount of bromine water
necessary to react with the 0·25 gram of pure phenol is thereby
obtained, and from this number the phenol-equivalent for
every cubic centimetre of the bromine solution is calculated.
The equation representing the chemical change is

$$C_6H_5OH + 3Br_2 = C_6H_2Br_3.OH + 3HBr.$$

The experiment is then repeated with the sample of phenol
which is being analysed, and we thus obtain the strength of the
phenol.

**The Lancet Acetone-baryta (L.A.B.) method of the
chemical analysis of phenol disinfectants.**

The majority of the liquid coal tar disinfectants are mixtures
of varying quantities of phenolic bodies with inert tar oils, in
many cases with soap or resins or other emulsifying agents such
as dextrin or gelatin, etc. In connection with The Standardization of Disinfectants, a very full account is given in the
Lancet for Nov. 13, 20 and 27, 1909, by Professor Sims Woodhead, Dr C. R. Ponder, Mr S. A. Vasey and Mr J. E. Purvis,
the members of the Commission appointed by the *Lancet* to
investigate the conditions of standardization. The inquiry
consisted of two parts, (*a*) the chemical analysis of disinfectants and (*b*) the bacteriological examination of disinfectants.

The methods of the chemical examination only are described here.

(a) Fluids containing soaps and resins as emulsifiers. The basis of the method is that the soaps and resins must be decomposed or made insoluble before there can be a complete separation of the phenoloid bodies in a pure state. This may be done by converting the soaps or resins, which are commonly of soda or potash, into insoluble combinations by the addition of a strong solution of barium hydroxide. Also, phenol, cresol, and the phenolic bodies generally are soluble in this alkaline solution. Lime water may be used, but calcium hydroxide is considerably less soluble in water than barium hydroxide. If a few grams of the disinfectant, which is made by amalgamating phenol bodies with soaps or resin (the constitution of most of the disinfectants sold), be first hydrolysed by stirring with water and then an excess of baryta water added, the actual germicidal body is completely dissolved in the baryta, and there is a rapid separation of the resins or soaps in the form of insoluble baryta compounds.

The method is to weigh out 10 grams of the disinfecting fluid (composed of phenol bodies, soaps or resins, and neutral oils); shake well with 100 grams of distilled water; add 15 grams of barium hydrate crystals; place the mixture in a large conical flask attached to a reflux condenser; heat for half an hour at 100° C. by immersing it in a vessel of boiling water; shake the flask at frequent intervals; allow to cool. In most cases the baryta solution can be decanted almost clear without filtering; but it is best to pour it upon a moistened asbestos plug in a glass funnel which is attached to a water-pump. The residue in the flask is then washed with warm baryta solution, and the whole filtered. Make up the filtrate to 300 c.c.; 50 c.c. of this are treated in a separating funnel with hydrochloric acid, calcium chloride added, and the liberated phenols extracted and washed with ether, and the ether evaporated off. The residue which consists of the phenol bodies is weighed. Then dissolve in sodium hydroxide and add excess of a solution of bromine in caustic soda, the amount of bromine present in the solution being ascertained previously by Koppeschaar's process (p. 269); the bromine is liberated by adding hydrochloric acid; the bromine absorbed by the phenol is thereby found. Care should be taken that the bromine is in excess, and the excess is determined by influxing it with iodine by the addition of a few crystals of potassium iodide, and estimating the iodine by N/10 thiosulphate of soda in the usual way. The amount of bromine which has reacted with the phenol body is thus determined and calculated in terms of its equivalent of carbolic acid according to the equation:

$$C_6H_5OH + 3Br_2 = 3HBr + C_6H_2Br_3OH.$$

If the phenol body present is carbolic acid, the percentage figure obtained in the bromine experiment will approximate to the percentage weight of carbolic acid found by drying the ether extraction of the acidified baryta solutions. If there is no agreement between these figures carbolic acid as such is not present but one or other of its homologues or a phenoloid, the bromine absorption of these bodies being lower. When, in fact, the difference is wide, the conclusion may be justified that carbolic acid is absent. The residues after treatment with baryta, which are generally of a viscous description when soap is present but hard and firm when resins are present, contain the neutral hydrocarbon oils, the fatty acids and the resins. To this residue add 200 c.c. of acetone; separation gradually follows, and the neutral hydrocarbon oils dissolve in the acetone, the soaps and resins are insoluble. Thoroughly rub down the insoluble matters with acetone, and filter and wash with acetone; treat the insoluble matter with hydrochloric acid and shake up with ether; evaporate the ether, and weigh the fatty acids or resins thus obtained. To the acetone solution add 10 per cent. solution of caustic soda and mix well, and then add about 20 c.c. of petroleum (white spirit) to facilitate the removal of oils, and finally add about 500 c.c. of water; shake and allow to stand; draw off the aqueous liquid and filter through a wetted filter paper; add hydrochloric to the filtrate till it is acid, and exhaust with ether; the residue consists of the resins or fatty acids which were not retained in the baryta residue. The amount is usually small and should be added to the weight of the fatty acids or resins found in the barium residue.

Any water present may be determined by taking 25 grams of the disinfectant fluid, adding exactly 10 c.c. of a 10 per cent. solution of sulphuric acid and then 25 c.c. of petroleum spirit; shaking thoroughly and allowing to rest. When the separation is complete, the clear liquid below is drawn off with a narrow and accurately graduated glass cylinder and its volume read; the excess over the 10 c.c. of aqueous sulphuric acid added is regarded as the water present in 25 grams of the sample.

The alkalis are estimated by obtaining the ash and titrating the solution of this residue with standard acid.

(b) Fluids containing neither soaps nor resins as emulsifiers.

The germicidal agent of these disinfectant fluids is brought into uniform suspension by means of gelatine or gum. In such cases the use of baryta is unnecessary. The method is to take 10 grams of the fluid and add excess of absolute alcohol or acetone which dissolves the phenoloid, but precipitates the gelatine or dextrin; thoroughly exhaust the insoluble mass with successive washings of acetone and finally dissolve in water; evaporate the solution to dryness, and then weigh the residue of gelatine or gum so obtained. The alcohol or acetone containing the phenoloids (and neutral oils if present) is then shaken up with a 10 per cent. solution of sodium hydroxide and diluted freely with water. Any neutral oils present are thus set free, and this may be promoted by adding 20 c.c. of petroleum (white spirit). The alkaline solution is then drawn off and filtered, and the filtrate made up to a known volume. Part of this is acidified and calcium chloride added; exhaust the separated phenoloids with ether; evaporate off the ether; and weigh the phenoloid. After weighing the phenoloid, dissolve in sodium hydroxide and examine for its bromine value as described above.

The water in these preparations is determined in the same way as in the analysis of disinfectants containing soaps and resins, but a longer time is required for the complete separation of the water from the phenoloids and oils owing to the difficulty of breaking up the emulsions.

(See also the *British Medical Journal*, October 16, 1920, for an article on disinfectants by Professor Sir German Woodhead.)

CHAPTER XIII

AIR—COAL GAS—OTHER GASES

AIR

AIR consists of a mixture of oxygen, nitrogen, carbon dioxide and water vapour, together with small quantities of the inert gases, argon, krypton, neon, xenon, etc. There are present in the air about 20 per cent. of oxygen, and 80 per cent. of nitrogen. Air has been examined from the tops of mountains, from the middle of large cities, from the depths of valleys and from the open prairie and from many other places, but the proportions of oxygen and nitrogen remain practically the same in all places. The carbon dioxide, on the other hand, varies considerably, and is influenced by the local conditions; respiration of animals removes oxygen and adds carbon dioxide, expired air containing about 5 per cent. of carbon dioxide; coal, gas, wood, etc., when burned use up the oxygen and add carbon dioxide. One litre of pure air at 0° C. and 760 mm. pressure weighs 1·29366 grams, and the air nearer the surface of the earth is more dense than that further away since it is subjected to greater pressure.

Ozone. There are usually only traces of ozone present in air and reliable methods for its determination are not known. A qualitative test for the presence of ozone has been proposed by Engler and Wild (*Ber.* 1896, XXIX, 1940), in which a large volume of the sample is passed first over chromic acid to remove the hydrogen peroxide, and then over manganese sulphate paper and thallous oxide paper; if both papers are coloured brown, ozone is present.

Test for ammonia. Ammonia is present in the atmosphere in traces from the putrefaction of organic matter containing nitrogen. For a qualitative test, large quantities of the sample are passed over moist litmus or turmeric paper, when, in the presence of ammonia, the litmus paper becomes blue, and the turmeric paper brown. A rough estimation of the amount of ammonia in the air may be obtained by passing a large volume of the sample through distilled water and estimating the ammonia, absorbed by the water, with Nessler's reagent as described under water analysis (p. 3).

Estimation of organic matter. A known volume of the sample is passed through a tube in which is placed a plug of clean glass wool, which is then stirred into 100 c.c. of potassium permanganate solution (containing 0·395 gram per 100 c.c.), and 100 c.c. of dilute sulphuric acid (1 in 3); the mixture is then digested for 1 hour at 60° F., 10 c.c. of the potassium permanganate solution are then titrated with the standard oxalic acid solution (p. 6); a blank experiment is at the same time performed, and the number of c.c. of the standard oxalic acid solution used in the actual estimation deducted from the number of c.c. used for the blank gives the number of c.c. of potassium permanganate solution used in the estimation. Each c.c. of potassium permanganate solution used = 0·0001 gram of oxygen absorbed by the organic matter in the sample. The results are expressed in terms of oxygen absorbed and are only comparative.

Estimation of dust. A large and definite volume of air is aspirated through a weighed tube containing cotton wool; the increase in weight represents dust.

Nitrogen. Nitrogen is always determined by difference and is left as a residue after the removal of all the other constituents.

Estimation of oxygen. *Solution required:* An alkaline solution of pyrogallol containing 5 grams of pyrogallol and 120 grams of potassium hydrate in 100 c.c. of water.

The process. The determination is made in Bunte's burette, which consists of a graduated cylinder closed by a tap at both ends; the tap at one end has a double bore, one of which connects with an inlet tube and the other with a glass cup; the burette is placed in a vessel of mercury with both taps open and is thus filled with mercury; the holder containing the sample is connected by a piece of rubber tubing to the inlet tube and the burette is raised partially out of the trough; the mercury in the burette sinks and draws the air from the holder into the burette; the tap at the inlet tube is now closed and the holder is disconnected; the volume of the gas in the burette is ascertained by raising or lowering the burette in the mercury until the levels of the mercury inside and outside the burette are the same; the volume is then read off on the graduations, and the temperature of the surrounding air is noted and also the height of the barometer. The alkaline pyrogallol solution is now placed in the cup, which is connected with the burette, and the solution allowed to run in, care being taken that no air enters with it; both taps are now closed and the burette is removed from the mercury trough and shaken to mix thoroughly the solution and the air; the burette is replaced in the mercury and the bottom tap opened, when the mercury will rise in the burette to take the place of the absorbed oxygen; the tap is again closed, and the contents of the burette shaken until the mercury ceases to rise on opening the tap; the levels of the mercury inside and outside the burette are then adjusted, and the volume of the residual gas noted and also the temperature and the barometric pressure; the volume is then reduced to 0° C. and 760 mm. pressure; the decrease in volume represents oxygen.

Carbon dioxide. Since carbon dioxide is one of the products of respiration it will accumulate in the air of closed and occupied rooms. It is necessary, therefore, to have a simple method of determining the proportion of carbon dioxide in air in order that a judgment may be formed of the efficiency of the ventilation. This is done by the well-known Pettenkofer's process.

Solutions required: Saturated lime water solution. Standard oxalic acid solution containing 2·8636 grams of pure dry crystallized oxalic acid per 1000 c.c. Each c.c. of this solution represents 0·001 gram of carbon dioxide.

The process. A glass bottle, holding about 8 to 10 litres and closed with a tight-fitting rubber bung, is obtained and the exact volume of the bottle is determined by filling it with water and measuring the volume of the water contained. The bottle, which must be perfectly clean and dry, is then filled with the air to be tested; 100 c.c. of the lime water are run into the bottle and the bung at once inserted and the temperature and pressure noted; the lime water is then mixed with the air in the bottle by shaking, and this is repeated occasionally during one hour; the lime water is then rapidly poured into a stoppered 200 c.c. flask; the bottle is rinsed once or twice with distilled water, free from carbon dioxide; the washings are added to the flask and the whole is made up to 200 c.c. with distilled water, free from carbon dioxide; 50 c.c. of this solution are then titrated with the standard oxalic acid solution, using phenol phthalein as an indicator, until the pink colour is just discharged; the number of c.c. of the standard oxalic acid solution used multiplied by four gives the number of c.c. required for the 100 c.c. of lime water taken. 50 c.c. of the original lime water are now similarly titrated with the standard oxalic acid solution and the number of c.c. used multiplied by two gives the number of c.c. required for 100 c.c. of the solution. The difference in the volume of acid used before and after the experiment is thus obtained; and this difference multiplied by 0·001 gives the weight of carbon dioxide in the volume of air taken. Care must be taken that throughout the experiment the lime water does not absorb any carbon dioxide from the breath or the surrounding atmosphere.

Example: The capacity of the bottle was 10,300 c.c.; the temperature of the sample was 20° C. and the pressure 750 mm.; 100 c.c. of the original lime water required 95·8 c.c. of the standard oxalic acid solution and after the experiment 88·7 c.c., then $95·8 - 88·7 = 7·1 \times 0·001 = 0·0071$ gram of carbon dioxide. 44 grams of carbon dioxide occupy 22,400 c.c. at 0° C. and 760 mm., therefore the volume of the carbon dioxide

$$= \frac{0·0071 \times 22,400}{44} = 3·61 \text{ c.c.} \text{ at } 0° \text{ C. and } 760 \text{ mm., therefore}$$

the volume at 20° C. and 750 mm. $= \dfrac{3·61 \times 293 \times 760}{273 \times 750} = 3·92$ c.c.,

then $\dfrac{3·92 \times 100}{10,300} = 0·038$ per cent. of carbon dioxide in the sample.

Haldane's method. A small and compact instrument has been devised by Haldane to determine the amount of carbon dioxide in air. It requires a little practice to get accurate results. The method consists in absorbing the carbon dioxide from 25 c.c. of air by caustic potash, and then measuring the decrease in volume under the same conditions of temperature and pressure. Each of the graduated parts of the burette is divided into 1/10,000 part of the whole capacity of the burette, so that the results are read off in parts per 10,000. The chemical change is, of course,

$$2KOH + CO_2 = K_2CO_3 + H_2O.$$

It is obvious that great care must be taken in the experiment with such small changes in volumes.

Lunge and Zeckendorf's method (Zeitsch. Angew. Chem. 1888, 1, 395). This is an excellent rapid method for the approximate determination of carbon dioxide, especially when it is present in large quantities.

Solutions required: N/10 sodium carbonate solution containing 5·3 grams of sodium carbonate, and 0·1 gram of phenol phthalein in 1000 c.c.

Dilute sodium carbonate solution; 2 c.c. of the above solution are placed in a 100 c.c. graduated flask, and made up to the mark with distilled water, free from carbon dioxide, and the flask instantly closed; this dilute solution will not keep for more than 12 hours.

The process. A wide-mouthed bottle, of 110 c.c. capacity, is fitted with a stopper in which are two holes through which pass two glass tubes, one reaching to the bottom of the bottle and attached to a rubber bulb of 70 c.c. capacity; fill the bottle with some of the air to be examined by compressing the rubber bulb several times; then place in the bottle 10 c.c. of the dilute sodium carbonate solution and immediately replace the stopper; the contents of the rubber bulb are now driven through the solution in the bottle, and the contents of the bottle are shaken; this is continued until the pink colour has been discharged; the amount of carbon dioxide is then obtained from the following table by noting the number of compressions of the bulb required to discharge the pink colour.

Compressions	CO_2 in parts per 1000	Compressions	CO_2 in parts per 1000	Compressions	CO_2 in parts per 1000
2	3·00	11	0·87	20	0·62
3	2·50	12	0·83	22	0·58
4	2·10	13	0·80	24	0·54
5	1·80	14	0·77	26	0·51
6	1·55	15	0·74	28	0·49
7	1·35	16	0·71	30	0·48
8	1·15	17	0·69	35	0·42
9	1·00	18	0·66	40	0·38
10	0·90	19	0·64	48	0·30

Aqueous vapour. The dew-point, or the temperature at which the aqueous vapour in the air begins to be deposited, is determined by Daniel's hygrometer or by a wet-and-dry bulb thermometer. In the latter instrument the temperature of the dry bulb is noted, together with the temperature of the other bulb upon which the film of moisture was first seen to be deposited. Certain factors have been worked out by Glaisher, and by means of his tables it is easy to calculate from the temperature observations the amount of aqueous vapour by weight in a definite volume of air. These details are given in most books dealing with the general principles of hygiene.

Ground air. There is a considerable amount of carbon dioxide in ground air with small quantities of ammonia and also various hydrocarbons, and sulphuretted hydrogen. The gases may be collected by Hesse's method. A narrow steel cylinder with a sharp point, and perforated with numerous holes just above the point, is forced into the earth to varying depths as required. The outside end of the tube is connected with a large glass vessel of 8 to 10 litres capacity, and this is connected in turn with an aspirator. The jar is first emptied of its air by means of the aspirator and the connection between the steel tube and the glass vessel is re-established by opening the stopcocks. The ground air is then aspirated into the glass vessel and the sample analysed for carbon dioxide as described above. Another series of experiments by aspirating the ground air through pure water will dissolve the ammonia and this can be determined by Nessler's solution in the usual way. The organic matter in the ground air can also be determined similarly by passing the gases through a known strength of a dilute solution of potassium permanganate, as described on p. 274.

Carbon monoxide. Vogel (*Ber. Chem. Gesellsch.* XI, 235) was the first to use the well-known spectrum of blood charged with carbon monoxide as a means for detecting the gas. The method is to take 2 or 3 c.c. of blood, dilute it with water till only a very faint red colour is seen; place in a dry bottle and aspirate about 10 litres of the suspected air through it. When carbon monoxide is present the blood at once becomes rose coloured, and upon the addition of two drops of a freshly prepared and colourless solution of ammonium sulphide and shaken the well-known absorption bands do not disappear; in blood which is free from carbon monoxide the absorption bands are replaced by a broad and weakly defined band. The ammonium sulphide should always be prepared as it is wanted, by passing sulphuretted hydrogen through a solution of ammonia. The comparison of the two spectra is best effected by placing the two solutions in test-tubes, and using the test-tubes as condensing lenses. One is placed in front of the slit end of the spectroscope, and the other in front of a small reflecting prism which covers the slit about half its length. Two small fish-tail burners are used as the sources of light, and these are placed end on and not with their broad fronts facing the slit; then, by carefully adjusting the two test-tubes containing the fluids, two sharp images can be easily obtained, and the spectra examined. The slit should not be too wide, otherwise the light is scattered and overlaps the absorption bands and their sharpness is lessened.

Haldane's method of detecting and estimating carbon monoxide in air (*Jour. of Physiology*, vol. XVIII, p. 461). The method depends upon the fact that when a hæmoglobin solution is well shaken with air containing CO, the proportion of the hæmoglobin, which finally combines with the CO, varies with the percentage of CO present in the air. By estimating colorimetrically the proportion of the hæmoglobin which has combined with the CO it is thereby possible to infer the percentage of CO present in the air. In employing hæmoglobin for the purpose Haldane proceeds as follows: "The sample is collected by sucking two or three litres of the air through a clean and dry bottle of about 100 to 200 c.c. capacity. The bottle is closed by means of a doubly tubulated cork, previously soaked in paraffin. Each of the pieces of glass tubing which pass through the cork is securely closed by means of a stopper made of about an inch of rubber tubing, into one end of which fits a piece of glass rod. For the determination of the CO about 5 c.c. of a solution of defibrinated ox blood diluted to 1/100th with water are introduced into the bottle in the following manner. A pipette having been filled with the blood solution one of the pieces of glass rod is removed, the rubber tubing being at the same time compressed, so as to prevent air from passing into the bottle. The end of the pipette is now inserted into the rubber tubing, and the blood solution allowed to flow into the bottle. As the increase of pressure within the bottle prevents more than a part of the blood solution from entering, it is necessary to allow some of the air inside to escape. This is easily effected by pinching the rubber tubing which fits in the other glass stopper, and so opening a small channel for the passage outwards of the air. The pipette having been removed and the glass stopper again inserted without letting any air in the bottle is now gently shaken for about 10 minutes, at the end of which time the hæmoglobin will have taken up all the CO which it is capable of taking up from the contained air. With vigorous shaking the time required is much less, but the solution may become turbid from mechanical coagulation of albumin and hæmoglobin, so that gentle shaking for a longer time is to be preferred. When the shaking is complete the solution is removed with a pipette into one of three narrow test-tubes of exactly equal diameter (about $\frac{3}{8}$ or $\frac{1}{2}$ inch), and each capable of holding at least 12 c.c. Into another of the test-tubes exactly 5 c.c. of the original blood solution are measured by means of a pipette. The third test-tube is filled with some of the same blood solution, the hæmoglobin of which has been already saturated with CO. The saturation is effected by placing some of the blood solution in a small bottle or flask, the air in which is then washed out with coal gas. When the bottle is full of coal gas it is quickly closed with the thumb, and then shaken for 2 or 3 minutes so as to saturate the hæmoglobin with CO, of which coal gas contains about 5 per cent.—a quantity sufficient to produce (particularly in the absence of oxygen) rapid and absolutely complete saturation. The test-tube containing the saturated blood should be filled

full and corked if it is to be kept any time, as otherwise the
CO escapes from the solution. The tints of the solutions in the
test-tubes are now compared. If more than 0·01 per cent. of
CO was present in the sample of air the blood solution which
has been shaken with the air will be pinker than the original
solution contained in the second tube. If more than 3 per cent.
of CO was present the tint will be sensibly equal to that of the
solution saturated with coal gas. An approximate estimate of
the saturation may even be made by simply comparing the
three tubes, and from this estimate the percentage of CO in
the sample of air may be roughly estimated from the table on
p. 283.

"Standard carmine solution is now added from a burette
to the solution in the second test-tube, until its tint is exactly
equal to that of the solution which was shaken with the air.
When the tints are nearly equal not more than 0·25 c.c. of
carmine solution are added at a time. The points are noted at
which there is just not enough, and just too much carmine, the
mean being taken as the correct result. The quantity of carmine required to produce equality of tint with the saturated
solution is also determined or redetermined at the same time.
The carmine solution is prepared as follows. One gram of pure
carmine is mixed in a mortar with a few drops of ammonia
and dissolved in 100 c.c. of glycerine. This solution is preserved
and a standard solution prepared from it when required by
diluting 5 c.c. of the glycerine solution to 500 c.c. with water.
It will be found that when about 5 c.c. of this standard carmine
solution are added to 5 c.c. of ox blood diluted to 1/100th, the
tint of the resultant solution is the same both in quality and
intensity as that of the diluted blood when saturated with
CO or coal gas. Before making a determination, however, it
is well to ascertain that the two solutions actually correspond.
If in order to produce equality in intensity as well as quality
of tint it is necessary to add water to either test-tube, the stock
of blood solution or carmine solution must be diluted accord-
ingly. It will be found that the amount of standard carmine
solution required to produce the saturation tint varies slightly
as the tint of the daylight changes. For this reason the amount
should be determined each time the solution is used. The

standard carmine solution should be prepared fresh when required, as it distinctly loses strength when kept for a few days.
The blood solution must also be freshly prepared, although
the blood itself may be kept for a long time in a corked bottle.
A blood solution may be so far altered as to be unfit for use
even when the oxyhæmoglobin bands, and no others, are visible
on spectroscopic examination. A solution thus altered does not
change colour to the usual extent when saturated with CO.

"From the results of the titration with carmine solution the
percentage saturation of the hæmoglobin with CO may be
easily calculated in the manner illustrated by the following
example. To 5 c.c. of blood solution 6·2 c.c. of standard carmine were required to be added to produce the tint of blood
solution shaken with the air under examination. In the former
case the carmine was in the proportion of 6·2 to 11·2; in the
latter case in the proportion of 2·2 to 7·2. The percentage
saturation of the hæmoglobin in the blood shaken with the air
was thus

$$\frac{2 \cdot 2}{7 \cdot 2} \times \frac{11 \cdot 2}{6 \cdot 2} \times 100 = 55 \cdot 2.$$

"The method will only give correct results when the oxygen
percentage in the air is nearly normal. A deficit of two or
three per cent. of oxygen will hardly influence the result appreciably, and may therefore be disregarded. A deficit of 5 per
cent. in the oxygen of the air will, however, cause the results
to be almost a third too high, so that, for example, half saturation of the blood solution would apparently indicate 0·15 per
cent. when in reality only 0·11 per cent. was present."

Also, when there is more than 0·5 CO per cent. present in
the air, or when there is little or no oxygen present, the sample
must be suitably diluted with air. Coal gas, for example,
would require to be diluted 1/40th or 1/50th with air.

In a later paper (*Jour. of Physiology*, vol. XX, 521) Haldane
states that daylight has a marked influence on the stability of
carboxyhæmoglobin, and therefore recommends that the blood
solution and sample of air must be covered with a cloth during
the process of shaking, and a very bright light should be
avoided during the process of titration with the carmine solution. The following table gives as nearly as possible the values

when the bottle is protected from light during the shaking, and from this table the percentage of CO in the sample of air may be calculated.

Percentage saturation of hæmoglobin in blood solution	Percentage of CO in the air	Percentage saturation of hæmoglobin in blood solution	Percentage of CO in the air
5	0·006	55	0·11
10	·012	60	·135
15	·019	65	·160
20	·026	70	·21
25	·034	75	·27
30	·043	80	·36
35	·054	85	·51
40	·066	90	·81
45	·078	95	1·70
50	·090		

Atmospheric pollution

The following method for the determination of atmospheric pollution is taken from the 1st Report of the Committee for the Investigation of Atmospheric Pollution (*Lancet Supplement*, February, 1916; and *Analyst*, 1916, XLI, 113):

Standard gauge. This is a galvanized iron stand, supporting a circular enamelled iron vessel of 4 square feet collecting area; the vessel has a conical bottom, which communicates with a group of bottles connected together, and of sufficient size to hold one month's rainfall; these bottles are removed once a month for analysis. The gauge should be placed on the ground in an open space, and should be washed down with some of the collected water, using a brush and squeegee of standard pattern. The bottles are to be allowed to remain at rest in the laboratory for several days until the contents have settled. The volume of the contents should be noted at the time of receipt.

Undissolved matter. All the collected water is to be used for the estimation. The bed of a Gooch crucible is prepared by heating a tared filter paper (12·5 cm. in diameter) with about 200 c.c. of the sample water, which has been specially syphoned off, and shaking until the paper is reduced to a pulp; a portion of this is collected in the crucible, which is supported in a graduated bottle and connected with a filter pump; the whole of the sample is then passed through the filter under pressure;

the contents of the bottle are shaken up towards the end, and poured on to the filter, and the bottle is rinsed with some of the filtrate; the remainder of the paper pulp is added and the contents of the crucible are washed, dried at 105° C. and weighed.

Tarry matters. The crucible and contents are extracted with carbon disulphide in a Soxhlet apparatus; dried and re-weighed; the loss in weight represents tarry matters.

Ash. The residue from the estimation of tarry matters is carefully ignited and reweighed.

Dissolved matter. 250 c.c. of the filtrate are evaporated to dryness for the determination of total solids, as described under water analysis (p. 5); the residue is gently ignited and weighed; the loss in weight represents organic matter, and the difference between total solids and organic matter represents mineral matter.

Sulphates. One litre of the filtrate is concentrated and the sulphates precipitated as barium sulphate as described under water analysis (p. 23).

Chlorides. 500 c.c. of the filtrate are titrated with N/10 silver nitrate solution, using potassium chromate solution as an indicator, as described under water analysis (p. 5). Each c.c. of N/10 silver nitrate solution used represents 0·00355 gram of chlorine.

Ammonia. 1000 c.c. of the filtrate are slightly acidified with sulphuric acid, evaporated to 100 c.c., and the resulting solution is distilled, after the addition of alkali; the ammonia is determined by means of Nessler's reagent, as described under water analysis (p. 3). Or the ammonia may be determined by "Nesslerizing" 10 to 25 c.c. of the water direct, without distillation.

Lime is determined on 1 litre of the filtrate, as directed under water analysis (p. 21).

Alkalinity is expressed as ammonia, and is determined by titrating 500 c.c. of the filtrate with N/100 sulphuric acid, using methyl orange as an indicator. Each c.c. of N/100 sulphuric acid used represents 0·00017 gram of ammonia.

Acidity is expressed as sulphuric acid, and is determined by titrating 500 c.c. of the filtrate with N/100 sodium hydroxide

solution, using methyl orange as an indicator. Each c.c. of
N/100 sodium hydroxide solution used represents 0·00049
gram of sulphuric acid.

All results are expressed as a percentage of the total solids
and calculated as metric tons per square kilometre. A metric
ton is 1000 kilograms.

Classification. The following units have been decided
upon in metric tons per square kilometre per month:

Total deposited solids	5 tons
Insoluble matter, tar	0·05 ton
carbonaceous matter other than	
tar	1 ton
ash	2 tons
Soluble matter, loss on ignition	0·75 ton
ash	1·5 tons
total solids	5 tons
sulphates	1 ton
chlorine	0·3 ton
ammonia	0·05 ton

All values below these units are grouped as Class A. Class B
includes 1 to 3 units; Class C, 3 to 5 units; and Class D above
5 units.

COAL GAS

The analysis of coal gas may be accomplished by means of
Hempel's gas apparatus. It consists of a burette, which includes a measuring tube and a pressure tube, and a pipette
used as an absorbing vessel for the various constituents. The
gaseous mixture is subjected to the action of suitable absor-
bents in turn in a series of the pipettes, whereby the proportions of the constituent gases in the mixture can be estimated.

The burette is filled with the gas and connected with the
pipette. The stopcock between the burette and the pipette is
opened; the pressure tube connected with the former is raised,
and the gas flows into the pipette; turn off the stopcock when
the water in the burette has reached the required mark in the
capillary tube connecting the burette with the pipette; shake

the pipette gently for a minute or two and repeat the operation; transfer the gas back to the burette by opening the stopcock, and read off the volume of gas after bringing the height of the water in the pressure tube to the same height as that in the burette. Subsequent absorptions are repeated similarly, each constituent gas being absorbed by a special reagent. A separate pipette is kept for each reagent. In coal gas the constituent gases are absorbed in the following order:

(1) Carbon dioxide, by caustic potash solution.

(2) Olefines, by saturated bromine water; and then remove the bromine vapour by caustic potash solution in a separate pipette.

(3) Benzene, by fuming nitric acid; and then remove the oxides of nitrogen by the caustic potash pipette.

(4) Oxygen, by a solution of alkaline pyrogallic acid.

(5) Carbon monoxide, by a freshly made solution of ammoniacal cuprous chloride.

(6) The residual gas is transferred to a pipette charged with water, and the hydrogen and methane are estimated by mixing with oxygen and sparking in a special form of Hempel explosion pipette. The gases are thus burnt to carbon dioxide and water.

(7) Nitrogen and the argon series of gases are estimated as a residue.

Estimation of ammonia and total sulphur. The gas is tested qualitatively for ammonia and sulphuretted hydrogen by passing it over moist lead acetate paper, and moist red litmus paper; in the presence of sulphuretted hydrogen the lead acetate paper becomes dark brown or black, and, in the presence of ammonia, the red litmus paper becomes blue.

Quantitative determination. The gas is first passed through a cylinder, containing glass beads, which have been moistened with a known quantity of N/10 sulphuric acid; during the passage through this cylinder the ammonia combines with the sulphuric acid to form ammonium sulphate. The gas is then passed through a burner and burned at the rate of 0·5 cubic foot per hour until 10 cubic feet have been burned; the burner is surrounded by pieces of solid ammonium carbonate and the gases formed by the combustion are passed through a trumpet tube into a cylinder filled with glass balls which are kept moist; the cylinder is connected with a long glass chimney in which the final condensation takes place; the sulphur dioxide formed by the combustion of the sulphur in the gas dissolves in the water and passes to the bottom of the cylinder, and through the bottom of the cylinder into a glass beaker; after the combustion is completed the cylinder is washed out with distilled water and the washings are heated with a few drops of bromine to complete the conversion of all the sulphur into sulphate; the liquid is then made acid with hydrochloric acid and an excess of barium chloride solution is added; the precipitated barium sulphate is collected on a filter paper, washed with distilled water, dried in a water oven, incinerated and weighed. The weight of barium sulphate obtained multiplied by 0·1373 gives the amount in grams of total sulphur in 10 cubic feet of the gas. The sulphur is usually returned as grains of sulphur per 100 cubic feet of gas.

Estimation of ammonia. The first cylinder, containing the N/10 sulphuric acid, is washed out with distilled water, and the excess of N/10 sulphuric acid is determined by titration with N/10 sodium hydroxide solution. The number of c.c. of N/10 sulphuric acid neutralized during the passage of the gas multiplied by 0·0017 gives the number of grams of ammonia in 10 cubic feet of the gas.

Estimation of sulphuretted hydrogen. Somerville (*Jour. Gas. Light*, 1912, CXII, 29). *Solutions required:* N/1000 iodine solution. Starch solution.

The process. 10 c.c. of the N/1000 iodine solution and 10 c.c. of the starch solution are placed in a 100 c.c. wash bottle, and the gas is passed through the mixture by means of an aspirator until the blue colour disappears; the volume of the gas used is determined by measuring the volume of the water run out of the aspirator. A second determination is then made in which the gas is first passed through a scrubbing tower, containing lead carbonate, which removes all the sulphuretted hydrogen; the apparent sulphuretted hydrogen obtained in the second experiment is subtracted from the amount obtained in the first experiment, as this apparent sulphuretted hydrogen is due to the unsaturated compounds, hydrogen cyanide, etc., present in the gas, which combine with the iodine. 10 c.c. of the N/10 iodine solution represent 0·01122 c.c. of sulphuretted hydrogen.

Determination of illuminating power. *Apparatus required:*

(1) Standard light, which is a 10 candle power pentane lamp.

(2) Standard burner, which is a Number 2 Argand burner.

(3) Standard photometer, which is a bar photometer, or a jet photometer.

The process. The pentane lamp and the standard burner are fixed at opposite ends of the photometer in such a manner that the tops of the two flames are equidistant from the table; the pentane lamp is lighted and allowed to burn for 15 minutes; the argand burner is then lighted, and the gas consumption regulated to 5 cubic feet per hour; a box containing a piece of paper on which is a grease spot between the two lights is then moved about on the bar until the grease spot is equally illuminated on both sides, which is shown by the grease spot becoming invisible; the illuminating power is then read off on the bar in candle power.

Calorific value of coal gas. Coal gas is now largely used for heating and cooking purposes, and its calorific value is usually determined by the Public Analyst. The calorific value is the amount of heat given out by the complete combustion of a known volume or mass of the gas. The unit employed is known as the *calorie,* and it is defined as the amount of heat necessary to raise 1 kilogram of water from 0° to 1° C. Another unit is called the *British Thermal Unit* and it is defined as the amount of heat required to raise 1 lb. of water 1° F. One calorie is equal to 3·9683 British Thermal Units.

The calorific value is determined experimentally by burning a definite volume of the gas under conditions whereby measurements can be made as to the amount of heat given off when it is burnt. The gas is conducted through an experimental meter and it is burnt at rates varying from 3 to 30 cubic feet per hour. Coal gas is usually burnt at about 6 cubic feet per hour. The burner is placed within the cavity of a double-walled cylinder, and the burnt gases escape through tubes which pass through the space between the walls of the cylinder. The space round the cylinder contains water which flows in at the bottom and out at the top, so that it is in contact with the tubes down which the burnt gases descend. Delicate thermometers indicate the temperatures of the incoming and outgoing water. The rate at which the water is supplied is regulated so that the exit water is from 10° to 20° warmer than the water which enters. A large measuring cylinder of 2 litres capacity is used to collect the water. The temperature of the outflowing water is observed till it remains constant, and the long hand of the experimental meter is noted till it is just passing the zero mark, when the water is collected in the 2-litre measuring flask. The temperature of the outflowing water is observed six times while the glass is filling, and the temperature of the inflowing water about twice. After 2 litres of the water have been collected, the gas supply is cut off and the meter is read. This gives, therefore, the amount of gas which has been burnt during the filling of the flask. The average temperature of the water which goes in and that which comes out is also known; and therefore we can estimate by how many degrees the combustion of a definite volume of the gas has raised the two litres of water. To find the calorific value of unit volume of the gas, twice the mean rise in temperature of the water is divided by the volume of the gas which has been burnt. As the gas is usually measured in cubic feet, the result is the calorific value of a cubic foot of gas.

The water condensed from the combustion of the gases collects at the bottom of the apparatus, and it is run off and measured in a small measuring cylinder. For every c.c. of water so condensed per cubic foot of gas burnt, a deduction of 0·6 calorie is made from the calorific value previously found. This is to eliminate the value of the heat given off on the condensation of the steam to water; because the water produced by the combustion of gas escapes as steam with the other products of combustion, and therefore its latent heat is not available for use.

The following analyses of an illuminating gas have been kindly supplied by Mr J. West Knights.

	(1)	(2)	(3)	(4)
Hydro-carbons (ethylene, etc.)	4·0	4·6	3·5	3·8
Oxygen	·5	·2	·5	·7
Carbon monoxide	5·7	6·2	5·6	5·6
Carbon dioxide	nil	nil	nil	nil
Methane	33·9	30·8	34·0	32·6
Hydrogen	51·8	56·1	51·6	52·7
Nitrogen	4·1	2·1	4·8	4·6
	100·0	100·0	100·0	100·0

Sulphur, in grains per 100 cubic feet.

Aug. 1911	17·32 grains	⎫ The sulphur in these
Jan. 1912	24·10 „	⎬ three instances is very
„ 1913	10·40 „	⎭ high.
„ 1914	7·95 „	

There was no sulphuretted hydrogen present.

Illuminating power.

Aug. 1912	17·22 candles
Jan. 1913	16·82 „
Sept. 1913	17·08 „
Jan. 1914	16·33 „

The legal standard is 16 candles.

CHAPTER XIV

RAG FLOCK—URINE

EXAMINATION OF RAG FLOCK

THE Rag Flock Act, 1911, provides that "it shall not be lawful for any person to sell or have in his possession for sale flock, manufactured from rags, or to use for the purposes of making any article of upholstery, cushions or bedding, flock manufactured from rags, or to have in his possession flock manufactured from rags intended to be used for any such purpose unless the flock conforms to such standard of cleanliness as may be prescribed by the regulations to be made by the Local Government Board." The Rag Flock Regulations, 1912, were issued by the Local Government Board under the above Act and came into force on July 1st, 1912, they provide that "Flock shall be deemed to conform to the standard of cleanliness for the purposes of the Rag Flock Act, when the amount of soluble chlorine in the form of chlorides, removed by thorough washing with distilled water at a temperature not exceeding 25° C. from not less than 40 grams of a well-mixed sample, does not exceed 30 parts of chlorine per 100,000 parts of flock." Warburton has shown (*Reports to the Local Government Board on Public Health and Medical Subjects*, No. 27) that "lice and their eggs may pass through the flocking machine without being crushed. The lice themselves are incapable of surviving more than 3 or 4 days without food, and it is extremely unlikely that any of them would be alive when the flock was converted into bedding. Their eggs however may take a month or more to hatch and it is quite possible that living eggs might be present in the bedding."

Chemical examination of rag flock. Garrett (*Reports to the Local Government Board on Public Health and Medical Subjects*, No. 27) adopts the following process: The flock is spread out to dry at the temperature of the room; and, after 24 hours, the moisture is determined by drying at 105° C. for 90 minutes.

100 grams of the sample are then placed in a large beaker, and 3000 c.c. of water are added; the mixture is allowed to stand for 39 minutes with frequent stirring; the flock is then strained and wrung out; the liquid is filtered and the filtrate examined as if it were a sample of water; the total solid matter, chlorine and free and albuminoid ammonia are estimated.

Estimation of soluble chlorine. Parkes (*Chem. News*, 1913, CVIII, 177). *Solution required:* Silver nitrate solution. Weigh out 4·8 grams of silver nitrate, dissolve it in water, and make the solution up to 1000 c.c. Each c.c. of this solution represents 0·001 gram of chlorine.

The process. 50 grams of the well-mixed sample are placed in a large beaker and 500 c.c. of water are added; the flock is allowed to steep for 4 hours and is then drained; pressed by hand and washed with successive quantities of water (of 100 c.c. each) until 1000 c.c. of washings are obtained; the washings are then filtered and 100 c.c. of the filtrate (= 5 grams of flock) are evaporated to dryness in a porcelain dish with a minute quantity of lime; the residue is then charred, cooled, extracted with water and filtered; a few drops of potassium chromate solution are added to the filtrate, and the standard silver nitrate solution drop by drop from a burette until a permanent red colour is obtained. Each c.c. of silver nitrate solution used multiplied by 20 gives the parts of chlorine per 100,000 parts of flock. In the case of unwashed flock it is advisable to add a few drops of phenol solution as a vermicide.

Example: Treated as described above the filtrate from a sample of rag flock required 17·3 c.c. of the standard silver nitrate solution; then 17·3 × 20 = 346 parts of soluble chlorine per 100,000 parts of flock.

Black's method (*Analyst*, 1913, XXXVIII, 409). *Solutions required:* N/10 silver nitrate solution. N/10 potassium sulphocyanide solution.

The process. 40 grams of the flock are placed on a Buchner funnel fitted to a 58 oz. flask, and thoroughly wetted with distilled water until the mass can be pressed down as a thick felt; the mass is then covered with water and allowed to stand; after standing the water is passed through the flock by pressure and the washing continued until the filtrate reaches 2000 c.c.;

to 500 c.c. of the filtrate a few drops of perhydrol are added
and the mixture is evaporated to small bulk; 5 c.c. of concentrated nitric acid, and 20 c.c. of the N/10 silver nitrate solution, are then added; the mixture is heated to 90° C., cooled,
agitated and filtered; the precipitate is washed, and the filtrate
titrated with the N/10 potassium sulpho-cyanide solution,
using a saturated solution of iron alum as an indicator, until a
permanent red colour is obtained. Each c.c. of silver nitrate
solution used represents 0·00355 gram of soluble chlorine.

URINE

Urine has a yellow colour, if normal; in the presence of
blood it has a brownish yellow smoky appearance and, in the
presence of bile, a green colour; turbidity is sometimes due
to the presence of urates, phosphates or mucus. It is essential
that the amount of urine daily voided should be known, for
the analysis of urine to be of any value and the sample should,
if possible, consist of the whole of the urine voided during a
period of 24 hours; if this is not possible care should be taken
that the sample is not obtained during a shorter period than
3 hours after a meal. The complete analysis of urine is a matter
of very great difficulty, but the most important constituents,
urea, chlorides, sugar and albumen, can be determined with
sufficient accuracy. A normal adult passes about 1500 c.c. of
urine during the 24 hours.

Qualitative examination. *Reaction.* Normal urine should
be acid to litmus but it quickly becomes alkaline owing to the
formation of ammonium carbonate by the fermentation of the
urea.

Albumen. Make a few c.c. of the urine faintly acid with
acetic acid and boil, albumen is precipitated, and appears as
a faint cloud; proteoses, etc., may be precipitated but redissolve on heating.

Picric acid test. To a few c.c. of the urine add an equal
quantity of picric acid solution (containing 10 grams of picric
acid and 20 grams of citric acid in 1000 c.c.); in the presence
of albumen an immediate precipitate is formed.

Detection of sugar. 5 c.c. of the urine (boiled and filtered in the presence of albumen) are mixed with 5 c.c. of mixed Fehling's solution and raised to boiling; in the presence of sugar a red precipitate of cuprous oxide is obtained. Or 5 c.c. of the urine may be mixed with 5 c.c. of saturated picric acid solution, and 2 c.c. of a 6 per cent. solution of potassium hydroxide added; the mixture is then heated to boiling, when, if the urine is, for clinical purposes, free from sugar a bright red colour appears in the transparent solution when held up to the light; but, in the presence of sugar, the colour becomes so intense as to cause the solution to be quite opaque.

Detection of bile. 5 c.c. of the urine are mixed cautiously with 5 c.c. of concentrated sulphuric acid and cooled; a small quantity of powdered cane sugar is added and the solution mixed and slightly warmed; in the presence of bile a reddish violet colour is produced. Or some of the urine may be filtered through a white filter paper, and the paper allowed to dry, when dry a drop of yellow nitric acid is applied from the end of a glass rod to the centre of the paper; in the presence of bile, colour rings of violet, red, green, and yellow appear on the paper.

Detection of blood. A reddish smoky appearance in urine is characteristic of the presence of blood. To 5 c.c. of the urine add 5 c.c. of freshly prepared tincture of guaiacum (made from unoxidized resin), and 5 c.c. of an ethereal solution of hydrogen peroxide; in the presence of blood a deep blue colour is produced. Too much reliance must not be placed on this test as many other organic bodies will produce the colour.

Detection of chlorides. The sample of urine is filtered and boiled to remove any albumen present; to a portion of the filtrate an equal bulk of a 3 per cent. solution of silver nitrate and a few drops of nitric acid are added; in the presence of the normal amounts of chlorides an abundant white precipitate of silver chloride appears immediately.

Detection of acetone. To 200 c.c. of urine a small quantity of phosphoric acid is added and the whole is distilled; to the distillate a few drops of a 10 per cent. solution of potassium hydroxide are added, and, after gently warming, a few drops of a solution of iodine in potassium iodide, until the solution

becomes straw coloured; a few drops of potassium hydroxide
solution are then added; in the presence of acetone a yellow
crystalline precipitate of iodoform is obtained, which is easily
recognized by its odour.

Examination of the deposit. Some of the urine is allowed
to stand in a conical glass and the deposit, which is generally
simple in character, examined by the following tests.

1. Warm a little of the deposit in the urine, if it dissolves
it consists entirely of urates.

2. If the deposit does not dissolve on warming, allow it to
settle; pour off the urine and warm the deposit with acetic
acid; if it dissolves it consists of phosphates.

3. If the deposit is insoluble in acetic acid, add a little
hydrochloric acid and warm again; if it dissolves it is calcium
oxalate.

4. If the deposit is still insoluble, it is probably uric acid;
to a fresh portion of the deposit add a few drops of potassium
hydroxide solution, uric acid will dissolve; or place a small
quantity of the deposit in a small white dish, add a few drops
of concentrated nitric acid and evaporate to dryness; cool and,
when cold, add to the dry residue a drop of ammonia solution;
in the presence of uric acid a purple colour is produced which
turns to violet on the addition of a drop of potassium hydroxide solution.

The deposit should also be examined microscopically; this
examination requires a large experience to be of any value,
but the general characteristics of some of the deposits are as
follows:

Uric acid. These crystals are flat plates, dumb-bell-shaped,
stellate, needle-shaped or rosetted; if a drop of potassium
hydroxide solution is inserted under the cover slip, they dissolve.

Ammonium urate. It occurs in small tufts of needle-shaped
crystals; these should be dissolved in a drop of water on the
slide and a drop of acetic acid added; the mixture warmed
slightly and allowed to cool, when the characteristic uric acid
crystals will be obtained.

Calcium oxalate. The crystals are generally small and octa-
hedral; if a drop of acetic acid is inserted under the cover

glass they do not dissolve but will do so with a drop of hydrochloric acid.

Magnesium ammonium phosphate. The crystals appear in
the form of stellate plates immediately the urine becomes, or
is made, alkaline.

Cystin appears as flat hexagonal crystals which are soluble
in ammonia.

Blood may be recognized by the circular red corpuscles
which are sometimes angular in old or stale urine.

Pus corpuscles are light coloured and slightly larger than
those of blood and appear in the deposit as a light coloured
layer.

Quantitative Examination of Urine

Determination of specific gravity. 10 c.c. of the urine
are measured out into a weighed beaker and weighed; the
weight of the urine multiplied by 100 gives the specific gravity;
or it may be taken with a good hydrometer.

Example: 10 c.c. of a sample of urine weighed 10·249 grams;
then the specific gravity of the sample was

$$10 \cdot 249 \times 100 = 1024 \cdot 9.$$

Estimation of total solid matter. An approximate
estimate of the total solid matter is obtained by deducting
1000 from the specific gravity, and multiplying the result by
0·233.

Example: The specific gravity of a sample of urine was
1024·9, then the percentage of total solid matter in the sample
was

$$1024 \cdot 9 - 1000 = 24 \cdot 9 \times 0 \cdot 233 = 5 \cdot 80.$$

Estimation of the chlorides. 10 c.c. of the urine and 1
gram of pure powdered ammonium nitrate are evaporated to
dryness and thoroughly charred; the char is extracted with
hot water, filtered and well washed on the filter paper; the
filtrate is acidified with dilute acetic acid to destroy the soluble
carbonates; and the excess of acetic acid is neutralized with
calcium carbonate; a drop or two of potassium chromate solution are added, followed by N/10 silver nitrate from a burette

until a permanent red colour is obtained. Each c.c. of N/10 silver nitrate used = 0·005845 gram of sodium chloride.

Example: 10 c.c. of urine required 11·7 c.c. of N/10 silver nitrate solution to produce a permanent red colour; then 11·7 × 0·005845 = 0·0683885 × 100 = 6·84 parts of sodium chloride per 1000 parts of urine.

Estimation of urea. Russell and West (*Journ. Chem. Soc.* 1859, XII, 749) devised an exceedingly simple apparatus consisting of a decomposition tube 9 ins. long and about half an inch in diameter, with a constriction near the closed end, and the open end fitted into a pneumatic trough, supported on legs; and a measuring tube, holding about 40 c.c.

Solution required: Solution of sodium hypobromite is obtained by dissolving 100 grams of sodium hydroxide in 250 c.c. of water; and, just before the experiment, mixing 25 c.c. of this solution with 2·5 c.c. of bromine.

The process. 5 c.c. of the urine are carefully placed in the decomposition tube and rinsed in with water, until the bulb is full; the constriction is then plugged with a glass rod; the hypobromite solution is now run into the tube and the measuring tube is filled with water and inverted in the trough; the glass rod is removed and the measuring tube instantly placed over the decomposition tube, the hypobromite reacts with the urea to form nitrogen, which escapes into the measuring tube; at the end of 15 minutes, the volume of gas in the measuring tube is noted, and this volume divided by 371 gives the number of grams of urea in the 5 c.c. of urine taken. This method obviates calculation for temperature and pressure, as Russell and West found that 0·1 gram of urea constantly gave 37·1 c.c. of nitrogen at ordinary temperatures and pressures.

Example: In an experiment 5 c.c. of urine evolved 27·3 c.c. of nitrogen, then $\frac{27\cdot3}{371}$ = 0·0736 × 200 = 14·72 grams of urea in 1000 parts of urine.

In the absence of sugar and albumen, an approximate determination of the percentage of urea is made by subtracting 1000 from the specific gravity and dividing the remainder by 10.

Example: The specific gravity of a sample of urine was 1024·9, then the percentage of urea in the sample was

$$\frac{1024·9 - 1000}{10} = 2·49 \text{ per cent.}$$

$$= 24·9 \text{ parts of urea per 1000 parts of urine.}$$

Estimation of sugar. *Solution required:* Pavy's solution. 60 c.c. of Fehling's copper solution (p. 109) and 60 c.c. of Fehling's alkaline solution are mixed with 300 c.c. of ammonia solution (specific gravity 0·880) and 10 c.c. of a 10 per cent. solution of sodium hydroxide in a 1000 c.c. flask, and made up to the mark with water. Each c.c. of this solution corresponds to 0·0005 gram of sugar calculated as glucose.

The process. 100 c.c. of the Pavy solution are placed in a boiling flask, fitted with an outlet tube, to which is attached a piece of rubber tubing leading out of the window or into a fume cupboard to carry away the fumes of ammonia. 10 c.c. of the filtered urine are placed in a 200 c.c. flask, and made up to the mark with water; this diluted urine is cautiously delivered from a burette, which is attached to the boiling flask by means of a piece of rubber tubing, into the boiling Pavy solution until the solution is colourless; the volume of diluted urine required to decolorize the Pavy solution is noted, and this contains 0·05 gram of sugar calculated as glucose.

Example: 35 c.c. of diluted urine were required to decolorize 100 c.c. of Pavy's solution; then 35 c.c. of the diluted urine contain 0·05 gram of sugar, therefore the original urine contains $\dfrac{0·05 \times 200 \times 100}{35} = 28·57$ parts of sugar calculated as glucose per 1000 parts of urine.

Estimation of albumen. *Solution required:* Esbach's solution; 10 grams of picric acid, and 20 grams of citric acid, per 1000 c.c.

The process. Esbach's albumenometer is a specially graduated tube with two marks U and R; the urine is poured into the tube to the mark U followed by the Esbach's solution to the mark R; the tube is then closed by a rubber bung and the contents are gently mixed, but not shaken; the tube is now set aside for 24 hours and the height of the coagulum read off

on the graduations, which represent parts of dry albumen per
1000 parts of urine. If the percentage of albumen is high, an
equal volume of water should be added to the urine, and the
result multiplied by two. If the urine is alkaline, it should
be made acid with acetic acid. The albumen in a urine with
less than 0·5 part per 1000 cannot be accurately estimated by
this method.

Alternative process. A quantity of the urine is filtered; made
faintly acid with acetic acid, and the specific gravity taken;
the acidified urine is boiled and filtered and the specific gravity
of the filtrate taken; the specific gravity of the unboiled urine
less the specific gravity of the boiled urine multiplied by
four gives the number of grams of albumen in 1000 parts of
urine.

Example: The specific gravity of an unboiled urine was 1029;
and the specific gravity of the boiled urine was 1022; then
$(1029 - 1022) \times 4 = 28$ parts of albumen per 1000 parts of
urine.

Estimation of total phosphates. *Solutions required:*
Standard uranium nitrate solution containing 35·5 grams of
uranium nitrate in 1000 c.c. Each c.c. of this solution = 0·005
gram of phosphate (as P_2O_5).

Acid sodium acetate solution; 100 grams of sodium acetate
and 100 c.c. of glacial acetic acid in 1000 c.c.

Tincture of cochineal.

The process. 50 c.c. of urine and 5 c.c. of the acid sodium
acetate solution are heated to 80° C.; to the hot solution a few
drops of the tincture of cochineal are added and the standard
solution of uranium nitrate is run in from a burette until the
red colour of the tincture of cochineal is changed to green.
The number of c.c. of the uranium nitrate solution used multiplied by 0·005 multiplied by two gives the amount of phosphate
(as P_2O_5) in 100 c.c. of the urine.

Example: 50 c.c. of a sample of urine required 25 c.c. of the
uranium nitrate solution, then the amount of phosphate (as
P_2O_5) in the sample was

$25 \times 0·005 \times 2 = 0·25$ gram per 100 c.c.

$= 2·5$ parts of phosphate (as P_2O_5) per 1000 c.c.

Estimation of phosphate combined with calcium and magnesium. 200 c.c. of the urine are made alkaline with ammonia and allowed to stand for 12 hours; the mixture is then filtered and the precipitate washed with dilute nitric acid (1 in 3); the precipitate is then dissolved in a few c.c. of acetic acid; 5 c.c. of the acid sodium acetate solution are added, and the whole made up to 50 c.c.; the phosphate is then determined as described above. The total phosphate less the phosphate combined with calcium and magnesium gives the phosphate combined with the alkalies.

Estimation of sulphate. 100 c.c. of the urine are placed in a beaker; 5 c.c. of concentrated hydrochloric acid are added and the mixture is boiled; to the boiling solution, excess of barium chloride solution is added and the precipitate is allowed to settle; the precipitate is then filtered off, washed with hot water, dried in a water oven, incinerated and weighed; the weight of barium sulphate obtained multiplied by 0·412 gives the weight of sulphate (as SO_4) in 100 c.c. of the urine.

Estimation of uric acid. *Solution required:* N/10 potassium permanganate solution containing 1·581 grams of potassium permanganate in 1000 c.c.

The process. To 100 c.c. of the urine add 25 grams of ammonium chloride; stir the mixture briskly until the ammonium chloride is dissolved; add 2 c.c. of strong ammonia solution and allow the solution to stand until the precipitate of ammonium urate has settled; filter and wash the precipitate with ammonium chloride solution; transfer the precipitate with boiling water (not more than 20 to 30 c.c.) to a beaker; add 1 c.c. of concentrated hydrochloric acid and heat the solution to boiling; allow the solution to stand until the uric acid has crystallized out (generally overnight); filter; measure the volume of the mother liquid; wash the precipitate with cold water; transfer it to a beaker and dissolve it in 1 c.c. of a 10 per cent. hot solution of sodium carbonate, and 100 c.c. of distilled water; to the solution add 20 c.c. of concentrated sulphuric acid, and titrate the mixture with the standard solution of potassium permanganate, with vigorous agitation, until a permanent pink colour is obtained. Each c.c. of the

XIV]   URINE   301

potassium permanganate solution used represents 0·00375 gram of uric acid; to the amount of uric acid obtained must be added 0·001 gram for each 15 c.c. of mother liquor.

Example: The uric acid obtained from 100 c.c. of a urine required 20·1 c.c. of the standard potassium permanganate solution to produce a permanent pink colour; and 20 c.c. of mother liquor were obtained; then

$$(20 \cdot 1 \times 0 \cdot 00375) + (0 \cdot 001 \times 20/15) = 0 \cdot 0767 \text{ gram}$$

of uric acid in 100 c.c. of the urine.

CHAPTER XV

TOXICOLOGY

CANDIDATES for the examination of the Institute of Chemistry in branch (e) are required to have a knowledge of the application of the principles of toxicological analysis and the detection of blood stains. It would be out of place in a book of this nature to attempt to give an exhaustive account of this subject and the following methods, due to Seyda (*Analyst*, 1890, xv, 69), are put forward solely as a basis upon which the student can work; for details of particular methods for each poison he must consult larger works, a list of which is given in the bibliography (p. 314). The poisons discussed in this chapter are those usually met with, and which are more or less within easy reach of the general public.

Preliminary tests. The acid or alkaline reaction of the material should be noted, and the material should be examined for any particular odour, or phosphorescence in the dark; if the reaction is alkaline, any phosphorescence cannot be due to phosphorus; if the material is solid, an aliquot portion is digested with alcohol, the residue examined microscopically, and the alcoholic solution tested for oxalic acid.

Chemical examination. *Volatile bodies;* A portion of the material is cut into small pieces, and distilled with water by immersing the flask in boiling water for several hours; to the residue in the distilling flask, a little tartaric acid is added and the mixture is distilled with steam. In this way two fractions are obtained; the first containing easily volatile bodies such as alcohol, aldehyde, acetone, chloroform, nitrobenzol, turpentine, camphor and amines or their sulphur derivatives; the second containing phenol, hydrocyanic acid, phosphorus, etc. (if chloral hydrate or hydrocyanic acid are suspected, the material should first be made alkaline with potassium hydroxide or sodium bicarbonate respectively); the reaction, colour, odour and volume of the distillates should be noted.

The first distillate. The distillate should be tested with:

(*a*) Silver nitrate.

(*b*) Ammoniacal silver nitrate solution (for aldehyde).

(*c*) Sodium nitroprusside and ammonia (for aldehyde, acetone).

(*d*) Alkaline permanganate as follows: mix 10 c.c. of the distillate with a few drops of potassium hydroxide solution, and 1 c.c. of a saturated solution of potassium permanganate, and allow the mixture to stand for 12 hours in a closed vessel, filter and test the filtrate for aldehyde. A large increase in the amount of aldehyde points to the presence of alcohol.

(*e*) With iodine and potassium hydroxide solution, iodoform reaction (for alcohol).

(*f*) With resorcin and potassium hydroxide solution (for chloroform) as follows: to 10 c.c. of the distillate, a pinch of resorcin and 3 drops of a 30 per cent. solution of potassium hydroxide are added, and the mixture is gently warmed, when, in the presence of chloroform, an intense red colour of rosolic acid is obtained.

(*g*) With zinc dust and hydrochloric acid (for nitro-benzene) as follows: to 10 c.c. of the distillate, 10 c.c. of 90 per cent. (by weight) alcohol, a little zinc dust, 1 c.c. of hydrochloric acid and 1 drop of platinic chloride solution are added; the mixture is allowed to stand for 3 hours, and is then decanted from the zinc, the alcohol is evaporated off on the water bath, the residue is diluted with water, made alkaline with potassium hydroxide solution and extracted with ether; the ethereal extract is evaporated, part of the residue is tested for aniline with freshly prepared solution of bleaching powder, which will produce a dirty violet blue colour changing to indigo on the addition of ammonia; the remainder of the residue is warmed with an alcoholic solution of potassium hydroxide and a drop or two of chloroform, when, in the presence of aniline, the characteristic odour of phenyl isonitrile is obtained. On account of the very small quantity of material, a quantitative estimation of the volatile bodies is generally impracticable.

The second distillate. (*a*) Phenol; the distillate is tested for phenol with Millon's reagent, which gives a red colour or precipitate with phenol; care should be exercised in the use of this reagent, as the reaction is also given by other substances, which are due to putrefaction, and a slight reaction is generally obtained. The phenol is estimated by carrying on the distillation until the distillate gives no colour with ferric chloride; the distillate is then filtered and extracted with pure ether, the ethereal extract is allowed to evaporate spontaneously, and the phenol is estimated with bromine water and sodium thiosulphate solution (p. 269).

(b) Hydrocyanic acid; the distillate is tested with a piece of filter paper dipped first in a very weak solution of copper sulphate, and then in a freshly prepared tincture of guaiacum; in the presence of prussic acid, a blue colour is obtained; when this colour is obtained, the prussian blue and sulphur tests may be applied.

In the prussian blue tests, care must be taken not to add excess of ferrous sulphate, otherwise the prussian blue colour may be obscured. The residue in the retort should always be tested for ferrocyanides, when these reactions have been obtained. The hydrocyanic acid may be quantitatively estimated by precipitation from nitric acid solution with silver nitrate solution.

(c) Phosphorus; if phosphorescence is obtained, on distillation from acid solution in the dark, phosphorus is certainly present; phosphorus in any quantity is usually easily detected by its odour. The material is placed in a flask with water, acidulated with sulphuric acid, and distilled in a dark room; in the presence of phosphorus, the inner portion of the condenser becomes luminous; this is a very delicate test and will detect even minute traces of free phosphorus. The distillate is received in nitric acid, and the resulting phosphoric acid is precipitated with ammonium nitromolybdate, and weighed as magnesium pyrophosphate in the usual way. The amount of phosphorus estimated is usually not above half that actually present. The residue in the retort should always be tested for phosphorous acid.

Alkaloids. The extraction of alkaloids is very difficult and the best method is that due to Stas (*Jour. Pharm. Chem.* 1851, XXII, 281). The material, if a solid, is digested with twice its weight of 95 per cent. alcohol at 35° C. for 24 hours; if a liquid, it is digested with twice its volume of 95 per cent. alcohol; the liquid is then filtered and the residue is extracted for 24 hours with 95 per cent. alcohol, and a few c.c. of acetic acid, and filtered, and again digested with acidified alcohol until no further colouring matter is extracted; the neutral and acidified extracts are separately warmed to 75° C., and immediately cooled and filtered; the filtrates are separately evaporated to small bulk, care being taken that the acidified extract remains only just acid; the liquids thus obtained are separately extracted with absolute alcohol until no further colour is extracted; the two alcoholic solutions so obtained are separately evaporated at a low temperature, filtered and mixed; the mixed filtrates are extracted with ether in a separating funnel; the water layer is transferred to another separating funnel, made alkaline with ammonia and extracted with chloroform several times; the chloroform solution is then extracted with water containing a very small quantity of sulphuric acid; the sulphuric acid solution is made alkaline with ammonia, and re-extracted with chloroform; the chloroform solution is then carefully evaporated and the residue of alkaloid is dried and weighed.

Morphine is not extracted in the above process and in order to remove it, the residue from the first extraction with chloroform is extracted with hot amyl alcohol.

The residue is then tested for alkaloids by the following general tests.

Alkaloid reactions

Atropine

Concentrated sulphuric acid gives no colour.
Nitric acid gives no colour.
Erdmann's reagent gives no colour.
Frohde's reagent gives no colour.
Vitali's reaction; fuming nitric acid produces a violet colour changing to red on the addition of a drop of alcoholic potassium hydroxide solution.

When warmed with concentrated sulphuric acid and a crystal of potassium bichromate, atropine gives an odour of bitter almonds.

Aconitine

Mallanneh's test (*Analyst*, 1921, XLVI, 193) is practically the only test for this alkaloid; if a minute particle of potassium ferricyanide be placed close to a minute portion of the alkaloid (or a small portion of the powdered root of aconite) and a drop of formic acid added, a green coloration is immediately produced.

Brucine

Concentrated sulphuric acid produces no colour.

Nitric acid produces a blood red colour, changing to purple on the addition, drop by drop, of stannous chloride solution; the colour is destroyed by excess of the reagent.

Erdmann's reagent gives a red colour changing to yellow.

Frohde's reagent gives a red colour changing to yellow.

Concentrated sulphuric acid and a crystal of potassium bichromate produce a deep red colour.

Brucine is completely oxidized by warming with nitric acid, and the residue may be extracted with ammonia and chloroform and tested for strychnine.

Caffeine

Concentrated sulphuric acid produces a violet colour when warmed.

Nitric acid produces no colour.

Erdmann's reagent produces no colour.

Frohde's reagent produces no colour.

This alkaloid is precipitated by tannic acid but not by Mayer's reagent. When warmed with a drop of chlorine water or dilute nitric acid and a drop of potassium hydroxide solution is added to the residue, caffeine gives a violet colour changing to bright red on the addition of ammonia.

Cocaine

The aqueous solution of cocaine should not be heated for any length of time and never in the presence of acid or alkali.

A 1 per cent. solution of potassium permanganate produces a violet precipitate with cocaine hydrochloride.

Theobromine

Concentrated sulphuric acid produces no colour.

Nitric acid produces no colour.

Erdmann's reagent produces no colour.

Frohde's reagent produces no colour.

Theobromine gives a violet colour when warmed with a drop of chlorine water or dilute nitric acid, followed by a drop of potassium hydroxide solution; this colour changes to bright red on the addition of ammonia.

Quinine

Sulphuric acid produces no colour.

Nitric acid produces no colour.

Erdmann's reagent produces no colour.

Frohde's reagent produces no colour.

Quinine gives the thalleioquin reaction; weak chlorine water or bromine water is added drop by drop (avoiding excess) to an acid solution of the alkaloid until a permanent faint yellow colour is obtained; ammonia is at once added drop by drop, when a dark green colour or precipitate is obtained which changes to red on acidification with hydrochloric acid.

The solution of the sulphate of quinine exhibits a characteristic fluorescence.

Cinchonine

This alkaloid does not give the thalleioquin reaction.

Strychnine

Concentrated sulphuric acid produces no colour.

Nitric acid produces a doubtful yellow colour.

Erdmann's reagent produces no colour.

Frohde's reagent produces no colour.

Treated with concentrated sulphuric acid and a crystal of potassium bichromate, a blue colour changing to violet and red, and finally a yellow is produced.

Treated with concentrated sulphuric acid, and a trace of manganese carbonate, a violet and finally rose colour is produced.

Morphine

Concentrated sulphuric acid produces no colour.

Nitric acid produces a deep red colour unaffected by stannous chloride solution.

Erdmann's reagent produces a red colour changing to violet.

Frohde's reagent produces a purple colour changing to violet.

Ammonium vanadate produces a yellow colour changing to faint violet.

Neutral ferric chloride solution produces a deep blue colour, which is discharged by acid.

Nitric acid added to a solution of morphine in sulphuric acid produces a carmine colour.

Concentrated sulphuric acid and a crystal of potassium bichromate produce a green colour.

Emetine

Concentrated sulphuric acid produces a greenish brown colour.

Nitric acid produces no colour.

Erdmann's reagent gives a greenish brown colour.

Frohde's reagent gives a violet to deep blue colour.

Neutral ferric chloride gives no colour.

Bleaching powder added to an acetic acid solution produces an orange to yellow colour.

Veratrine

Concentrated sulphuric acid produces a blood red colour.

Nitric acid produces a yellow colour.

Erdmann's reagent produces an orange colour.

Frohde's reagent produces a yellow colour changing to red.

Metallic poisons. The residue from the alcoholic extraction is mixed with boiling water and the alcohol evaporated off; the organic matter is then destroyed by heating with potassium chlorate and hydrochloric acid, excess of chlorine is expelled, and a little tartaric acid is added to keep the antimony in solution; the whole is then set aside for 24 hours; the mixture is filtered and the residue is washed with water until the washings are colourless, with alcohol, and finally with ether, and the residue so obtained is incinerated and the ash is tested for silver, lead, barium and strontium. The soluble filtrate is made up to 500 c.c.

Mercury. 50 c.c. of the filtrate are neutralized with potassium hydroxide solution in a platinum dish; a small coil of

clean brass is introduced and the whole is warmed for 15
minutes; the coil is washed with water, alcohol and ether, and
dried, and finally placed in a combustion tube; the combustion
tube is partially filled with coarse copper oxide, and one end
is drawn out so as to form a small bulb between two capillary
tubes; a slow current of air is drawn through and the tube is
heated, the mercury volatilizes and condenses in the bulb
between the two capillary tubes; these are then broken off
and a small quantity of iodine is introduced and gently
warmed, when the characteristic red colour of mercuric iodide
will be obtained. For the quantitative estimation, the mercury
is precipitated from the acid solution as sulphide, the precipitate is digested in nitric acid and the mercury precipitated as
chloride, in the presence of phosphorous acid, after 24 hours'
standing.

Antimony. 50 c.c. of the filtrate are saturated with sulphuretted hydrogen and allowed to stand for 3 days; the
excess of sulphuretted hydrogen is removed by boiling; the
precipitate filtered off, washed with a very dilute solution of
ammonium acetate and then dissolved in sodium hydroxide
solution; sulphuretted hydrogen is passed through this liquid
until the precipitated antimony is redissolved; any insoluble
matter is filtered off and the liquid is made slightly acid with
hydrochloric acid and boiled; after standing for 24 hours, the
precipitate is filtered off, washed, oxidized with nitric acid
and weighed as oxide.

Tin. 50 c.c. of the filtrate are made alkaline with sodium
hydroxide solution, and then acidified with acetic acid, heated
to boiling and saturated with sulphuretted hydrogen; the
solution is made alkaline with sodium carbonate and filtered;
the precipitate is washed with sodium sulphide solution until
the washings are colourless; the filtrate is acidified with hydrochloric acid, boiled and saturated with sulphuretted hydrogen;
after standing for 24 hours the precipitate is filtered off and
washed with ammonium acetate solution; the sulphide of tin
is then converted into oxide and weighed.

Detection of Arsenic. The material is finely minced and
evaporated to dryness; when dry, it is digested in the cold for
at least 24 hours with concentrated hydrochloric acid; the

mixture is then distilled from a sand bath, the distillate being collected in a receiver containing a small quantity of distilled water, the process is repeated at least 3 times; all the arsenic will be found in the distillate as arsenic chloride and is detected and estimated by Reinsch's test and Marsh's test (pp. 255, 256). Great care should be exercised in carrying out this test, especially in being quite sure that all the materials used are free from arsenic.

Detection of acids and alkalis. If the material gives a strongly acid or a strongly alkaline reaction, it should be tested for sulphuric, nitric or hydrochloric acids; or for potassium hydroxide, sodium hydroxide or ammonia.

Estimation of strychnine in the presence of quinine. Simmonds (*Analyst*, 1914, XXXIX, 81). The mixed alkaloids, obtained by extraction in the usual way, are weighed and dissolved in 50 c.c. of a 10 per cent. solution of sulphuric acid; 5 c.c. of a 4 per cent. solution of potassium ferrocyanide are added drop by drop from a burette, and the mixture is set aside for a few hours; the precipitate is then filtered off and washed three times with 3 c.c. of a 5 per cent. solution of sulphuric acid, and then washed into a small separating funnel with 10 c.c. of 10 per cent. ammonia, and extracted three times with 15 c.c., 10 c.c. and 10 c.c. of chloroform; the alkaloids are extracted from the chloroform solution with 30 c.c., 10 c.c., and 10 c.c. of 20 per cent. sulphuric acid, and the precipitation with potassium ferrocyanide solution is repeated; the chloroform solution so obtained is carefully evaporated and the residue of strychnine is dried at 100° C. and weighed. The quinine is estimated in the mixed filtrates by precipitation with ammonia and extraction with chloroform. The solution extracted should not contain more than 0·1 gram in 50 c.c. of the acid.

Detection of colocynth. Seyda (*Analyst*, 1890, XV, 94). The material is extracted in the way described for alkaloids; the residue is mixed with a pinch of powdered potassium bichromate, and one drop of concentrated sulphuric acid; in the presence of colocynth a violet red colour is obtained; or, if ammonium vanadate be used instead of potassium bichromate, a blue colour changing to violet-red appears. The residue also gives a fine red colour with concentrated sulphuric acid, and a cherry red colour with Frohde's reagent.

Detection of savin. Maurelli and Ganassini (*Anal. Chem. Appl.* 1910, xv, 373).

Ferric chloride gives a black precipitate.

Silver nitrate gives a reddish precipitate as also does lead acetate.

Nessler's reagent gives a brown precipitate.

Phosphomolybdic acid gives a deep blue colour.

Savin produces a red stain on linen, which gives the guaiacum test; this can be distinguished from blood by the following colours given by savin:

Hydrochloric acid (specific gravity 1·05)	cream colour
Alum (10 per cent. solution)	light yellow
Ferric chloride solution	green yellow
Nitric acid	yellow ochre
Potassium bichromate and sulphuric acid	deep yellow
Sodium sulphide	yellow changing to lilac

Detection of antipyrine (phenazone). Lander and Winter (*Analyst*, 1913, xxxviii, 97). The material is extracted as described for alkaloids and the residue is evaporated to dryness with 5 c.c. of Steensma's reagent, antipyrine gives a rose-red colour, which is discharged by heating with sulphuric acid but reappears on cooling; commercial amyl alcohol and rectified spirit give a pink colour.

Reagents used:

Millon's reagent. 10 grams of mercury are gently warmed with 10 grams of nitric acid (specific gravity 1·40) until all the mercury is dissolved, the solution is then diluted with 20 grams of distilled water.

Erdmann's reagent. To 20 grams of concentrated sulphuric acid are added 10 drops of a solution of 6 drops of nitric acid (specific gravity 1·25) in 200 c.c. of water.

Frohde's reagent. 1 gram of sodium molybdate is dissolved in 100 c.c. of concentrated sulphuric acid, this solution must always be freshly prepared.

Mayer's reagent. Dissolve 13·55 grams of mercuric chloride, and 50 grams of potassium iodide, in 1000 c.c. of distilled water. This solution gives a precipitate with most alkaloids.

Dragendorff's reagent. Dissolve 5 grams of bismuth iodide in 20 c.c. of a concentrated solution of potassium iodide (1 : 1), cool, and filter the solution; to the filtrate add a further 20 c.c. of the potassium iodide solution.

Sonnenschein's reagent. 10 grams of sodium phosphomolybdate are dissolved in 100 c.c. of 30 per cent. nitric acid. This solution gives a precipitate with most alkaloids.

Steensma's reagent. Dissolve 1 gram of *p*-dimethyl-amino-benzaldehyde in 100 c.c. of a solution of 5 c.c. of 25 per cent. hydrochloric acid in 100 c.c. of absolute alcohol.

Detection of blood. *Guaiacum test.* Shrewsbury (*Analyst*, 1913, XXXVIII, 186).

Preparation of the reagent. 1 gram of guaiacum resin is washed three times with rectified spirit, and the residue is shaken with 100 c.c. of rectified spirit until the extract is pale straw-yellow in colour. This solution must be freshly prepared for each test.

The test. The fabric is placed on a filter paper in a flat-bottomed porcelain dish and moistened with two or three drops of distilled water (the surrounding filter paper is examined for red stains); if the stain is on metal, it is gently rubbed with wet filter paper; one or two drops of the guaiacum solution are added and if no colour is produced in a few seconds then add a drop or two of hydrogen peroxide (20 volumes). If blood only is present, no colour is produced after the addition of the guaiacum solution alone, but a characteristic blue colour is obtained within one second of the addition of the hydrogen peroxide. The reaction must occur within one second, any colour developed after that time being disregarded. This reaction is given by clothing, which has been stained by blood, even after it has been well washed.

Benzidine test. Willcox (*Analyst*, 1913, XXXVIII, 190).

Reagent. A saturated solution of benzidine in glacial acetic acid, diluted with four times its volume of 10 per cent. hydrogen peroxide; the hydrogen peroxide must be perfectly pure and must not contain free acid; this reagent is not so liable to decompose as tincture of guaiacum.

The test. A few drops of the reagent are placed upon the stain, when in the presence of blood, a magnificent blue colour is obtained.

Ruttan and Hardisty (*J. Can. Med. Assoc.* 1912) claim that a 4 per cent. solution of o-toluidine in acetic acid, in the presence of hydrogen peroxide is a much more sensitive reagent than either of the above.

If a positive reaction is obtained with either of the above tests, the material should always be examined microscopically, for blood corpuscles, and hæmin crystals, and also spectroscopically. The stain is dissolved off the material either with distilled water, or with dilute salt solution, a drop of the solution is examined microscopically for blood corpuscles, which are round bi-concave discs without nucleus in all mammals (the blood of different mammals cannot be differentiated) and cannot be detected in very old stains as they become disintegrated with age. In order to obtain crystals of hæmin, a few drops of the saline solution of the stain are placed on a glass slide, a few drops of glacial acetic acid are added and the whole is gently warmed until the mixture boils; it is then allowed to cool and examined under the microscope; hæmin crystals show a characteristic dark brown colour and are rhombic in shape. For the spectroscopic examination, the stain is dissolved in dilute potassium hydroxide solution with gentle heat, one drop of ammonium sulphide solution is added to the solution and the resulting liquid is examined in the spectroscope, when an absorption band will appear between the lines D and E and another band just at the side of the line E.

Detection of semen. Dominicis (*Analyst*, 1913, xxxviii, 29). The stained fabric is stretched on a glass slide and extracted with a few drops of distilled water; to the solution so obtained a few drops of a concentrated solution of gold bromide are added; the liquid is covered with a glass slip, carefully warmed, allowed to cool and then examined under the microscope; in the presence of semen, garnet coloured, cruciform or square crystals, due to cholin, and also elongated yellowish crystals are formed. If the stain is not fresh, rectangular brown crystals are obtained.

APPENDIX

THE SALE OF FOOD ORDER 1921—STRENGTH OF SPIRITS IN IRELAND

The Sale of Food Order 1921. This Order has been issued by the Board of Trade in exercise of their powers under The Ministry of Food (Continuance) Act 1920 and The Ministry of Food (Cessation) Order 1921 and provides for the following standards:

Jam shall contain a water soluble extract of not less than 65 per cent. of the jam; not more than 10 per cent. of the jam by weight shall consist of added fruit juice.

Marmalade shall consist only of citrous fruits, citrous fruit juices and sugar or other sweetening substances.

Dripping shall be manufactured by a process other than the acid process from raw-beef or raw-mutton fat or beef or mutton bones and shall not contain more than 2 per cent. of free fatty acids nor more than 1 per cent. in all of water and substances other than fat.

Edible fats other than butter, margarine or dripping, shall not contain more than 0·5 per cent. of free fatty acids nor more than 0·5 per cent. in all of water and substances other than oil or fat.

Margarine shall contain at least 80 per cent. of fat.

Strength of Spirits in Ireland. As The Licensing Act 1921 does not apply to Ireland, section 6 of The Sale of Food and Drugs Act 1879 is therefore not repealed in that Kingdom, and, in consequence, the alcoholic strength of whiskey, brandy and rum must not be diluted beyond 25 degrees under proof and the alcoholic strength of gin must not be diluted beyond 35 degrees under proof.

Calculation of excess water in a sample of whiskey, brandy or rum, sold in Ireland. In order to obtain the percentage of excess water in a sample of whiskey, brandy or rum, multiply the number of degrees under proof over 25 by 4/3.

Example. A sample of whiskey was 37 degrees under proof, then the percentage of excess water in the sample was:

$$(37 - 25) \times 4/3 = 16 \text{ per cent.}$$

BIBLIOGRAPHY

In addition to the various references to periodicals, memoirs and reports in the preceding pages, the following list gives the titles of books which have been consulted from time to time during the laboratory experience of the authors of this book. The list does not profess to mention the names of all the volumes and memoirs which have been published dealing with the different subjects, but it probably contains the most useful.

ALLEN, A. H. *Commercial Organic Analysis.*
AMERICAN PUBLIC HEALTH ASSOCIATION. *Standard Methods for the Examination of Water and Sewage.*
ATACK, F. W. *The Chemist's Year Book*, vols. I and II.
BARWISE, S. *Purification of Sewage.*
BOLTON, E. R. and REVIS, C. *Fatty Foods, their practical examination.*
BOOTH, W. P. *Water Softening.*
CLAYTON, E. G. *A Compendium of Food Microscopy.*
CLOWES, F. and COLEMAN, J. B. *Quantitative Chemical Analysis.*
COHN, A. J. *Indicators and Test Papers.*
COSTE, J. H. *The Calorific Power of Gas.*
CROOKES, Sir W. *Select Methods of Chemical Analysis.*
DIBDIN, W. J. *The Purification of Water and Sewage.*
DON and CHISHOLM. *Modern Methods of Water Purification.*
ELLIS, C. *The Hydrogenation of Oils.*
FOLIN, O. *Preservatives and Other Chemicals in Food.*
FRYER AND WESTON. *Oils, Fats and Waxes.*
FULLER, G. W. *Water Purification.*
FULLER, H. C. *Chemistry and Analysis of Drugs and Medicines.*
GRANT, J. *The Chemistry of Breadmaking.*
GREENISH, H. W. *The Microscopical Examination of Foods and Drugs.*
GREENISH, H. W. and COLIN, E. *An Anatomical Atlas of Vegetable Powders.*
GRIFFITHS, W. *The Principal Starches used in Food.*
HALDANE, W. *Methods of Air Analysis.*
HAZEN, A. *The Filtration of Public Water Supplies.*
HEMPEL, W. *Methods of Gas Analysis.*
HILL, J. W. *The Purification of Public Water Supplies.*
HOLDE, D. *The Examination of Hydrocarbon Oils.*
HOLLAND, J. W. *Medical Chemistry and Toxicology.*
HOUSTON, Sir A. C. *Studies in Water Supplies.*
—— *Reports to the Metropolitan Water Board.*
HUMBER, W. *Water Supply of Cities and Towns.*
JAGO, W. and W. C. *The Technology of Breadmaking.*
JAGO, W. *Manual of Forensic Chemistry.*
JOHNSON, A. E. *Analyst's Laboratory Companion.*
KENWOOD, H. R. *Public Health Laboratory Work.*
KINICUTT, L. P., WINSLOW, C. E. and PRATT, R. W. *Sewage Disposal.*
LEACH, A. E. and WINTON, A. L. *Food Inspection and Analysis.*
LEFFMAN, H. and BEAM, W. *Select Methods in Food Analysis.*
LEWKOWITSCH, J. *Chemical Technology of Oils, Fats and Waxes.*
LLOYD, C. F. *Bell's Sale of Food and Drugs Acts.*
LUNGE, G. and KEANE, C. A. *Technical Methods of Chemical Analysis.*
MASON, W. P. *Examination of Water.*
MERCK and SCHENK, H. *Chemical Reagents.*

PARRY, E. J. *Foods and Drugs*; vol. I, Chemistry and Analysis of Foods and Drugs.
RACE, J. *The Examination of Milk.*
RICHARDS, E. H. *Laboratory Notes on Industrial Water Analysis.*
RICHARDS, E. H. and WOODMAN, A. C. *Air, Food and Water.*
RICHMOND, H. DROOP. *Dairy Chemistry.*
RIDEAL, S. *Disinfection and Preservation of Food.*
—— *Sewage and the Bacterial Treatment of Sewage.*
RIDEAL, S. and E. K. *Water Supplies: their Purification, Filtration and Sterilization.*
RIDSDALE, C. H. and N. D. *Analyst and Client.*
SAVAGE, W. G. *Milk and the Public Health.*
SMITH, F. J. *Lectures on Medical Jurisprudence.*
STEIN, M. F. *Water Purification Plants and their operation.*
STEVENSON, Sir T. *Taylor's Principles and Practice of Medical Jurisprudence.*
SUTTON, F. *Volumetric Analysis.*
THORPE, Sir E. *Dictionary of Chemistry.*
THRESH, J. C. *The Examination of Water and Water Supplies.*
THRESH, J. C. and PORTER, A. E. *Preservatives in Food and Food Examination.*
WANKLYN, J. A. *Water Analysis.*
WILEY, H. W. *Foods and their Adulteration.*
—— *Beverages and their Adulteration.*
WINTER BLYTH, A. and M. *Foods: their Composition and Analysis.*
—— *Poisons: their Effect and Detection.*
WINTON, A. L. *The Microscopy of Vegetable Foods.*
WOODWARD, H. B. *The Geology of Water Supply.*

ADDENDA

Table of atomic weights.

1919

International Atomic Weights.

	$O = 16$			$O = 16$
Aluminium	Al 27·1	Lithium	Li 6·94
Antimony	Sb 120·2	Magnesium	Mg 24·32
Arsenic	As 74·96	Manganese	Mn 54·93
Barium	Ba 137·37	Mercury	Hg 200·6
Bismuth	Bi 208·0	Nickel	Ni 58·68
Boron	B 10·9	Nitrogen	N 14·01
Bromine	Br 79·92	Oxygen	O 16·00
Cadmium	Cd 112·40	Phosphorus	P 31·04
Calcium	Ca 40·07	Platinum	Pt 195·2
Carbon	C 12·00	Potassium	K 39·10
Chlorine	Cl 35·46	Silicon	Si 28·3
Chromium	Cr 52·0	Silver	Ag 107·88
Cobalt	Co 58·97	Sodium	Na 23·00
Copper	Cu 63·57	Strontium	Sr 87·63
Fluorine	F 19·0	Sulphur	S 32·07
Gold	Au 197·2	Thallium	Tl 204·0
Hydrogen	H 1·008	Tin	Sn 118·7
Iodine	I 126·92	Titanium	Ti 48·1
Iron	Fe 55·84	Uranium	U 238·5
Lead	Pb 207·20	Zinc	Zn 65·37

Table containing the percentages of absolute alcohol by volume and weight obtained from a determination of the specific gravity at 15° C.

Specific gravity at 15° C.	Vols. per cent.	Weight per cent.	Specific gravity at 15° C.	Vols. per cent.	Weight per cent.
1·0000	0	0	·9362	49·00	41·55
·9999	0·05	0·05	·9343	50·00	42·50
·9998	0·15	0·10	·9324	51·00	43·45
·9991	0·55	0·45	·9303	52·00	44·40
·9985	1·00	0·80	·9283	53·00	45·35
·9970	2·00	1·60	·9263	54·00	46·25
·9956	3·00	2·40	·9242	55·00	47·25
·9942	4·00	3·20	·9221	56·00	48·20
·9929	5·00	3·95	·9199	57·00	49·20
·9915	6·00	4·80	·9178	58·00	50·20
·9902	7·00	5·65	·9157	59·00	51·15
·9890	8·00	6·40	·9134	60·00	52·20
·9878	9·00	7·25	·9111	61·00	53·20
·9866	10·00	8·05	·9089	62·00	54·15
·9854	11·00	8·90	·9066	63·00	55·15
·9843	12·05	9·75	·9043	64·00	56·20
·9832	13·00	10·50	·9020	65·00	57·20
·9821	14·00	11·35	·8996	66·00	58·25
·9811	15·00	12·15	·8971	67·00	59·30
·9800	16·00	13·00	·8949	68·00	60·30
·9790	17·00	13·80	·8923	69·00	61·40
·9780	18·00	14·65	·8899	70·00	62·50
·9770	19·00	15·45	·8874	71·00	63·50
·9760	20·00	16·30	·8848	72·00	64·65
·9750	21·00	17·10	·8824	73·00	65·65
·9739	22·05	17·95	·8797	74·00	66·75
·9730	23·05	18·80	·8772	75·00	67·90
·9719	24·00	19·60	·8744	76·00	69·00
·9709	25·00	20·45	·8719	77·00	70·10
·9698	26·00	21·30	·8692	78·00	71·25
·9688	27·00	22·10	·8664	79·00	72·40
·9677	28·05	23·00	·8638	80·00	73·50
·9666	29·00	23·80	·8610	81·00	74·70
·9654	30·00	24·70	·8580	82·00	75·85
·9643	31·00	25·05	·8553	83·00	77·00
·9630	32·05	26·45	·8524	84·00	78·25
·9619	33·00	27·20	·8493	85·00	79·45
·9605	34·00	28·10	·8465	86·00	80·65
·9592	35·00	28·95	·8433	87·00	81·90
·9578	36·00	29·85	·8402	88·00	83·10
·9564	37·00	30·70	·8369	89·00	84·45
·9549	38·00	31·60	·8337	90·00	85·65
·9533	39·05	32·50	·8304	91·00	87·00
·9519	40·00	33·35	·8269	92·00	88·35
·9503	41·00	34·25	·8237	93·00	89·60
·9487	42·00	35·15	·8199	94·00	91·00
·9470	43·00	36·05	·8160	95·00	92·45
·9453	44·00	36·95	·8123	96·00	93·80
·9436	45·00	37·85	·8081	97·00	95·30
·9417	46·00	38·80	·8036	98·00	96·85
·9406	47·00	39·70	·7988	99·00	98·40
·9381	48·00	40·60	·7938	100·00	100·00

Table showing the volumes of oxygen and nitrogen absorbed from the atmosphere by distilled water and by sea-water at 760 mm., and at various temperatures. The numbers are in c.c. per litre.

Temperature °C	Dittmar (*Challenger Reports*, Physics and Chemistry, vol. 1, p. 160).				Roscoe and Lunt (*Jour. Chem. Soc.* 1889, p. 552).	
	Sea-water		Distilled water		Distilled water	
	Oxygen	Nitrogen	Oxygen	Nitrogen	Oxygen	Nitrogen
− 5	9·42	17·85				
− 4	9·14	17·35				
− 3	8·89	16·37				
− 2	8·63	16·43				
− 1	8·40	16·00				
0	8·18	15·60	10·24	19·30		
+ 1	7·97	15·21	9·97	18·86		
2	7·77	14·85	9·71	18·35		
3	7·58	14·50	9·46	17·91		
4	7·39	14·18	9·22	17·50		
5	7·22	13·86	8·99	17·09	8·68	
6	7·05	13·56	8·78	16·72	8·49	
7	6·90	13·26	8·57	16·36	8·31	
8	6·74	12·99	8·37	16·02	8·13	
9	6·59	12·73	8·18	15·69	7·95	
10	6·45	12·47	8·00	15·37	7·77 (7·87)	(15·47)
11	6·31	12·23	7·82	15·07	7·6	
12	6·19	11·99	7·66	14·77	7·44	
13	6·06	11·77	7·50	14·49	7·28	
14	5·94	11·56	7·35	14·22	7·12	
15	5·83	11·34	7·20	13·96	6·96 (7·09)	(13·83)
16	5·72	11·14	7·06	13·71	6·82	
17	5·61	10·95	6·92	13·47	6·68	
18	5·51	10·76	6·78	13·25	6·54	
19	5·41	10·58	6·66	13·01	6·40	
20	5·31	10·41	6·53	12·80	6·28 (6·44)	(12·76)
21	5·22	10·24	6·41	12·60	6·16	
22	5·13	10·07	6·30	12·39	6·04	
23	5·04	9·92	6·18	12·20	5·94	
24	4·95	9·77	6·07	12·01	5·84	
25	4·87	9·62	5·97	11·83	5·76 (5·91)	(11·78)
26	4·79	9·48	5·87	11·65	5·68	
27	4·71	9·34	5·77	11·48		
28	4·64	9·20	5·68	11·31		
29	4·55	9·07	5·58	11·15		
30	4·50	8·94	5·495	10·955		
31	4·43	8·82	5·41	10·84		
32	4·36	8·70	5·32	10·69		
33	4·30	8·58	5·24	10·55		
34	4·23	8·47	5·16	10·41		
35	4·17	8·36	5·08	10·28		

Table for calculating the deficiency of fat in milk from the percentage of fat found.

Fat	Deficiency	Fat	Deficiency	Fat	Deficiency
2·9	3·33	1·9	36·66	0·9	70·00
2·8	6·66	1·8	40·00	0·8	73·33
2·7	10·00	1·7	43·33	0·7	76·66
2·6	13·33	1·6	46·66	0·6	80·00
2·5	16·66	1·5	50·00	0·5	83·33
2·4	20·00	1·4	53·33	0·4	86·66
2·3	23·33	1·3	56·66	0·3	90·00
2·2	26·66	1·2	60·00	0·2	93·33
2·1	30·00	1·1	63·33	0·1	96·66
2·0	33·33	1·0	66·66	0·0	100·00

For each additional 0·01 per cent. of fat deduct 0·33 per cent. in the deficiency; thus a sample of milk contained 1·85 per cent. of fat, then the deficiency was

$$40·00 - (0·33 \times 5) = 38·35 \text{ per cent.}$$

MILK TABLES

Table for calculating the percentage of added water from the solids-not-fat found in a sample of milk.

Solids-not-fat	Percentage of added water	Solids-not-fat	Percentage of added water
8·4	1·18	4·4	48·24
8·3	2·35	4·3	49·41
8·2	3·53	4·2	50·59
8·1	4·71	4·1	51·76
8·0	5·88	4·0	52·94
7·9	7·06	3·9	54·12
7·8	8·24	3·8	55·30
7·7	9·41	3·7	56·47
7·6	10·59	3·6	57·65
7·5	11·76	3·5	58·83
7·4	12·94	3·4	60·00
7·3	14·12	3·3	61·18
7·2	15·29	3·2	62·36
7·1	16·47	3·1	63·53
7·0	17·65	3·0	64·71
6·9	18·82	2·9	65·89
6·8	20·00	2·8	67·06
6·7	21·18	2·7	68·24
6·6	22·35	2·6	69·42
6·5	23·53	2·5	70·59
6·4	24·71	2·4	71·77
6·3	25·88	2·3	72·95
6·2	27·06	2·2	74·12
6·1	28·24	2·1	75·30
6·0	29·41	2·0	76·48
5·9	30·59	1·9	77·70
5·8	31·76	1·8	78·83
5·7	32·94	1·7	80·00
5·6	34·12	1·6	81·18
5·5	35·29	1·5	82·36
5·4	36·47	1·4	83·53
5·3	37·65	1·3	84·71
5·2	38·82	1·2	85·89
5·1	40·00	1·1	87·06
5·0	41·18	1·0	88·24
4·9	42·35	0·9	89·42
4·8	43·53	0·8	90·59
4·7	44·71	0·7	91·78
4·6	45·88	0·6	92·95
4·5	47·06	0·5	94·12

For each additional 0·01 per cent. of solids-not-fat deduct 0·118 per cent. of added water.

Table for calculating the percentage of added water from the solids-not-fat found in a sample of skimmed or separated milk.

Solids-not-fat	Percentage of added water	Solids-not-fat	Percentage of added water
8·6	1·14	4·6	47·12
8·5	2·29	4·5	48·27
8·4	3·44	4·4	49·42
8·3	4·59	4·3	50·57
8·2	5·74	4·2	51·72
8·1	6·89	4·1	52·87
8·0	8·04	4·0	54·02
7·9	9·19	3·9	55·17
7·8	10·34	3·8	56·32
7·7	11·49	3·7	57·47
7·6	12·64	3·6	58·62
7·5	13·79	3·5	59·77
7·4	14·94	3·4	60·91
7·3	16·09	3·3	62·06
7·2	17·24	3·2	63·21
7·1	18·39	3·1	64·36
7·0	19·54	3·0	65·51
6·9	20·68	2·9	66·66
6·8	21·83	2·8	67·81
6·7	22·98	2·7	68·96
6·6	24·13	2·6	70·11
6·5	25·28	2·5	71·26
6·4	26·43	2·4	72·41
6·3	27·58	2·3	73·56
6·2	28·72	2·2	74·71
6·1	29·88	2·1	75·86
6·0	31·03	2·0	77·01
5·9	32·18	1·9	78·16
5·8	33·33	1·8	79·31
5·7	34·48	1·7	80·45
5·6	35·63	1·6	81·60
5·5	36·78	1·5	82·75
5·4	37·93	1·4	83·90
5·3	39·08	1·3	85·05
5·2	40·23	1·2	86·20
5·1	41·37	1·1	87·35
5·0	42·52	1·0	88·50
4·9	43·67	0·9	89·65
4·8	44·82	0·8	90·80
4·7	45·97	0·7	91·95

For each additional 0·01 per cent. of solids-not-fat deduct 0·115 per cent. of added water.

Formulae for converting different statements of alcoholic strength. (Liverseege, *Analyst*, 1919, XLIV, 167.)

$$\text{Per cent.} = \frac{0.79359 \times v/v}{S} = \frac{w/v}{S} = \frac{0.45257 \times P}{S}.$$

v/v = Per cent. × $1.2601S$ = $1.2601w/v$ = $0.5710P$.

w/v = Per cent. × S = $0.79359v/v$ = $0.45257P$.

P = Per cent. × $2.2096S$ = $1.753v/v$ = $2.2096w/v$.

S = specific gravity at 60° F.

Per cent. = grams of absolute alcohol per 100 grams.

v/v = c.c. of absolute alcohol per 100 c.c.

w/v = grams of absolute alcohol per 100 c.c.

P = c.c. of proof spirit per 100 c.c.

Corrections for Specific Gravity of Alcohol to 15·5° C., expansion of Glass included.
(Richmond, Analyst, 1920, XLV, 222.)

Temp.		Specific gravity on hydrometer or Westphal balance														
		0·99	0·985	0·98	0·975	0·97	0·965	0·96	0·955	0·95	0·94	0·93	0·92	0·9	0·88	0·85-0·79
10	Subtract	0·6	0·75	1·2	1·7	2·25	2·85	3·15	3·35	3·7	3·9	4·1	4·15	4·35	4·45	4·6
11		0·5	0·65	1·0	1·35	1·85	2·3	2·6	2·75	3·05	3·2	3·35	3·45	3·6	3·65	3·8
12		0·4	0·5	0·8	1·05	1·45	1·8	2·0	2·15	2·35	2·5	2·6	2·7	2·8	2·85	2·95
13		0·3	0·35	0·55	0·75	1·0	1·3	1·45	1·55	1·7	1·8	1·9	1·95	2·0	2·05	2·15
14		0·15	0·2	0·35	0·45	0·6	0·75	0·85	0·95	1·05	1·1	1·15	1·2	1·25	1·25	1·3
15		0·05	0·05	0·1	0·1	0·2	0·25	0·3	0·35	0·35	0·4	0·4	0·46	0·45	0·45	0·45
16	Add	0·05	0·1	0·1	0·2	0·2	0·25	0·25	0·25	0·3	0·3	0·35	0·35	0·35	0·35	0·35
17		0·2	0·25	0·35	0·5	0·55	0·7	0·8	0·85	0·9	1·0	1·05	1·1	1·15	1·15	1·2
18		0·35	0·4	0·6	0·8	0·95	1·15	1·3	1·45	1·5	1·65	1·75	1·85	1·95	1·95	2·05
19		0·5	0·6	0·85	1·1	1·3	1·6	1·85	2·0	2·15	2·35	2·5	2·6	2·7	2·8	2·9
20		0·7	0·8	1·1	1·4	1·7	2·0	2·35	2·6	2·75	3·0	3·2	3·35	3·5	3·6	3·75
21		0·9	1·05	1·35	1·7	2·05	2·45	2·8	3·15	3·35	3·7	3·9	4·1	4·25	4·4	4·6
22		1·1	1·25	1·65	2·0	2·4	2·85	3·3	3·7	3·95	4·35	4·6	4·85	5·05	5·2	5·45
23		1·35	1·45	1·9	2·3	2·8	3·3	3·8	4·25	4·55	5·0	5·35	5·6	5·8	6·0	6·3
24		1·55	1·7	2·2	2·6	3·15	3·75	4·25	4·8	5·2	5·65	6·05	6·35	6·6	6·8	7·15
25		1·8	1·95	2·45	2·9	3·55	4·15	4·75	5·35	5·8	6·3	6·75	7·1	7·4	7·6	8·0

Factors for use in Volumetric Analysis.

Normal Acid Solution

Ammonia (NH₃)	0·017
Borax (Na₂B₄O₇10H₂O)	0·191
Lime (CaO)	0·028
Calcium hydroxide (Ca(OH)₂)	0·037
Calcium carbonate (CaCO₃)	0·050
Magnesia (MgO)	0·020
Magnesium carbonate (MgCO₃)	0·042
Potash (K₂O)	0·047
Potassium hydroxide (KOH)	0·056
Potassium carbonate (K₂CO₃)	0·069
Cream of tartar (KHC₄H₄O₆)	0·188
Sodium hydroxide (NaOH)	0·040
Sodium carbonate (Na₂CO₃)	0·053
Sodium bicarbonate (NaHCO₃)	0·084

Normal Alkali Solution

Acetic acid (HC₂H₃O₂)	0·060
Citric acid (H₃C₆H₅O₇H₂O)	0·070
Tartaric acid (H₂C₄H₄O₆)	0·075
Lactic acid (HC₃H₅O₃)	0·090
Oxalic acid (H₂C₂O₄2H₂O)	0·063
Boric acid (H₃BO₃)	0·062
Hydrochloric acid (HCl)	0·0365
Nitric acid (HNO₃)	0·063
Sulphuric acid (H₂SO₄)	0·049

N/10 Silver Nitrate Solution

Chlorine (Cl)	0·00355
Sodium chloride (NaCl)	0·00585
Sodium bromide (NaBr)	0·01029
Potassium chloride (KCl)	0·00746
Potassium bromide (KBr)	0·01190
Potassium iodide (KI)	0·01660
Potassium cyanide (KCN)	0·01302

N/10 Iodine Solution

Sulphur dioxide (SO₂)	0·0032
Sulphurous acid (H₂SO₃)	0·0041
Sodium sulphite (Na₂SO₃7H₂O)	0·0126
Potassium sulphite (K₂SO₃2H₂O)	0·0097
Sodium thiosulphate (Na₂S₂O₃5H₂O)	0·0248

N/10 Sodium Thiosulphate Solution

Iodine	0·0127
Bromine	0·0080
Chlorine	0·00355

N/10 Potassium Dichromate Solution

Iron (ferrous)	0·0056
Ferrous oxide (FeO)	0·0072
Ferrous carbonate (FeCO₃)	0·0116
Ferrous sulphate (FeSO₄)	0·0152

Table containing some useful constants.

1 cubic centimetre = 16·9 minims.
1 minim = 0·059 c.c.
1 grain = 64·8 milligrammes.
1 metre = 39·37 inches.
1 cubic centimetre = 0·061 cubic inch.
28·35 cubic centimetres = 1 fluid ounce.
1000 cubic centimetres = 1 litre.
1 litre = 35·3 ounces = 1·765 pints.
1 gram = 15·432 grains.
1 ounce = 28·35 grams.
16 ounces = 453·6 grams.
1 gallon of water = 4·536 litres = 10 pounds.
1 litre of hydrogen at 0° C. and 760 mm. weighs 0·0896 gram.
1 c.c. of distilled water at 4° C. and 760 mm. weighs 1 gram.
To convert pints into litres, × 0·568.
To convert grains to grams, × 0·0648.
To convert Centigrade scale to Fahrenheit scale, × 9 ÷ 5, and add 32.
To convert Fahrenheit scale to Centigrade scale, subtract 32, ÷ 9 × 5.
To convert grammes per 100 c.c. into grains per ounce × 4·375.
To convert grammes into ounces (av.) × 0·03534.
To convert cubic feet into litres × 28·3.
To convert cubic inches into gallons × 0·0036.
To convert litres into gallons × 0·22.
To convert grammes per c.c. into grains per gallon × 70,000.
To convert parts per 100,000 into grains per gallon × 0·7.
To convert grains per gallon into parts per 100,000 ÷ 0·7.
To convert metres into feet × 3·281.
To convert kilometres into miles × 0·6214.
To convert miles into kilometres × 1·6093.
1 metrical ton = 1000 kilogrammes = 0·9842 tons.

INDEX

abrastol, detection of, in milk, 124
absolute alcohol, percentages of, table of, 317
Acer saccharinum, 220
acetic acid, estimation of, in vinegar, 239, 240
acetic acid solution in estimation of arachis oil in olive oil, 168
acetone, detection of, in urine, 294
acetyl value of edible oils, determination of, 166
acid mercuric nitrate solution, in estimation of cane sugar and lactose in condensed milk and lactose in milk, 110, 139, 140
acid silver nitrate solution for estimation of formaldehyde in milk, 120
acid sodium acetate solution in estimation of total phosphates in urine, 299
acidity of water, 2
acids and alkalies, detection of, 310
aconitine, 306
Adam on action of cream with Schardinger's reagent, 130; on detection of hydrogen peroxide in milk, 124
Adams' process for determination of fat in milk and cream, 105, 127
added water in milk, tables for calculating percentage of, 320, 321
Adeney, Dr W. G., on dilution method of sewage disposal, 93
Adeney, Dr W. E., and Professor Letts, experiments of, on sea-water, 77–79, 92
agar-agar, detection of, in jam, 226
Agriculture, Board of, Sale of Milk Regulations of, 101, 117
air, 273–84
    aqueous vapour in, 278
    contents of, 273
    detection and estimation of carbon monoxide in, 278–83; Haldane's method of, 279–83; Vogel's method of, 278, 279
    determination of carbon dioxide in, 275–78; Haldane's method of, 276, 277; Lunge and Zeckendorf's method of, 277; of nitrogen in, 274; of ozone in, 273
    estimation of dust in, 274; of or-

ganic matter in, 274; of oxygen in, 274, 275
    ground, 278; carbon dioxide in, 278; gases in, collected by Hesse's method, 278
    solutions required for determination of carbon dioxide in, 275, 277; estimation of oxygen in, 274; test for ammonia in, 273
albumen, estimation of, in urine, 298, 299
albumenometer, Esbach's, in estimation of albumen in urine, 298
albuminoid ammonia, estimation of, in water, 4, 5, 29, 30
albuminoids, determination of, in meat extract, 246
alcohol, estimation of, in beer, 236; specific gravity of, corrections for, 323
alcoholic beverages, 228–37
alcoholic hydrochloric acid solution in estimation of arachis oil in olive oil, 168
alcoholic potash solution in estimation of arachis oil in olive oil, 168
alcoholic potassium hydroxide solution in determination of saponification value of edible oils, 163
alcoholic solution in butter tests, 145
alcoholic solution of turmeric for determination of boric acid in butter, 153
alcoholic strength of spirits, calculation of, from the total solid matter and the specific gravity, 230; conversion of, formulae for, 322; estimation of, 229, 230
alkalies, estimation of, in water, 22
alkaline permanganate solution in water tests, etc., 4, 303
alkalinity of water, 2; determination of, 20, 21
alkaloid reactions
    aconitine, 306
    atropine, 305
    brucine, 306
    caffeine, 306
    cinchonine, 307
    cocaine, 306
    emetine, 308
    morphine, 307

alkaloid reactions—*contd.*
  quinine, 307
  strychnine, 307
  theobromine, 306
  veratrine, 308
alkaloids, extraction of, 304, 305
allyl isothiocyanate in mustard, 215
almond oil, 171
alum in bread, 204, 205
aluminium sulphate, use of, in purification of water, 28
aminoazo-benzene, 13
ammonia, estimation of, in coal gas, 286, 287; test for, in air, 273, 274; free and saline, estimation of, in water, 2–4
ammonia method in estimation of nitrogen as nitrates in water, 8, 10, 31
ammoniacal lead acetate solution in detection of cane sugar in dried milk, 133
ammoniacal silver nitrate solution in toxicology, 303
ammonium carbonate solution in detection of alum in bread, 204
ammonium chloride solution in water tests, 3
ammonium picrate, formation of, 9
ammonium salts in water, 4
ammonium urate in urine, 295
ammonium vanadate in toxicology, 308
α-naphthylamine in determination of nitrite in wheat flour, 195; in water tests, 13
Ancholme, River, Lincoln, analysis of water from, 45
annatto in milk, 117
antimony, 309
antipyrine (phenazone), detection of, 311
Apis mellifica, 223
apple pulp, detection of, in jam, 225, 226
aquatic plants and river-water, etc., 73, 74, 92
aqueous vapour in air, 278
arachidic acid, 168, 169
Arachis hypogæa, 171
arachis oil, 167–9, 171
army rations, tinned, 250; typical analyses of, 251
Arnaud and Hawley, cocoanut oil and butter-fat calculations of, 148
Arnold on detection of sesamé oils in fats containing colouring matter, 170
arrowroot starch, 209

arsenic in beer and foods, 252; apparatus, solutions and reagents required for B.P. test for, 256, 257, 259; detection and estimation of, 235, 255–8, 309, 310; general test for, 257, 258; in water, 18; preparation of standard deposits of, 256; standard stains of, 258
arsenic solution in tests for arsenic in foods, 257
Arsenical Poisoning, Royal Commission on, 1903, 252, 259
Arthur, C., analysis of water by, 37
artificial vinegar, 238, 239
Ashton-under-Lyne, Stalybridge and Dukinfield, water supply, analysis of, 42
atmospheric pollution, classification, 285; determination of, 283–5; estimation of acidity, alkalinity, ammonia, ash, chlorides, dissolved matter, lime, sulphates, tarry matters, undissolved matter, 283–5; standard gauge used in, 283
Atmospheric Pollution, Report of the Committee for the Investigation of, 283
atomic weights, table of, 316
atropine, 305
Aylesbury Dairy Company, analyses of milk of, 102

Bacillus acidi lactici, 100
Bacillus coli, presence of, in the Cam water, 74–6
bacterial analyses of the Cam water, 74, 75; sea-water, mixtures of sea-water and sewage, 81–84, 86–90
Baier and Neumann's method in cream tests, 129
Baker, J. L., methods of analysis of, of infants' foods, 210
Baker and Hulton on estimation of cocoa shell, etc., in cocoa, 190–3
baking powder, 200–4
  adulterations of, 200
  composition of, 200
  estimation of calcium in, 203; carbon dioxide in, 201–3; of sulphates in, 203; of tartaric acid in, 203
"baking soda," 201
Ballard, analyses of coffee by, 184
barium chloride solution, 94
barium salts, presence of, in natural water, 49
barley starch, 209
"barley sugar," 220

Baudouin's test for sesamé oil, 169
bean starch, 210
Becchi's reaction for cottonseed oil, 170
beef fat, 158
beef stearine, detection of, in lard, 157, 158
beef tea, evaporated, 245
beer, 232–6
  adulterations of, 233
  arsenic in, 252
  detection of hop substitutes in, 235
  determination of acidity of, 233; original gravity of, 233
  estimation of alcohol in, 236; of arsenic in, 235; of salt in, 235; of sulphites in, 236
  manufacture of, 232, 233
  solution required in determination of acidity of, 233
  spirit indication for acidity of, 233, 234
beet, cane sugar from, 220
Belfield's microscopical method for detection of beef stearine in lard, 157, 158
Bell Bros., of Manchester, water analyses of, 23–7, 41
benzidine test for detection of blood, 312
benzoates, detection of, in milk, 122
benzoic acid, detection of, in dried milk, 135; in meats, 262; in milk, cream and butter, 261, 262
Beta vulgaris, 220
bile, detection of, in urine, 294
Birmingham City Water Supply, analysis of, 36
biscuits, estimation of sugar in, 296
Bismarck-brown, 13
bisulphite as a food preservative, 265
Black's method of estimation of soluble chlorine in rag flock, 292, 293
black malt, 180
black pepper, 213
black tea, 176
Blackpool Water Supply, analysis of, 37, 52
bleaching of wheat flour, 194, 196
Blichfeldt's method for fat estimation, 150
blood in urine, detection of, 294, 296
blood stains, detection of, 302, 312, 313
Blyth, Winter, on chicory in coffee, 181
Bohea tea, 176

Bolton and Revis, butter fat, calculations of, 148
borax and boric acid in butter, cream, dried milk, meat, milk, sausages, etc., detection and estimation of, 118, 119, 127, 129, 135, 152, 153, 251, 261
boric acid solution in determination of boric acid in butter, 153
boron, compounds of, in butter and milk, 118, 153
brandy, adulteration of, 229; alcoholic strength of, 229, 314; dilution of, 229
Brassica campestris, 172
Brassica juncea, 215
Brassica nigra, 215
Brazilian coffee, 180
bread, 204–7
  adulteration of, 204
  composition of, 204
  detection and estimation of alum in, 204, 205; of potato starch in, 205
  estimation of sugar in, 206
  solutions required in detection of alum in, 204
Bristol City Water Supply, analysis of, 36, 37
British Channel, analysis of water from, 77
British Thermal Unit of coal gas, 288
bromide of tin test for rosin oil, 175
brominated hydrochloric acid in tests for arsenic in foods, 257
bromination, heat of, of butter, cocoanut oil and margarine, 143
bromine, solution of, in tests for arsenic in foods, 257, 258
Brown, Professor J. Campbell, analyses of water by, 36–8, 48; on analysis of pepper, 214
brucine, 306
Buchanan and Schryver on determination of tin in canned foods, 252
Bunte's burette in estimation of oxygen in air, 274, 275
Burchard's modification of Lieberman-Storch test for rosin oil, 175
Burrell, B. A., analysis of water by, 49
Burton-on-Trent, analyses of waters from, 36, 50
Bury Water Supply, analysis of, 43
butter, 141–55
  adulteration of, 141, 142
  analysis of, 142
  borax and boric acid in, 152, 153
  detection of benzoic acid in, 261, 262; of coal-tar dyes in 154; of cocoanut oil in, 145, 146; of colouring matter in, 153, 154

butter—*contd.*
    determination of boric acid in, 152,
    153; of curd in, 142; of fat in, 142,
    152; of heat of bromination of,
    143; of salt in, 142; of the
    Reichert-Wollny number of, 143,
    144; of the Shrewsbury and
    Knapp number of, 144, 145; of
    water in, 142
    fat in, examination of, 143
    margarine in, 143
    preservatives in, 152
    reagents required in estimation of
    boric acid in, 153
    salt in, 142
    solutions required in determination
    of the Reichert-Wollny number
    of, 144; of the Shrewsbury and
    Knapp number of, 144, 145
    sorting test for samples of, 142, 143
    typical analyses of, 154
    water in, 141
butter and margarine, detection of
    fluorides in, 262, 263
Butter and Margarine Act, 1907, 141
buttermilk, 117, 118
Buxton, analysis of water from, 47

cacao bean, analysis of germ of, 193
cacao butter, 171
caffeine, 306; in coffee mixtures, 183
calcium, estimation of, in baking
    powder, 203
calcium and magnesium sulphates in
    water, 15
calcium bisulphite as a preservative
    in foods, 260
calcium chloride solution in water
    tests, 14, 15
calcium hydroxide in tests for arsenic
    in foods, 257
calcium oxalate in urine, 295, 296
calcium phosphate in baking powder,
    200
calcium sulphate, determination of, in
    self-raising flour, 197, 198
calculation method for determination
    of fat in milk, 106
calorie unit of coal gas, 288
calorific value of coal gas, 288, 289
Cam, River, and the sewage effluent
    of Cambridge, oxygen content of,
    66–72; chemical and bacterial
    analyses of, 74–76
Cambridge Sewage Farm, experiments
    on sewage from, 85
cane sugar, 220, 221
    adulteration of, 220
    detection of dyed crystals in, 221;
    of ultramarine blue in, 220, 221

estimation of, in cocoa, 187; in con-
    densed milk, 138, 139; in golden
    syrup and treacle, 222; in infants'
    foods, 211
    in cream, 128
    in dried milk, detection of, 132,
    133
    in honey, 223, 224
    process of manufacture of, 220
    specific rotatory power of, 222
canned foods, determination of tin in,
    252–4
    solutions required in determination
    of tin in, 252
caper tea, 176–8
capsicum, detection of, for ginger, 218
Capsicum annum, 215
Capsicum fastigiatum, 215
Capsicum frutescens, 215
caramel, 220; in rum, 229; in vinegar,
    238
caraway seeds, 217
carbon dioxide, determination of, in
    air, 275–7; by Haldane's method,
    276, 277; by Lunge and Zecken-
    dorf's method, 277; estimation
    of, in baking powder, 201–3
carbon monoxide in air, 278–83
carbonates of calcium and magnesium
    in water, 15
carmine solution, employment of, in
    detecting and estimating carbon
    monoxide in air, 281–3
Carum carui, 217
cassia, 217
castor oil, 170
catechu in tea, 177
caustic potash-potassium iodide solu-
    tion in determination of dissolved
    oxygen in sewage effluents, 62, 63
cayenne, 215
    adulteration of, 215
    typical analysis of, 215
cellulose, estimation of, in infants'
    foods, 212
Chalk formation, analysis of water
    from the, 35–7, 39, 40, 48, 51
Chapman on detection of hop substi-
    tutes in beer, 235, 236; on deter-
    mination of creatin in meat ex-
    tract, 247
Cheddar cheese, 159
cheese, 159–61
    analysis of, 159
    calculation of composition of cream
    (or milk) in making, 161
    composition of, 159
    determination of ash in, 160; of fat
    in, 159, 160; of proteids in, 160;
    of water in, 160

cheese—*contd.*
  estimation of chlorides in, 160, 161
  examination of the fat of, 160
  test for starch in, 160
  typical analyses of, 162
chemical analyses of the Cam water, 74, 75
chemicals, use of, in reducing hardness of water, 16, 28
Cheshire cheese, 159
Chicorium intybus, 181
chicory in coffee mixtures, 181–3; analyses of the ash of, 184
chloride of lime as disinfectant, 265
chlorides, detection and estimation of, in cheese, 160, 161; in urine, 294, 296; in water, 5, 30
chlorine, estimation of, in chloride of lime, 266; in rag flock, 292; solutions required for estimation of, in chloride of lime, 266
cider, 236–7
  detection of spurious, 237
  typical analyses of, 237
cinchonine, 307
Cinnamomum cassia, 217
Cinnamomum zeylanicum, 217
cinnamon, 217, 218
  adulteration of, 217
  typical analyses of, 218
citric acid, estimation of lead in, 203, 204; in lime juice, estimation of, 243; in tests for arsenic in foods, 257
Citrus medica acida, 242
Citrus medica limonum, 242
Claremont, C. L. L., analysis of water by, 36, 37, 48
Clark's soap solution in estimating hardness of water, 14
cloves, 217; adulteration of, 217
coal gas, 285–90
  analyses of, 290
  analysis of, by Hempel's apparatus, 285, 286
  constituent gases of, 286
  determination of calorific value of, 288, 289; illuminating power of, 288
  estimation of ammonia and total sulphur in, 286, 287; of sulphuretted hydrogen in, 287
  solutions required in estimation of sulphuretted hydrogen in, 287
coal-tar disinfectants, 267–72
coal-tar dyes in butter and margarine, detection of, 154; in milk, 117
cocaine, 306
cochineal, tincture of, in estimation of total phosphates in urine, 299

cocoa, 184–93
  adulteration of, 185
  analysis of, 185–93
  detection of red sandars wood in, 192
  determination of the ash of, 187, 188; of the cold water extract of, 185
  estimation of added cane sugar in, 187; of added starch in, 188; of alkalinity of the ash of, 188; of cocoa shell in, 190, 191; of crude fibre in, 189, 190; of fat in, 185, 186; of fibre in, 191; of nitrogen in, 192; of soluble ash of, 188; of starch in, 188, 189; preparation of, 184, 185
  typical analyses of, 192
cocoa butter, detection of "green butter" in, 186, 187
cocoanut oil, 143; heat of bromination of, 143; Reichert-Wollny number of, 244
Coffea arabica, 180
Coffea liberica, 180
coffee, 180–4
  adulteration of, 180, 181
  analyses of, 184
  analyses of the ash of, 184
  chicory in a mixture of, 181
  detection and estimation of chicory in, 181, 182
  estimation of caffeine in, 183
  preparation of, 180
  varieties of, 180
coffee and chicory mixtures, 183; analyses of, 184
coffee extracts, 181
Colne Valley district, analysis of water from the, 52
colocynth, detection of, 310
colorimetric method in estimation of nitrogen as nitrates in water, 8, 9, 30, 31
colouring matter in butter, 153, 154
condensed milk, 136–40
  analyses of, 140
  determination of lactose in, 139; of proteids in, 137, 138
  estimation of ash in, 137; of cane sugar in, 138, 139; of fat in, 137; of milk sugar in, 138; of total solids in, 137
  methods of analysis, 137
  misrepresentation regarding, 137
"Condy's fluid," 267
Congou tea, 176
constants, table of some useful, 325
constants of oils and fats, table of, 174

copper, determination of, in preserved peas, 254; in foods, 252; presence and estimation of, in water, 18–20, 31

copper sulphate solution in estimation of boric acid in cream, 129

copper-zinc couple in estimation of nitrogen as nitrates in water, 10, 11

Cornelison's method for determination of colouring matter in butter, 154

Cornish and Golding on estimation of chlorides in cheese, 160, 161

"corrosive sublimate," 267

Corylus avellana, 171

cottonseed oil, 170; Becchi's reaction for, 170; in lard, 155; solutions required for Becchi's reaction for, 170

cottonseed stearine, 170

County Memoirs of the Geological Survey, 55

Coutts, Dr, report of, on condensed milks, 140; on dried milk, 131, 136

Coutts, Dr, and Baker, J. L., reports of, on proprietary foods, 140

Coutts, Dr, and Winfield, G., on dried milks, 140

cow dung in milk, test for, 116

cow's milk, 100, 101; natural variations in, 126

Cranfield on Kirschner and Polenske fat values, 149

cream, 126–31

  adulterations of, 126
  detection of benzoic acid in, 261, 262; of fluorides in, 129; of hydrogen peroxide in, 130; of viscogen in, 128
  estimation of boric acid in, 129; of fat in, 127
  fat content of, 126
  preservatives in, 126, 127, 129, 130; regulations as to, 126, 127
  solutions required for detection of hydrogen peroxide in, 130; for test for gelatine in, 127, 128; in estimation of boric acid in, 129
  test for gelatine in, 127, 128; for starch in, 128
  typical analyses of, 130

cream cheese, 162

cream of tartar, estimation of lead in, 203, 204; in baking powder, 200, 201

creatin, determination of, in meat extract, 246, 247

creatinin, determination of, in meat extract, 246

Cribb on composition of cream cheese, 162

Cripps and Wright's method for estimation of sulphates in self-raising flour, 198

Crum's nitrometer in estimation of nitrogen as nitrates in water, 8

crystallized cane sugar, yellow, 220

Curtel on detection of phosphate "improver" in wheat flour, 196

cystin in urine, 296

Daniel's hygrometer in determination of dew-point, 278

deep well water, 28, 29, 34, 36–8, etc.

Delepine, Prof., on the bacterial content of dried milks, 140

Demerara sugar, 220; tin chloride in, 220

deodorizers, 267

Departmental Committee's Report on Milk and Cream Regulations, 1901, 126; Report on Preservatives and Colouring Matters in Food, 1901, 152, 252, 260, 263

deposit of urine, examination of, 295

Derbyshire, analyses of water from, 38

Derwent Valley, Langley Mill, analysis of water from the, 43, 52

dextrose, 220, 221, 223

dinitrodiphenylaminesulphoxide, preparation of, 252, 253

di-phenylamine solution in detection of cane sugar in dried milk, 133

disinfectants, 264–72
  coal tar, 267
  estimation of available chlorine in chloride of lime, 266; of available sulphur dioxide in, 265; of formaldehyde, 267; of hydrogen peroxide in, 264, 265; of phenol in coal tar, 268; "reverted" sulphur dioxide in, 265; of tar oils in coal tar, 268
  formaldehyde or "formalin," 267
  lime and chloride of lime, 265, 266
  mercuric chloride, 267
  permanganates of potassium and sodium, 266, 267
  phenol, 267–72
  standardization of, 269

Dobbie on detection of cane sugar in dried milk, 132; on detection of preservatives in dried milk, 135; on estimation of lactose in dried milk, 133

Dominicis on the detection of semen, 313

Dragendorff's reagent in toxicology, 312

dried milk, 131–6
  detection of benzoic acid in, 135;
    of boric acid in, 135; of cane sugar
    in, 132, 133; of fluorides in, 135;
    of preservatives in, 135; of sali-
    cylic acid in, 135; of sulphites in,
    135
  determination of fat in, 131, 132;
    of milk sugar in, 132; of moisture
    of, 131; of proteids in, 132
  estimation of lactose in, 133
  methods of analysis of, 131
  solutions required for detection of
    cane sugar in, 133
  typical analyses of, 136
dripping, 158; standard for, 314
Durham on sulphite in cider and
    perry, 260
dust, estimation of, in air, 274
dyed crystals, detection of, in cane
    sugar, 221
Dyer and Gilbard, analyses of cinna-
    mon by, 218; on adulteration of
    cinnamon, 217; on detection of
    exhausted ginger, 219

edible fats, standard for, 314
edible oils, 163–75
  cloud test of, 165, 166
  detection of rancidity of, 165
  determination of acetyl value of, 166;
    of bromine absorption of, 164,
    165; of iodine absorption of, 164;
    of Maumené number of, 165; of
    saponification value of, 163, 164;
    of specific gravity of, 163; of
    unsaponifiable matter in, 164
  general tests of, 163
  solutions required in determination
    of bromine absorption of, 164;
    in determination of saponifica-
    tion value of, 163
  test for acidity of, 163
Edinburgh district, analysis of water
    from, 50
Edmonton district, analysis of water
    from, 43
Elæis guineensis, 172
Elæis melanococca, 172
electrolytic test for detection of
    arsenic in foods, 255
Elsdon's method for estimation of
    sulphates in self-raising flour, 198;
    method for fat estimation, 150;
    on detection of cane sugar in
    milk, 111
Elsdon and Hawley on detection of
    adulteration in linseed oil, 173
Elsdon and Sutcliffe on detection of
    nitrates in milk, 122

Embrey, analysis of perry by, 237; on
    estimation of maize starch in self-
    raising flour, 199
emetine, 308
Engler and Wild's test for ozone in
    air, 273
Erdmann's reagent in toxicology,
    305–8, 311
Esbach's albumenometer and solution
    in estimation of albumen in urine,
    298
Etherow, River, Hollingworth, analysis
    of water from, 44, 53
ethyl alcohol, estimation of methyl
    alcohol in, 232
Eugenia caryophyllata, 217
excess water in whiskey, brandy or
    rum sold in Ireland, calculation
    of, 314
extract of meat, 245–7

fat in milk, table for calculating
    deficiency of, 319
Fehling's alkaline solution in estima-
    tion of sugar in urine, 298; copper
    solution in estimation of lactose
    in dried milk, 133; in estimation
    of sugar in urine, 298; method
    for determination of lactose in
    milk, 109; for determination of
    cane sugar in condensed milk,
    138; for estimating sugars in jam,
    225
Fendler and Kuhn's method for
    estimation of dirt in milk, 116
Fendler and Stüber on estimation of
    caffeine in coffee, 183
ferrous sulphate solution in determina-
    tion of dissolved oxygen in
    sewage effluents, 64, 65
Filsinger's levigation method in cocoa
    analysis, 190
filters, household, 27, 28
Fischer and Gruenert on detection of
    benzoic acid in meats, 262
fish oils, hydrogenized, detection of,
    151, 172; production of solid fats
    from, 141
flock, regulations concerning, 291
fluorides, detection of, in butter,
    cream, dried milk, margarine and
    sausages, 129, 135, 262, 263
Folin on determination of creatinin
    in meat extract, 246
formaldehyde or "formalin" as a dis-
    infectant, 267; estimation of, in
    meats, etc., 263, 267; in milk,
    118–22; in sausages, etc., 251
formaldehyde solution in determina-
    tion of aldehyde value of milk, 108

"formalin," 267; see also formaldehyde

formalin solution in milk tests, 121

Fowler, Dr, experiments of, on seawater and sewage, 92

Frederick's method in estimation of nitrates in water, 9, 10

free and saline ammonia, estimation of, in water, 29

Fresenius and Popp on estimation of boric acid in meat, 251, 261

Frohde's reagent in toxicology, 305–8, 311

furfural in spirits, 231; reagent in tests for sesamé oil, 169, 170

Fylde Water Board, analyses of water of the, 37, 44, 52

Garnett and Crier on detection of capsicum for ginger, 218

Garrett on chemical examination of rag flock, 291, 292

gasometric method in estimation of nitrogen as nitrates in water, 8, 30

Gastaldi's modification of Halphen's test for cottonseed oil in lard, 155

gelatine, determination of, in meat extract, 247; test for, in cream and sour cream, 127, 128

Geological Survey, County Memoirs of the, 55

Gilmour on detection of coal-tar dyes in butter and margarine, 154

Gilmour's method for fat estimation, 150, 151

gin, adulteration of, 229; alcoholic strength of, 229, 314; dilution of, 229

ginger, 218–9

adulterants of, 218

detection of capsicum for, 218; of exhausted, 219; of foreign starches, etc., in, 219

determination of ash of, 218; of cold water extract of, 218, 219

typical analyses of, 219

Glaisher's tables in calculating aqueous vapour in air, 278

Glasgow Water Supply, analysis of, 37, 49

glucose, estimation of, in jam, 225; specific rotatory power of, 225

gluten, estimation of, in wheat flour, 195, 196

glycerol-soda solution in butter examination, 144, 145

golden syrup and treacle, 221–3

adulteration of, 221

analysis of, 221

determination of the copper reducing power of, 223

estimation of cane sugar and starch glucose in, 222; of total solid matter in, 221; of water in, 223

Goldenberg's method for estimation of tartaric acid in baking powder, 203

Goode and Perkin's modification of Gutzeit test for arsenic in foods, 256

Gossypium herbaceum, 170

Gottlieb-Rose method for determination of fat in dried milk, infants' foods, milk and sour milk, 105, 106, 113, 131, 132, 211

gravimetric estimation of tin in canned foods, 254

"green butter," detection of, in cocoa butter, 186, 187

green tea, 176

Greenfield Valley, Saddleworth, analysis of water from, 42

"greening" of preserved vegetables, 252

Greensand, analysis of water from the, 40

ground air, analysis of, 278

Gryzedale Lea reservoir, analysis of water from the, 44

guaiacum test for detection of blood, 312

gunpowder tea, 176

Gutzeit test for arsenic in foods, 256; Goode and Perkin's modification of, 256

hæmoglobin, employment of, in detecting and estimating carbon monoxide in air, 279–83

Haldane's method of determining amount of carbon dioxide in air, 276, 277; method of detecting and estimating carbon monoxide in air, 279–83

Halphen's test for cottonseed oil, 155, 170

Hamill, Dr J. M., on the bleaching of flour, 196; on nutritive value of bread, 207; on presence of calcium sulphate in baking powder, etc., 204

hardness of water, 14–16

Harris, F. W., analysis of water by, 37, 49

Harris, L. J., on adulteration of milk, 113

Harry and Mummery's method for estimation of salicylic acid in beer, jam, wines, etc., 226, 261

Harting and Solling on detection of agar-agar in jam, 226

Hasses' method for detecting methyl alcohol in spirits, 231, 232

Hawley's method for determination of boric acid in butter, 153

hazel nut oil, 171

Hehner's test for formaldehyde in milk, 119, 122

Hempel's gas apparatus in analysis of coal gas, 285, 286

Hesse, A., on determination of fat in butter, 152

Hesse's method, gases in ground air collected by, 278

Hinks on detection of benzoic acid in milk, cream and butter, 261; on detection of cocoanut oil in butter, 145

Holde's method for detection of paraffin wax in lard, 157

honey, 223–4
    adulteration of, 223
    analysis of, 224

hop substitutes in beer, detection of, 235, 236

Houston, Sir A. C., Reports to the London Metropolitan Water Board, 7, 53, 54

Howard's modification of Elsdon's method for estimation of sulphates in self-raising flour, 198

Huddersfield Water Supply, analysis of, 42, 51

Hughes' method for estimation of fat in cocoa, 186

hydrochloric acid solution in determination of boric acid in butter, 153; in determination of dissolved oxygen in sewage effluents, 62, 63; in determination of saponification value of edible oils, 163; test for sesamé oil, 169; in tests for arsenic in foods, 257, 258; in water tests, 15

hydrocyanic acid, estimation of, 304

hydrogen peroxide, detection of, in cream, 127, 130; in milk, 124; estimation of, in disinfectants, 264, 265

hydrogenization of oils, 141

hydrogenized oils, detection of, 151, 172

hypochlorite in water, detection of, 17

hypochlorite solution in determination of dissolved oxygen in sewage effluents, 65

hyson tea, 176

Ilkeston, Derbyshire, analyses of water from, 38, 48

Ilkley Spa water, analysis of, 49

Ilosvay's method of estimating nitrites, 13

imperial tea, 176

"improvers" of wheat flour, 194, 196

Indian coffee, 180

indigo method in estimation of nitrogen as nitrates, 8, 11, 79

indigo solution in water tests, 11, 12

infants' foods, 210–12
    analysis of, 210
    estimation of cane sugar in, 211; of cellulose in, 212; of cold water extract of, 210, 211; of fat in, 211; of lactose in, 211; of mineral matter in, 211; of moisture of, 211; of proteins in, 211; of reducing sugar, other than lactose in, 211; of starch in, 210

international atomic weights, 316

invert sugar, specific rotatory power of, 222

iodine absorption of butter, edible oils and lard, 143, 156–8, 164

iodine solution, 303, 324

Irish Milk Commission, Report of the, 126

Irish Sea, analysis of water from the, 77

iron in water, 18; estimation of, 20, 21

jam, 224–7
    adulterations of, 224, 225
    detection of agar-agar in, 226; of apple pulp in, 225
    estimation of glucose in, 225; of insoluble matter in, 225; of salicylic acid in, 226, 227; of water in, 225
    standard for, 314

Jamaican coffee, 180

Jamieson, analyses of vinegar by, 242

Jones, E. W. T., analysis of, of golden syrup and treacle, 221; method for estimation of formaldehyde in milk, 121; method of analysis of coffee by, 182; on estimation of talc in rice, 207, 208

Jonescu's method for detection of benzoic acid in dried milk, 135

Jorissons' test for formaldehyde in milk, 119

Katrine, Loch, analysis of water from, 37

Kenwood and Kay-Menzies on seawater and sewage, 84

Kerr on detection of rancidity of edible oils, 165

Keuper Marl, analysis of water from, 50
Keuper Sandstone, analysis of water from, 36, 37
Kirschner fat values, 147–9
Kjeldahl's method for estimation of nitrogen, 106, 132, 138, 160, 192, 195, 211, 246, 248, 253
Kjeldahl-Jodlbaur method in sewage analysis, 57
Klimont and Meyer on detection of hydrogenized fish oils, 151
Knapp on detection of hydrogenized oils, 151
Knapp and McLellan's method for estimation of crude fibre, etc., in cocoa, 190
Knecht, titanous chloride method of, 12
Knights, J. West, analyses of, of butter, 154; of coffee and coffee mixtures, 184; of creams, 130; of illuminating gas, 290; of milk, 125; of rice, 208; of tea, 180; of water, 35, 39, 40, 51
Koppeschaar's method of estimating amount of phenol in coal-tar disinfectants, 269, 270

lactic acid, formation of, in milk, 100
lactose, determination of, in condensed milk, 139, 140; in dried milk, 133, 134; in infants' foods, 211; in milk, 108–11
lævulose, 220, 221, 223
Laird, Dr, milk analyses from, 125
Lancashire (south-west), analysis of water from, 36–8
Lancashire Moors, analysis of water from the, 37
Lancet Acetone - baryta (L. A. B.) method of the chemical analysis of phenol disinfectants, 269
Lander and Winter on detection of antipyrine (phenazone), 311
Lane-Claypon, Dr T. E., reports of, on boiled milk, 126
Langley Mill, analysis of water from, 43, 52
lard, 155–8
    adulterants of, 155
    detection of beef stearine in, 157, 158; of cocoanut oil in, 155; of cottonseed oil in, 155
    determination of the iodine absorption of, 156, 157
    gradation of, 155
    solutions required for detection of cottonseed oil in, 155; in deter-

mination of the iodine absorption of, 156
    test for paraffin wax in, 157
    water in, 158
Leach's method for determination of fat in condensed milk, 137
lead
    B.P. test for, in foods, 258, 259
    detection of, in foods, 255, 258, 259
    in water, 18; estimation of, 19, 31
    solution of, in test for lead in foods, 258, 259
    solutions required for B.P. test for, in foods, 258, 259
lead papers, 257
Ledent on total soluble matter in milk, 111
Leffman on detection of abrastol in milk, 124
Leffman-Beam process for determination of fat in cream, milk, etc., 103, 104, 127, 137, 144, 186
lemon juice, 242
lemon squash, 242; preservatives in, 243
Letts, Prof., experiments of, on *Ulva latissima*, 74; on decomposition of sewage in sea-water, 93
Letts, Prof., and Dr Adeney, Report of, on Sewage Disposal, 92
Letts and Blake on method of determining amount of oxygen dissolved in water, 64
Letts and Richards on sea-water and sewage, 84, 86, 93
Lewkowitsch on determination of acetyl value of edible oils, 166
Liberian coffee, 180
Licensing Act, The, 1921, 228, 229, 314
Lieberman-Storch test for palm oil and rosin oil, 172, 173
Liebig, meat extract popularized by, 245
lime, estimation of, in water, 21; use of, to soften water, 16, 17, 28
lime and chloride of lime as disinfectants, 265
lime and lemon juice, 242–4
lime juice, 242–4
    description of, 244
    detection of mineral acid in, 243
    estimation of combined citric acid in, 243; of free citric acid in, 243
    typical analyses of, 244
lime juice cordial, 242; preservatives in, 243
lime water, solution for determining proportion of carbon dioxide in air, 275

Linder's methods of analysis of works effluents, 94

Ling on detection of hypochlorite in water, 17

linseed oil, 173; detection of adulteration in 173

Linum usitatissimum, 173

Liscard, analysis of water from, 40, 41, 45, 46

Liverpool City Water Supply, analysis of, 37, 40, 41, 45, 46, 48

Liverseege, J. F., analysis of water by, 36, 46; on calculating percentage of skimmed milk, etc., 113; on conversion of alcoholic strength, 322

Local Government Board Annual Report, 1911–12, 238; Food Reports, 115, 122, 126, 131–3, 135, 136, 140, 194, 196, 200, 204, 207, 210, 251, 262; Public Health Regulations of, 118; Reports to the, on Public Health and Medical Subjects, 291

London Chalk, analysis of water from, 50

London Metropolitan Water Board, Reports to, 7, 53, 54

London water, chemical examination and mineral analyses of, 54

long pepper, 213

Lott, F. E., and Matthews, C. G., analyses of waters by, 36, 47

Lowe's method for estimation of dirt in milk, 116

Lower Greensand, analysis of water from the, 14, 29, 32, 33, 40, 51

Lower Keuper Sandstone, analysis of water from the, 36, 47

Lunge and Zeckendorf's method of determining carbon dioxide in air, 277

Lythgoe, formula of, for calculating proteins from the fat in milk, 108; method of, for detection of colouring matter in milk, 117

Macara's modification of Filsinger's levigation method in cocoa analysis, 190; on estimation of carbon dioxide in baking powder, 202

mace, 216

"machine skimmed milk," 131

magnesia, estimation of, in water, 21, 22

Magnesian Limestone, analysis of water from the, 33

magnesium ammonium phosphate in urine, 296

Maix-Trommsdorf method in estimation of nitrogen as nitrates in water, 11

maize oil, 172

maize starch, 209; detection and estimation of, in self-raising flour, 198, 199

maize vinegar, 242

Mallanneh's test for aconitine, 306

malt vinegar, 238, 239

adulteration of, 239

typical analyses of, 242

Manchester tap water, analysis of, 49, 50

manganous chloride solution in determination of dissolved oxygen in sewage effluents, 62, 63, 65

margarine, 141–55

butter fat in, 141

definition of, 141

detection of coal-tar dyes in, 154

estimation of butter fat and cocoanut fat in, 146

heat of bromination of, 143

Reichert-Wollny number of, 144

water in, 141

margarine cheeses, 159

Marl bed, analysis of water from the, 36, 47

marmalade, standard for, 314

Marsh's arsenic apparatus, 235, 310

Martelli on detection of poivrette in pepper, 214

Maumené number, determination of, of edible oils, 165

Maurelli and Ganassini on detection of savin, 311

Mayer's reagent in toxicology, 306, 311

McGowan, Dr, formula of, for calculating strength of sewage, 58; zinc-copper couple method of, 78, 79

meat extract, 245–7

adulteration of, 245

detection of starch in, 246

determination of albuminoids in, 246; of ash in, 245; of creatin in, 246, 247; of creatinin in, 246; of fat in, 246; of gelatine in, 247; of water in, 245

preparation of, 245

solutions required in determination of creatinin in, 246

meat pastes, 250; typical analyses of, 251

meats

detection of benzoic acid in, 262

estimation of boric acid in, 261; of formaldehyde in, 263

mercuric chloride as a disinfectant, 267
mercuric chloride papers, 257
mercury, 308
Mersey, River, analysis of water from, 45
metallic poisons
antimony, 309
mercury, 308, 309
tin, 309
metaphenylene-diamine method, use of, for determining nitrites, 13, 79
methyl alcohol, detection of, in spirits, 231, 232; estimation of, in ethyl alcohol, 232
milk, 100–26
adulteration of, 100; calculation of, 112
ash of, 103
boiled, chemical changes in, 126
colouring matter in, 117
cow dung in, test for, 116
detection of abrastol in, 124; of added water in, 113, 115; of benzoates in, 122; of benzoic acid in, 261, 262; boric acid and borax in, 118, 119; of cane sugar in, 111; of formaldehyde in, 119–22; of hydrogen peroxide in, 124; of mystin in, 122; of nitrates in, 122; of non-fatty solids in, 111; of salicylic acid, 123
determination of aldehyde value of, 108; of fat in, 103–6; of milk sugar in, 108–11; of total proteids in, 106, 107; of total soluble matter in, 111
estimation of dirt in, 116; of formaldehyde in, 120; of total solid matter in, 103
fat standard of, 101
government laboratory method of analysis of, 114, 115
mineral matter of, 100
preservatives in, 118
proteids of, 100
skimmed, formulæ for calculating percentage of, 113
solutions and reagents required for detection of abrastol in, 124; for detection of hydrogen peroxide in, 124; for detection of nitrates in, 122, 123; for determination of aldehyde value of, 108; for determination of lactose in, 109, 110; for determination of total proteids in, 106; for estimation of formaldehyde in, 120–1
sour, analysis of, 113; estimation of fat in, 114

"sourness" of, 100
specific gravity of, 100; determination of the, 102
sterilized, chemical changes in, 126
typical analyses of, 125
Milk and Dairies Act, 1914, 101
Milk and Dairies (Consolidation) Act, 1915, 101
milk sugar, estimation of, in condensed milk, 138; in dried milk, 132; in milk, 108–11
Millon's reagent in toxicology, 303, 311
Millstone Grit formation, analysis of water from the, 37, 48, 49
mineral acid, detection and estimation of, in lime juice, 243; in vinegar, 240, 241
mineral analyses of water, 20, 46–53
Mocha coffee, 180
molybdate test for cane sugar in milk, 111
Monier-Williams, Dr G. W., on bleaching of flour, 196; on detection of added water in milk, 115, 116; on detection of fluorides in butter and margarine, 262; on mystin in milk, 122
Moor on standard for cream cheese, 162
moorland waters, 29
Moors of Lancashire and Yorkshire, analysis of water from, 37
Muestra, India, analysis of water from, 53
Muspratt, analysis of water by, 47
mustard, 215, 216
adulterants of, 215
detection of turmeric in, 216
estimation of oil in, 216
starch in, 215, 216
typical analyses of, 216
"mustard condiment," 215
Muter on estimation of available and "reverted" sulphur dioxide in disinfectants, 265; on estimation of tar oils, 268
mutton fat, 158
Mycoderma aceti, 238
Myristica fragrans, 216
mystin, detection of, in milk, 122

naphthylamine solution in determination of nitrite in wheat flour, 194; in water tests, 13
Nessler's reagent in ammonia determination, 2, 3, 11, 12, 115, 274, 278, 284; in detection of savin, 311
New Red Sandstone, analysis of water from the, 52

New York Metropolitan Sewage Commission Report, 64

Newmarket, analysis of water from near, 51

Newton, south-west Lancashire, analysis of water from, 38

nitrates and nitrites, detection and estimation of, in milk, 122, 123; in sewage and sea-water, 80, 81; in water, 8–14, 31; in wheat flour, 194, 195

nitric nitrogen in water, 11, 12

nitric oxide, formation of, 8

nitrogen, determination of, in air, 274; solubility of, in distilled water and sea-water, 65, 318; table of volumes of, absorbed from the atmosphere, 318

nitrometer, Crum's, in estimation of nitrogen as nitrates in water, 8

normal acid solution, 324

normal alkali solution, 324

North Barnacre reservoir, analysis of water from the, 44

nutmeg, 216, 217

oat starch, 209

Olea sativa, 167

olive oil, 167, 168
  solutions required in estimation of arachis oil in, 168
  test for and estimation of arachis oil in, 168

olive stones, ground, in pepper and cayenne, 213, 215

Olson, formula of, for calculation of proteins in milk, 108

organic matter, estimation of, in air, 274

Oriza sativa, 207

Ormskirk district, analysis of water from the, 52

oxalic acid solution in estimation of carbon dioxide in air, 275; in water and sewage tests, 5, 6, 10, 56

oxygen, estimation of, absorbed from potassium permanganate solution in water, 30; in air, 274, 275; in river-water and sewage, 66–76; in sewage and sewage effluents, 55, 56, 61–65; in water, 5–7, 17
  solubility of, in distilled water and sea-water, 65, 318
  table of volumes of, absorbed from the atmosphere, 318

ozone in air, 273; Engler and Wild's test for, 273

palm oil, 172

paraffin wax, test for, in lard, 157

Parkes on estimation of soluble chlorine in rag flock, 292

Parry on detection of turmeric in pepper, 214

Pavy's solution in estimation of sugar in urine, 298

pea starch, 210

peach kernel oil, 171

pearl barley, 208
  determination of talc in, 208
  estimation of rice powder in, 208

peas, preserved, determination of copper in, 254

pectin in fruit juice, 224

Pekoe tea, 176

Penot's method for estimation of available chlorine in chloride of lime, 266

pepper, 213, 214
  adulterants of, 213
  detection of adulteration of, 213, 214; of poivrette in, 214; of turmeric in, 214
  solution required in detection of turmeric in, 214
  standard for, 213
  typical analyses of, 214

pepperette, 213

permanent hardness of water, 15, 16

permanganates of potassium and sodium as disinfectants, 266, 267; estimation of strength of, 267

perry, 236; analysis of, 237

Pettenkofer's process for determining proportion of carbon dioxide in air, 275

Pharmacopœia Committee of the General Medical Council, 259

phenazone, detection of, 311

phenol, estimation of, 268, 269, 304

phenol disinfectants, chemical analysis of, 269–72

phenol sulphuric method, use of, in determining nitrates, 9, 10, 57, 79

phosphate, estimation of, in vinegar, 240

phosphate "improver" in wheat flour, 196

phosphorus, detection of, 304

Pickel's method in cocoa analysis, 190

picric acid, formation of, 9; in test for albumen in urine, 293

pimento, 217

Piper nigrum, 213

Plimmer, Dr, *Analyses and Energy Values of Foods* of, 207

poisonous metals in foods and in water, 18, 19, 252–9; detection of, 259

poisons
  preliminary tests for, 302
  volatile bodies, chemical examination of, 302
poivrette, detection of, in pepper, 214
Polenske's apparatus in estimation of fat values, 146–9
Pollard on detection of mineral oil in vegetable oil, 166
pond water, analysis of, 34
Ponder, Dr C. R., on standardization of disinfectants, 269
Pontius' method for estimation of available chlorine in chloride of lime, 266
Portsmouth Public Water Supply, analysis of, 36, 37, 48
potassium chlorate in tests for arsenic in foods, 257
potassium chloride in water tests, 13
potassium chromate solution in estimation of chlorine as chlorides in water, 5
potassium cyanide solution in estimation of formaldehyde in milk, 120; in test for lead in foods, 259
potassium dichromate solution, 324
potassium hydroxide solution in determination of dissolved oxygen in sewage effluents, 63; use of, in toxicology, 303
potassium iodide solution in determination of bromine absorption of edible oils, 164; in determination of iodine absorption of lard, 156; use of, in water tests, 6, 7
potassium nitrate, detection of, 250
potassium nitrate solution in water tests, 9, 11, 12
potassium nitrite solution in water tests, 13
potassium oxalate solution in determination of dissolved oxygen in sewage effluents, 62
potassium permanganate solution in determination of dissolved oxygen in sewage and sewage effluents and water, 5–7, 55, 62, 64, 65; in estimation of uric acid in urine, 300, 301
potassium persulphate "improver" in wheat flour, 196
potassium sulphocyanide solution in estimation of formaldehyde in milk, 120; in estimation of soluble chlorine in rag flock, 292
potato starch, 209; detection of, in bread, 205
preservatives in butter, 152; in cream, 129, 130; in dried milk, 135; in foods, 250, 251, 260–3; in milk, 122–4
Preservatives and Colouring Matters in Food, Report of the Departmental Committee on the use of, 1901, 152, 252, 260, 263
"preserved cream," 127
proof spirit, 228
proprietary foods, 140
proteids, determination of, in dried milk, 132; in milk, 106, 107
Prunus amygdalus, 171
Public Health (Milk and Cream) Regulations, 1912, 118, 126, 131; Amendment Order, 1917, 127
Public Health (Regulations as to Food) Act, 1907, 118, 126
purification of water, notes on, 23–28
Purvis, J. E., on standardization of disinfectants, 269
Purvis and Black on oxygen content of the river Cam, 66, 76
Purvis and Coleman on sea-water and sewage, 78, 79, 92
Purvis and Courtauld on sea-water and sewage, 78, 79, 92; on the copper-zinc couple method, 11
Purvis and Rayner, chemical and bacterial analyses of, of the Cam water, 74, 75
Purvis and Walker on sea-water and sewage, 85, 93
Purvis, Brehaut, and McHattie, investigations of boiled and sterilized milk by, 126
Purvis, Macalister, and Minnett on sea-water and sewage, 79, 84, 93
Purvis, McHattie, and Fisher, experiments of, on sea-water and sewage, 84, 93
pus corpuscles in urine, 296
pyrogallol, alkaline solution of, in estimation of oxygen in air, 274

quinine, 307

rag flock, chemical examination of, 291–3
  estimation of soluble chlorine in, 292
  regulations concerning, 291
  solutions required in estimation of soluble chlorine in, 292
Rag Flock Act, 1911, 291
Rag Flock Regulations, 1912, 291
rain-fall, effects of, on river-water, 73, 74
rape oil, 172
Ratzlaff's method for determination of fat in cheese, 159, 160

Red Sandstone, analysis of water from the, 40, 41, 46
Reichelman and Leuscher, on detection of red sandars wood in cocoa, 192
Reichert-Meissl fat values, 147–9
Reichert-Meissl-Polenske process, 150
Reichert-Meissl-Polenske-Kirschner process, 146, 158
Reichert-Wollny number, determination of the, of butter, 143, 144; of cheese, 160; of cocoanut oil, 144; of margarine, 144
Reinsch's test for detection of arsenic, 255, 310
resorcin and potassium hydroxide solution, use of, in toxicology, 304
resorcinol test for cane sugar in milk, 111
Revis on estimation of total solid matter in milk, 103
Revis and Bolton's modification of the Reichert-Meissl-Polenske-Kirschner process, 146; on detection of "green butter" in cocoa butter, 186, 187
Revis and Burnett on estimation of starch in cocoa, 188, 189
Revis and Payne's method for determination of cane sugar and lactose in condensed milk, 139, 140
Rhayader, Wales, analysis of water from, 36
rice, 207, 208; estimation of talc in, 207, 208
rice powder, estimation of, in pearl barley, 208
rice starch, 209
Richards, analysis of, of germ of cacao bean, 193
Richardson on estimation of boric acid in milk and cream, 129; typical analysis of, of cayenne, 215
Richmond, analysis of cream by, 130, 131; fat percentages of milk by, 102; formulæ and slide rule of, 106, 107; method of, for detection and estimation of boric acid in cream and milk, 119, 129; on calculation of cream (or milk) in making cheese, 161; on corrections for specific gravity of alcohol, 323; on determination of aldehyde value of milk, 108; determination of fat in dried milk, 132; on determination of specific gravity of sour milk, 114; on Kirschner and Polenske fat values, 149; on methods of analysis of dried milk, 131; typical analyses of dried milk by, 136

Ricinus communis, 170
Rideal and Stewart's modification of Winkler's method, 61
river-water and sewage, determinations of oxygen dissolved in, 66–76
Rivingstone Water Supply, analysis of, 37, 48
Romijn on estimation of formaldehyde in meats, etc., 263
Rose-Gottlieb process; see Gottlieb-Rose
rosin oil, Lieberman-Storch test for, 173, 175; bromide of tin test for, 175
Rothenfuser's method for detection of cane sugar in dried milk, 132
Rowbottom, J., and Raddin, G. H., analysis of water by, 42
Royal Commission on Arsenical Poisoning, 1903, 252, 259; on Sewage Disposal, 58, 60, 61, 64–66, 74, 76, 77, 79, 84, 92, 93, 99; on Whiskey and other Potable Spirits, 1908–9, 228
rum, 228, 229
adulteration of, 229
alcoholic strength of, 229, 314
dilution of, 229
estimation of the total solid matter in, 230
"impurities" in, 229
Russell, E., analysis of water by, 36, 37; on sorting test for butter samples, 142, 143
Russell and Barker, analyses of ciders by, 237; on detection of spurious cider, 237
Russell and Hodgson on vinegar analysis, 239
Russell and West on estimation of urea in urine, 297
Ruttan and Hardisty on reagents for detection of blood, 313
rye starch, 209

Saccharum officinarum, 220
sago starch, 209
Sale, analysis of water from, 45
Sale of Butter Regulations, 1902, 141
Sale of Food and Drugs Acts, 1879, 1899, 101, 137, 141, 176, 194, 200, 228, 229, 237, 242, 252, 314
Sale of Food Order, 1921, 314
Sale of Milk Regulations, 1901, 1912, 101, 117
Salford district, analysis of water from the, 41
salicylic acid as a preservative in beer, wines, etc., 261; detection of, in

dried milk and milk, 123, 135; estimation of, in jam, 226, 227; in lime juice cordial and lemon squash, 243

salt, estimation of, in beer, 235; in butter, 142; in sausages, etc., 250

saponification value, determination of, of edible oils, 163, 164

sausages, 247–9
  composition of, 247
  detection of fluorides in, 263
  determination of ash in, 248; of fat in, 248; of nitrogen in, 248; of water in, 248
  methods of analysis of, 247
  microscopical examination and calculations of, 248, 249
  typical analyses of, 251

savin, detection of, 311

Schardinger's reagent for detection of hydrogen peroxide in cream and milk, 124, 130

Schidrowitz's method in estimation of free mineral acid in vinegar, 241

Schiff's test for formaldehyde in milk, 120

Schoore's formula in calculation method for determination of fat in milk, 106

Schryver and Wood on estimation of methyl alcohol in ethyl alcohol, 232

Schutz and Wein on detection of potato starch in bread, 205

sea-water, analyses of, 77, 85

sea-water and sewage, 77–93; chemical and bacterial analyses of, 80–85; estimations of nitrates and nitrites in, 80

Seidenberg, A., on detection of gelatine in sour cream, 128

self-raising flour, 196–9
  detection and estimation of maize starch in, 198, 199
  determination of calcium sulphate in, 197, 198
  estimation of sulphates in, 198
  solutions required in estimation of maize starch in, 199

semen, detection of, 313

"separated milk," 131

sesamé oil, 169, 170
  Baudouin's test for, 169
  detection of, in fats containing colouring matter, 170
  solutions required in Baudouin's test for, 169; in Villavecchia and Fabri's test for, 169
  Villavecchia and Fabri's test for, 169

Sesamum Indicum, 169

Settimj on detection of soya bean oil, 172

sewage, 55–59
  estimation of free and albuminoid ammonia in, 55; of nitrogen as nitrates and nitrites in, 55; of oxygen absorbed in, 55, 56; of suspended matter in, 56, 57; of total organic nitrogen in, 57, 58
  method of sampling, 55
  solutions required in analysis of, 55–7
  strength of, 58, 59
  typical analyses of, 59

Sewage Disposal, Royal Commission on, Reports of, 58, 60, 61, 64–6, 74, 76, 77, 79, 84, 92, 93, 99

sewage effluents, 60–72
  determination of dissolved oxygen in, 61–5; of suspended matter in, 60, 61, 66, 73
  solution and reagents required in determination of dissolved oxygen in, 62, 64
  typical analyses of, 66

Seyda's methods, use of, in toxicology, 302; on detection of colocynth, 310

shallow well water, 29; analysis of, 33–36, 39, 41, 43, 45

Shrewsbury's method for detection of paraffin wax in lard, 157; on detection of blood, 312

Shrewsbury and Knapp's process in examination of butter, lard, milk etc., 121, 144, 145, 150, 155, 158, 251

Shrotter's carbon dioxide apparatus, 201

silica, determination of, in tea, 177, 178; in water, 20, 21

Silurian formation, analysis of water from the, 36, 46

silver nitrate solution, 324; in estimation of chlorine as chlorides in water, 5; of soluble chlorine in rag flock, 292; use of, in toxicology, 303

Simmonds on estimation of strychnine in the presence of quinine, 310

Sinapis alba, 215

Singapore pepper, 214

skimmed milk, 117; formulæ for calculating percentage of, 113

Smith, J. Woodhead, analysis of water by, 43

sodium arsenite solution in estimation of available chlorine in chloride of lime, 266

sodium benzoate used as a preservative of milk, 122
sodium bisulphite as a preservative in foods, 260
sodium carbonate solution in determination of carbon dioxide in air, 277; of dissolved oxygen in sewage effluents, 64; use of, to soften water, 16, 17, 28
sodium hydroxide solution in determination of aldehyde value of milk, 108; of total proteids in milk, 106; in examination of butter, 144, 145; use of, to soften water, 28; in water tests, 12
sodium hydroxide-potassium iodide solution in determination of dissolved oxygen in sewage effluents, 65
sodium hypobromite solution in estimation of urea in urine, 297
sodium nitroprusside, use of, in toxicology, 303
sodium permanganate solution, 266, 267
sodium sulphide solution in test for lead in foods, 259
sodium thiosulphate solution, 324; in determination of bromine absorption of edible oils, 164; of dissolved oxygen in sewage effluents, 62–65; of iodine absorption of lard, 156; in water tests, 6, 7
softening of water, 16, 17, 28
Soja hispida, 172
solid matter, determination of, in golden syrup and treacle, 221; in milk, 203; in sour milk, 113, 114; in spirits, 230; in vinegar, 239; in water, 5, 30
Somerville on estimation of sulphuretted hydrogen in coal gas, 287
Sonnenschein's reagent, use of, in toxicology, 312
Souchong tea, 176
sour cream, detection of gelatine in, 128
sour milk, analysis of, 113; determination of specific gravity of, 114; of total solids in, 113, 114; estimation of fat in, 104
South Barnacre reservoir, analysis of water from the, 44
South Downs, analysis of water from the, 36, 37, 48
Soxhlet apparatus in determination of fat, 105, 164, 211, 216, 246, 268, 284

soya bean oil, 172; detection of, 172
specific gravity of alcohol, 323; of edible oils, 163; of milk, 102; of urine, 296
specific rotatory power, 110; of glucose, 225; table of, of various sugars, 227
spirit indication for acidity of beer, 233, 234
spirits, 228–32
calculation of alcoholic strength of, from the total solid matter and the specific gravity, 230
detection of methyl alcohol in, 231
estimation of alcoholic strength of, 229, 230; of percentage of excess of water in, 230, 231; of total solid matter in, 230
strength of, in Ireland, 314
Sprinkmeyer and Wagner on detection of colouring matter in butter 153
spurious cider, detection of, 237
St Ann's well, Buxton, analysis of water from, 47
Staffordshire, South, analysis of water from, 41, 51
Stalybridge, analysis of water from, 53
stannous chloride solution in tests for arsenic in foods, 257, 258
starch, test for, in cheese, 160; in cocoa, 188, 189; in cream, 128; in infants' foods, 210
starch glucose, estimation of, in golden syrup and treacle, 221, 222; in honey, 223, 224
starch solution in estimation of sulphuretted hydrogen in coal gas, 287; in water tests, 6, 7
starches, 208–10; examination of, 208; microscopical appearance of the commoner, 209, 210
Stas' method of extraction of alkaloids, 304, 305
steatite in rice, 207, 208
Steensma's reagent, use of, in toxicology, 311, 312
sterilized sewage, chemical and bacterial analyses of, 89–91
Stockport, analyses of water supply of, 23–7
Stokes' method for detection of mystin in milk, 122; methods of analysis of meat pastes, sausages and tinned foods, 249, 250; typical analyses of sausages, etc., 251
strontium hydroxide solution in determination of aldehyde value of milk, 108

strychnine, 307; estimation of, in the presence of quinine, 310
Stubbs and More on the analysis of sausages, 247
Stutzer on determination of gelatine in meat extract, 247
suet, 158
sugar, detection and estimation of, in urine, 294, 298; estimation of, in bread and biscuits, 206, 207
sugar cane, 221
sugar maple, 220
sugars, various, table of specific rotatory powers of, 227; table of weights of, 227; typical analyses of, 224
sulphanilic acid solution in determination of nitrite in wheat flour, 194; in water tests, 13
sulphates, estimation of, in baking powder, 203; in self-raising flour, 198; in urine, 300; in water, 23
sulphite preservative, estimation of, in foods, 260; in lime juice cordial and lemon squash, 243
sulphites, estimation of, in beer, 236; in dried milk, 135
sulphuretted hydrogen, estimation of, in coal gas, 287, 288
sulphur dioxide as a disinfectant, 265; determination of, in sausages, etc., 251; estimation of, in disinfectants, 265
sulphuric acid solution in determination of dissolved oxygen in sewage effluents, 62, 64, 65; in determination of total proteids in milk, 106; in examination of butter, 144, 145; in sewage tests, 56; in water tests, 6, 11, 12, 13
sunshine, effect of, on river water, etc., 73, 74, 92
Swineshaw Valley, Stalybridge, analysis of water from the, 42

talc, estimation of, in pearl barley, 208; in rice, 207, 208
tallows and fats, titre test of, 167
tapioca starch, 209, 210
tar oils, estimation of, in coal-tar disinfectants, 268
tartaric acid, estimation of, in baking powder, 203; estimation of lead in, 203, 204
Tatlock and Thomson on estimation of lead in tartaric acid, etc., 203, 204; method of analysis of tea, 178
tea, 176-80
    adulteration of, 176, 177

analysis of, 178
    detection of catechu in, 177; of foreign astringent matter in, 177; of foreign leaves in, 177
    determination of alkalinity of the ash in, 178; of ash in, 177; of insoluble ash and silica in, 177
    estimation of caffeine in, 179; of exhausted leaves in, 178; of moisture of, 178, 179; of tannin in, 179; of water extract of, 179
    examination of, 177
    typical analyses of, 179, 180
    typical analysis of the ash in, 180
    varieties of, 176
temperature, changes of, effect of, on river water, etc., 73, 74, 92
temporary hardness of water, 15
Testoni on estimation of water in golden syrup and treacle, 223
Thea, 176
theobroma, oil of, 171
Theobroma cacao, 171, 184, 185
theobromine, 306, 307
Thirlmere, Lake, analysis of water from, 49, 50
Thompson's method for estimation of boric acid, 118, 119, 251
Thomson's method for estimation of sulphates in self-raising flour, 198
Thorp and Morton, analysis of, of water from the Irish Sea, 77
Thorpe on analysis of milk, 114
tidal estuaries, pollution of, 77
tin, 309; in foods, determination of, 252-4; in water, 18
tin chloride in cane sugar, 220
tinned foods, 250
titanous chloride solution in water tests, 8, 12
titre test of tallows and fats, 167
Tortelli and Jaffé on detection of hydrogenized fish oils, 172
toxicological analysis, 302-13
Trade Waste Waters, standards for, 99
treacle, see golden syrup and treacle
Trent Valley, analysis of water from the, 36, 47
turmeric, detection of, in mustard, 216; in pepper, 214
typical analyses of ash of tea, 179; of butter, 154; of cayenne, 215; of cheese, 162; of cider, 237; of cinnamon, 218; of cocoa, 192; of cream, 130; of ginger, 219; of lime juice, 244; of meat pastes, 251; of milk, 125; of mustard, 216; of pepper, 214; of sausages, etc., 251; of sewage, 59; of

sewage effluents, 66; of sugars, 224; of tea, 179, 180; of vinegar, 242; of water, 31–53; of wheat flour, 196

ultramarine blue, detection of, in cane sugar, 220, 221
Ulva latissima, 74
Upper Chalk, analyses of water from the, 32, 34
uranium nitrate solution in estimation of total phosphates in urine, 299
urea, estimation of, in urine, 297
uric acid, estimation of, in urine, 300
urine, 293–301
    albumen in, 293; picric acid test for, 293
    ammonium urate in, 295
    analysis of, 293
    blood in, 296
    calcium oxalate in, 295, 296
    cystin in, 296
    detection of acetone in, 294, 295; of bile in, 294; of blood in, 294; of chlorides, in 294; of sugar in, 294
    determination of specific gravity of, 296
    estimation of albumen in, 298, 299; of chlorides in, 296, 297; of phosphate combined with calcium and magnesium in, 300; of sugar in, 298; of sulphate in, 300; of total phosphates in, 299; of total solid matter in, 296; of urea in, 297, 298; of uric acid in, 300
    examination of the deposit of, 295
    magnesium ammonium phosphate in, 296
    pus corpuscles in, 296
    qualitative examination of, 293
    quantitative examination of, 296–301
    solutions required in estimation of albumen in, 298; of sugar in, 298; of total phosphates in, 299; of urea in, 297; of uric acid in, 300
    uric acid in, 295

Valenta Acetic-acid number in butter examination, 143
Vasey, S. A., on standardization of disinfectants, 269
vegetable oil, detection of mineral oil in, 166; production of solid fats from, 141
veratrine, 308
Villavecchia and Fabri's test for sesamé oil, 169

vinegar, 238–42
    calculation of original solids in, 240
    definition of, 238
    detection and estimation of free mineral acid in, 240, 241
    determination of ash in, 239; of total solid matter in, 239
    estimation of acetic acid in, 239, 240; of phosphate in, 240
    solutions required in estimation of free mineral acid in, 241
    typical analyses of, 242
    varieties of, 238
viscogen, detection of, in cream, 128
Vitali's reaction, use of, in toxicology, 305
Vivario on detection of methyl alcohol in spirits, 231
Vogel on detection of carbon monoxide in air, 278, 279
Volhard's method for estimation of formaldehyde in milk, 120
volumetric analysis, factors for use in, 324
Vyrnwy Water Supply, analysis of, 37, 48

Wallasey Water Supply, analysis of, 40, 41
walnut shells, cinnamon adulterated with, 217, 218
Warburton on rag flock, 291
Warren on detection of lead in foods, 255
water, 1–55
    acidity of, 2
    alkalinity of, 2, 20
    analysis of, 1–55; interpretation of results of, 28–31
    colours of, 2
    detection of hypochlorite in, 17; of poisonous metals in, 259
    estimation of albuminoid ammonia in, 4, 29, 30; of alkalies in, 22; of chlorine as chlorides in, 5, 30; of copper in, 31; of dissolved oxygen in, 17; of free and saline ammonia in, 2–4, 29; of iron in, 21; of lead in, 31; of lime in, 21; of nitrogen as nitrates in, 8–12, 30, 31; of nitrogen as nitrites in, 13, 14, 31; of oxygen absorbed from potassium permanganate solution in, 30; of permanent hardness of, 16; of poisonous metals in, 18, 19; of silica in, 20; of sulphates in, 23; of total hardness of, 15, 16; of total solid matter in, 5, 30
    hardness of, 14–16, 28; table of, 15
    method of sampling, 1, 2

water—*contd.*
mineral analysis of, 20–23
nitrogen in organic combination in, 4, 5
oxygen in, 5–7
physical characters of, 2
poisonous metals in, 18, 19
purification of, notes on, 23–8
reactions of, to litmus paper tests, 2
softening of, 16, 17
solutions required in analysis of, 2–6, 9–11, 13, 14, 19, 20
standard colours in estimation of ammonia in, 3, 4
typical analyses, 31–53
Werner-Schmidt process for determination of fat in milk, etc., 104, 113, 127, 131, 211, 249, 261
wheat flour, 194–6
adulteration of, 194
bleaching of, 194
detection of phosphate "improver" in, 196; of potassium persulphate "improver" in, 196
determination of nitrite in, 194, 195; of total nitrogen in, 195
estimation of gluten in, 195, 196; of total ash in, 195
solutions required in determination of nitrite in, 194
typical analyses of, 196
wheat starch, 209
whiskey, 228
adulteration of, 228
alcoholic strength of, 228, 314
dilution of, 228
"impurities" in, 228
manufacture of, 228
White, J., analyses of water by, 38, 48, 49; modification of, of Goldenberg's method for estimation of tartaric acid in baking powder, 203; on composition of baking powder, 200; on detection of maize starch in self-raising flour, 198, 199
white pepper, 213
Wij's iodine solution in determination of the iodine absorption of lard, 156
Wilkie, method of, for estimation of phenol, 99, 268
Wilkinson and Peter's method for detection of hydrogen peroxide in milk, 124, 130

Willard on determination of nitrite in wheat flour, 194
Willcox on benzidine test for detection of blood, 312
Winkler's method in determination of dissolved oxygen in sewage effluents, 61, 63, 65
Winton, Ogden and Mitchell on determination of the cold water extract of ginger, 218, 219
Wirral peninsula, analysis of water from the, 40, 41
Wollaston, T. R., analysis of water by, 46
"wood" vinegar, 238, 239; analysis of, 242
Woodhead, Prof. Sir German, on disinfectants, 272; on standardization of disinfectants, 269
works effluents, 93–99
determination of chlorine in the presence of thiocyanate in, 97; of CO_2 in, 96; of fat in, 93; of ferrocyanides in, 97; of fixed ammonia in, 96; of free ammonia in, 96; of hydrocyanic acid in, 97; of phenol in, 98; of sulphur as sulphates in, 94; of sulphur as sulphide in, 94; of sulphur as thiocyanate (sulphocyanide) in, 95; of total sulphur in, 94
estimation of sulphur as thiosulphate and sulphite in, 96
method of analysis of, 93, 94
putrescibility of, 93
standards of, 99
wort, specific gravity of, lost during fermentation, 234

yeast extracts, 245
Yorkshire Moors, analysis of water from the, 37

Zea mays, 172
Zeiss Butyro-refractometer number in butter examination, 143
zinc in tests for arsenic in foods, 257, 258; in water, 18
zinc-copper couple method, use of, to determine nitrates and nitrites, 78, 79
Zingiber officinale, 218
zoogloea masses of a filamentous bacillus in sewage effluents, 73

Printed in the United States
By Bookmasters